My Husband Betty

Love, Sex, and Life with a Crossdresser

Helen Boyd

SEAL PRESS

My Husband Betty:
Love, Sex, and Life with a Crossdresser

© 2003 by Helen Boyd

Published by Seal Press
A Member of the Perseus Books Group
1700 Fourth Street
Berkeley, CA 94710

Grateful acknowledgement is made to Dan Savage for permission to print "What You Don't Want" on pp. 183-184.

Library of Congress Cataloging-in-Publication Data

Boyd, Helen.
  My husband Betty : love, sex, and life with a crossdresser / Helen Boyd.
      p. cm.
  ISBN-13: 978-1-56025-515-4
  ISBN-10: 1-56025-515-3
  1. Transvestism. 2. Transvestites. 3. Transgender people. 4.
Man-woman relationships. I. Title.

HQ77.B63 2008
306.77'8--dc22

                              2007049505

Designed by Kathleen Lake, Neuwirth & Associates, Inc.

Printed in the United States of America
Distributed by Publishers Group West

My Husband Betty

"*My Husband Betty* is a frank and engaging look into the world of cross-dressers and their adjacent neighbors in the transgender community. Helen Boyd peers inside this world with an intent stare, fixating on the fact behind the façade. *My Husband Betty* gives even treatment to both crossdressers and their spouses, with hard candor and tender insight and empathy. Some readers may bristle at comments that perhaps hit too painfully close to home. However, it's done in the same vein as a mother would chasten her rambunctious child, with a swift swat followed by hug and reminder that she still loves and understands. Helen has observed what few have seen, and much fewer speak of openly. Thank you for penning such a wonderful and informative book!"

—Vanessa Edwards Foster, Chair and Co-Founder,
National Transgender Advocacy Coalition

"This book is about freedom—the freedom that comes from self-knowledge and self-acceptance. It's a very special gift to the transgender community in our times."

—Prof. Lynn Conway, University of Michigan

"Crossdressers are an important and underserved part of our American community. Cutting, incisive, sometimes maddening—*My Husband Betty* will help bring them back into the public debate."

—Riki Wilchins, Founding Executive Director of GenderPAC

"This is an insider's view of transvestism. It is sympathetic, understanding, but also realistic and critical. Essential reading for wives of transvestites, transvestites, and transgender individuals themselves. I know of no other book that gives such a realistic and all encompassing view. For those who are not involved in or with the transgender community, it ought to be a fascinating read about a group of people of whom they know little. I recommend it highly."

—Vern L. Bullough, SUNY Distinguished
Professor Emeritus, Past President of the
Society for the Scientific Study of Sex,
Honored with the Kinsey Award for his research,
and author of *Crossdressing, Sex, and Gender*

"The most thorough study on crossdressing I've ever read. A must for every transgendered person and their families. Helen Boyd speaks the truth, eloquently!"

—Gina Lance, *GIRL TALK* magazine

"Helen Boyd's insight, humor, and no-punches-pulled style provide a refreshing, spouse-eye-view of crossdressers and what makes them tick. She offers clear counsel and common sense perspectives for those who may be in conflict about this highly misperceived topic. *My Husband Betty* should be liquified, bagged, and plugged in as an IV drip for all self-questioning cross-dressers and those in their lives."

—Lacey Leigh, author of *Out & About*
and 7 *Secrets of Successful Crossdressers*

For my husband Betty, who makes me laugh

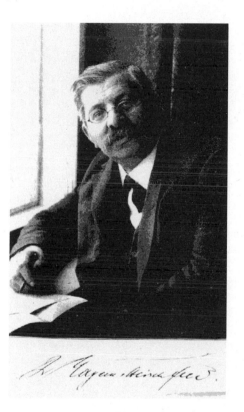

and

For Magnus Hirschfield,
for his light & work

Contents

CONTENTS

Preface

I NEVER THOUGHT I would write a book about crossdressing, but when the opportunity knocked, I couldn't resist. In my time as the girlfriend and then the wife of a crossdresser, I felt there were too many conversations going on among the women in the community that weren't addressed by crossdressing literature or websites. There was no real acknowledgement of the huge problems that came with being married to a crossdresser. The books all seemed to give advice based on the ideal crossdressing husband, someone who can communicate well, shows respect for his wife's feelings, and is absolutely sure he is a crossdresser and not transsexual. That advice didn't do a whole lot for me, and my experience is that most wives of crossdressers are not married to the "ideal crossdresser." We deal with men who have online habits that bother us, sexual fantasies that disturb us, and communication skills that are lacking.

Instead of putting a 'pretty face' on crossdressing, I think this book paints a more realistic picture. Many wives and crossdressers will not like what I have to report, and others, I hope, will appreciate my honesty.

The journey this book has taken me on has brought me toward a level of acceptance I previously didn't think was possible, and watching myself go through various phases gives me the idea that this book is only the beginning of my life with my husband Betty. I know that many women, especially when they first find out, cannot fathom ever really accepting this behavior, much less enjoying it. After I was deeply upset by my husbands' gender conflicts, I didn't think I would be able to do either. It has taken years for me to get to a point where I can conceive of really enjoying my husband's crossdressing, and I hope I will eventually get to the point that I don't have days of deep anxiety over it.

Our goal is for him to be able to crossdress without it causing tumult in both of our lives. Many couples share this goal, but how that happens is a matter of individual concern. My hope is that more women will learn to understand that their husband's gender identity is not necessarily something to fear or worry about. I also hope more women will find the courage to see their husbands dressed, to start asking questions about his sexuality, and to face some of the less pleasant realities of having a transgendered husband. Why? Not so they can be "good wives" and make their husbands happy, but because only fifty years ago women were demonized for wearing pants, and only a hundred years ago for wanting to learn to read. We genetic women are in an extraordinary position to see crossdressing as more than just a fetish or perversion; we can understand how it feels to be told what we can and cannot do. Understanding that our men are trying to access those parts of themselves that are restricted by deep cultural taboos is not easy—not by any stretch—but "we can do it," as Rosie the Riveter said.

Slowly, as a community, we will unearth more of our history. We have begun to find some of the people who were crossdressers—the Chevalier d'Eon, the Abbé de Choisy, Ed Wood. We now have Magnus Hirschfield's important and empathetic work to help us understand that even in acknowledging our sexuality we do not demean ourselves. We acknowledge Eddie Izzard as a role model, and we will find new leaders as more and more of us come out. It may seem inconceivable right now for crossdressers to live lives out in the open, but with a little work, and a little patience, I firmly believe that time will come. The couples I profile in this book are still rare, exceptions more than the rule, but more and more come out of the closet all the time.

We already have the community to create the movement. The most truly remarkable experience I have had writing this book is in meeting the people of the transgender community. Lacey, the crossdressing partner of Just Evelyn, the author of *Mom, I Need To Be A Girl*, wrote to me out of the blue when he heard about this book. Lynn Conway wrote me long, in-depth emails of her understanding of transgender history and science of the last thirty years. Jane Ellen Fairfax of Tri-Ess sent me e-mails answering any and all questions I asked. Other "known" members of the community— JoAnn Roberts, Lacey Leigh, Renee Reyes, Yvonne of Yvonne's Place, Gina Lance of *Girl Talk*, Bobbi Williams, the folks at Gender PAC, Angela Gardner of Renaissance, Dixie and Becca Nettle of the En Femme Getaways—all responded with enthusiasm and support and help, and often with information, too. Individual crossdressers—like Barbara Van Horn, Alyssa Davis, Dixie Darling, Becky Adams, Marti, and many others— engaged my continuing questions with thoughtfulness and open minds. Lisa Jackson loaned me the use of her lyrics. The groups I had the most contact with—MHVTA, Chi Delta Mu, and CDI—were all likewise welcoming and encouraging. I was overwhelmed some days with the warmth and solidarity within the community, and I want to apologize upfront for the fact that I may end up stepping on some toes by telling it like I see it.

To all the crossdressers who responded to my absurdly long and in-depth questionnaire—thank you! The honesty and bravery it took to answer some very difficult questions will always be appreciated.

To all the wives and girlfriends who responded to their version of the questionnaire—thank you! The sense of humor the partners of crossdressers manage—even in the midst of worry and unusual sexual requests—regularly blows my mind.

The ongoing process of running CDOD, the online support group for couples I started in February 2000, has been one of great affirmation and education (my own, that is). I have had some of the most remarkable and insightful and articulate people subscribe to CDOD, so much so that one recent member, George, described it as a "transgender think-tank." I could not even have considered writing this book without them. The crossdressers themselves shared their experiences and insights into their own predicament: Melissa, "perpetual lurker" Jan, Kyrie, Theresa, Donna T., Victoria, Lori, Becky, Carolyn, Caroline, Cheryl, Jamie, Margaret in India, and all the others of CDOD past and present. Ali, who is perhaps the wisest and kindest soul ever, provided support in unimagined ways.

The genetic women on the list were remarkable. They sent me URLs to useful websites, shared their fears and anxieties and concerns, and one woman—Lisa—even sent me a box full of books. Sue provided encouragement, Elizabeth input and critiques, Minna a sense of humor, Kathy her experience, and Myrna her soul. Bootz kept me sane and Liz shared her insight.

To all of the people whose names I never learned, or whom I have forgotten, but who helped in any small way, thank you. Of course I am especially grateful for the input of the six couples I profile in the Relationships chapter: Gidget and Jayne, Ali and Sue, Melissa and Denise, Victoria and Meredith, Minna and Heather, and Kathy and Amanda. Hearing both sides of each of their stories provided an inestimable opportunity to analyze how crossdressing affects relationships.

This book would not have happened without the instigation of Karen Auerbach. Her faith in this project, from Day One, was a source of ongoing enthusiasm. She answered innumerable questions, gave me feedback, and bolstered my self-esteem when it lagged. Dan O'Connor, my editor, provided the kind of enthusiasm and intelligence that got me excited about the work. He also let me go on endlessly about the insights I had, and caused a few new ones with his questions.

My friends were a similar source of support and encouragement: Sadie, Lara, Ming, Guy, "the other Helen," Willow, both Dougs, Jen, Xina & Christopher, Carey & Patrick, Estelle & Judy, Donna & Joanne, Brendan, and Brian. My friend Julie deserves a prize, or a crown, for her effort—she spent endless hours reading over the manuscript and providing critical feedback. I also have to thank my family, and especially my parents, for loving my husband nearly as much as I do. And though he'll probably never see this, I have to thank Rufus Wainwright for providing the soundtrack—days spent alone writing were far easier to bear with such a beautiful voice in my head.

I could not have written this book if I were not married to the most remarkable man on this planet, whose willingness to let me expose our lives and experiences reaffirms my belief that feminine men are certainly not lacking in courage. My husband Betty is the source of all my inspiration, a font of love and encouragement and comfort. En femme or as the boyish rock star he is, he is the most beautiful person I have ever known—inside and out.

Helen Boyd
May 14, 2003

Notes

FOR THOSE WHO are new to crossdressing, names will be confusing, as many crossdressers use femme names for themselves. Since most crossdressers are not out, most of the people I interviewed for this book opted to use their femme names as their pseudonym of choice. I have tried to indicate in the context of a sentence whether or not I am referring to a CD or his girlfriend.

Many of the wives and girlfriends also chose to use pseudonyms. Some of the transsexual women did likewise.

In Appendix B, Cast of Characters, there are brief descriptions of all the people mentioned in this book. If you are unclear as to who the person is while reading, please consult the list. It is alphabetized by last name if used, otherwise by first name.

There are a lot of words used in the crossdressing community that the average reader will not be familiar with. There is a glossary toward the end of the book to remedy that situation. If a reader more experienced in gender issues wants to know my "take" on a word that might be controversial, the glossary will serve as an explanation.

Both the use of femme names and the lingo will become familiar after a time.

Also, there is not much about FTM transgendered people in this book. These communities—like most groups within the TG community—tend to separate themselves. Some of this separation is more organic and determined by the starting identities of the individuals. For instance, many FTM transsexuals, and transmen, are in relationships with women and so identify—until transition—as lesbians. For reasons described in more detail in Chapter 8: Gendered Politics, the average straight crossdresser and the average transman do not naturally cross paths. As a result, I have not had as much contact with transmen, and so did not feel comfortable writing about their experiences. That said, I hope to. Having always been a tomboy myself, masculinity in people born as female is a topic of both personal and professional interest. My hope is that in my next book I will be able to discuss the lives and experiences of the FTM side of the spectrum. In the meantime, my decision not to discuss a subject I am only just learning about was made out of respect, not indifference.

"Sometimes I just like pretty shoes and pretty blouses,
but because I have a penis we have to
use big words to describe it."

—my husband Betty, evening of March 13, 2003

My Husband Betty

CHAPTER 1

Introduction

A SEXY YOUNG wife misses her husband so much she opens the closet and puts on one of his shirts. Turning the collar toward her cheek, she inhales his smell deeply. Her tan legs contrast nicely with the stiff white shirt, and her long hair falls over its starched collar. She steps gingerly toward the full-length mirror, sensually burying her toes in a white rug and holding yet another of his shirts, this one still on a hanger. She smiles. She spins. She collapses on the bed wearing one shirt and clutching the other, and the camera slyly gives us a glimpse of her upper thigh.

It could be an ad for sheets, cotton, or cologne. It could be the beginning of a porn film. In any case, it does not seem sexually deviant. We decide that the woman is missing her husband or boyfriend—wherever he is—and never consider the fact that she might be enjoying the clothes for the power they imply. It never crosses our minds that she could be single and trying these clothes on secretly just for a thrill. We give the whole scenario a comfortable meaning even when we are given nothing more than the images.

Now picture this: A sexy young husband misses his wife so much he opens the closet and puts on one of her silk dressing gowns. He turns the lace collar to his cheek and inhales her smell deeply. Taking a translucent slip out of her drawer he walks to the full-length mirror, where he presses it against himself, looks into the mirror wistfully, and collapses on the bed—wearing one negligee and clutching the other. The camera slyly gives us a glimpse of his upper thigh.

It would never happen. No advertising company would ever use it. The only chance we'd have of seeing such an image is if it were played for laughs, a skit on *Saturday Night Live* featuring the late Chris Farley. It certainly wouldn't be sexy.

Why is the woman in a man's shirt never a joke? Because she is sexy. We agree as a culture that women are sexy, and that they love men. It's okay for a woman to roll around in her husband's clothes because we understand she does so only because she misses him, loves him.

Even if the man in the ad were a handsome young man, a million objections instantly spring to mind. We would assume he was gay. We would assume he was a pervert.

Men across America would look forward to seeing that first ad, especially if the camera showed her body in glimpses: cleavage, thigh, naked painted toes, hair on the pillowcase. Not one of them would feel a homosexual panic for being attracted to her because she was wearing a man's shirt. No one would think she was wearing a man's shirt because she wanted to be a man, and almost none would assume that the shirt belonged to her butch lesbian lover.

A woman in a man's shirt is sexy, assumed to be straight, perfectly normal, and well-adjusted, while a man in a woman's negligee is assumed to be gay, sexually deviant, or comic. Somehow when a woman crossdresses (that *is* what she's doing when she puts on her husband's shirt) it's interpreted as either a positive thing or as insignificant. But if a man crossdresses, it's sick. The idea that any woman would find that man sexy—and sexy especially because he's wearing women's lingerie—is even sicker.

Recall how easily you envisioned the first image of the woman in her husband's shirt. You know what the woman looks like, how the room is decorated, and how the camera captures her. Even if it isn't an actual commercial, you can picture it easily because it's familiar, a standard image in our culture. You don't need to be told she misses her husband: you know it.

But the man in the slip you can't picture. It is difficult to imagine what kind of man might wear his wife's lingerie, or would want to. How would the camera present him? In lush strokes up his body as the woman was filmed, with tantalizing glances at his sexier parts (abdomen, nipple, biceps)? Perhaps one calls to mind a scene from *La Cage Aux Folles*: an effete man sitting at a vanity in feathered mules and plenty of mascara. Or Tim Curry in *Rocky Horror*, all garters, black stockings, and heels. If it's a young Richard Gere we remember the rumors about his homosexuality. Insert a purely masculine icon like Arnold Schwarzenegger in the scene and again it becomes comic. It's impossible to see this ad in your mind's eye because it's not a standard image in our culture; there is no template to work from.

Simply put, that's because crossdressing men are still a taboo. We know nothing about them—who they are, what they do, or why. For most of my life the word "transvestite" triggered a hazy image of a guy in a raincoat nervously running his hands through a lingerie drawer. Later on I learned about drag queens and transsexuals, but I'd never met a crossdresser.

When I met my future husband, I still didn't know I had met a crossdresser, but I had. Most people probably don't think they've met a crossdresser either, but odds are they have. Crossdressers pass under the radar. They go fishing, watch football, love their wives, and take care of their children. If they're single, they go to work, go on dates, and hang out at bars, as impressed as any regular Joe by a plunging neckline. In a private moment, they go into their bedrooms and put on that negligee and look at themselves in the mirror, and smile back at themselves, relieved and euphoric. What they see is beautiful and sexy. Their love of lingerie is a reflection of their love of all things feminine—including women—and a reflection of their own femininity. For most of them, every day is another chance to be caught: by a spouse who doesn't know, by a child who came back in because he forgot his hat, by a neighbor who looks out her window when he's leaving home "en femme" to go to a bar across town. What most people would not choose to see is a man who, for a few moments at a time, can revel in the fact that he loves pretty things, and who doesn't have to pretend brown is his favorite color. They could—but probably won't—see a man who would trade cottons and wool for the cool touch of silk; a man who likes to cross his legs or dance with his arms in the air; a man who enjoys donning his wife's negligee and for a few minutes—or a weekend—gets to feel what he imagines it's like to be a woman.

I ASKED MY husband out on our first date. That should have indicated to both of us how much gender roles—and their subversion—would play in our relationship, but we didn't have a clue. He had arrived in Manhattan a few months before from a small town in upstate New York, and was looking forward to being able to go out crossdressed more. My call had interrupted him doing his makeup: he held the phone in one hand and an eyeliner pencil in the other while listening to me stutter and stammer. He hadn't dated in years and knew full well that crossdressing was the main reason. He didn't like casual relationships, and couldn't face another rejection from a woman he truly liked. Long before, he had decided he could not be in a serious relationship where he concealed his crossdressing, so he reacted to my call with a mixture of excitement and dread: excitement because he'd been intrigued by me, too; dread, because he knew if he liked me and I liked him, he'd have to face that awful truth and tell me about his femme self. He agreed to meet me at the screening of a documentary film. He came to New York to start a new life, and start a new life he would.

I remember him looking at my lips intently when I first met him at the movie theater. He was probably checking out my lipstick technique, guessing the color and brand. I also remember forcing myself to wear a skirt on our second date (I'd worn trousers for the first, since my belief is that comfort and confidence are sexy, and I have never felt as confident or as comfortable in a skirt as I do in pants). Otherwise our courtship was typical: long conversations and long walks; remarkable discoveries of shared loves in music, art, and politics; nervous waits for phone calls; enthusiastic plans. The only thing that bothered me was that I couldn't immediately picture his face when I wanted to think dreamily about him, and I worried if my lack of recall meant he wasn't "the one."

We were blessed and cursed by an extraordinary circumstance: we had only three weeks together before he left town for four months. That time limitation forced us to have conversations we might not have had until much later. We each wanted to know whether the other felt convinced that this was something special, and we felt compelled to discuss whether either of us planned to date other people during those four months of separation. We talked about past dates and past flames, high school heartbreaks and longed-for lovers. He told me the story of how an ex-girlfriend and he decided a decade ago to dress for Halloween as King Louis and Marie Antoinette. I nodded and listened and held his hand. He stumbled a little over his words as he admitted that he had been the one to go as Marie Antoinette. His girlfriend had been King Louis.

I felt a pang of jealousy as he described how playful and fun their sex was that night, full of crinoline and corsets, and maybe that's why I failed to be shocked. I had seen *Dangerous Liaisons* just like everyone else and the thought of making love in those period costumes turned me on.

He repeated that he had gone as Marie Antoinette, waiting again for my shock.

"So you went as Marie Antoinette. *And?*" I wanted to hear more about the sex, the girlfriend; the writer in me wanted to hear the rest of the story. He looked a little surprised but he continued: they'd both been very turned on by the experience. He'd been surprised at how sexy she had found him in stockings and corset. The second surprise came when months later she came out as a lesbian, and left him for a woman.

He had thought he had found the crossdresser's dream: a woman who was not only okay with his crossdressing but found it erotic. Just as quickly, his dreams became a nightmare of rejection: he wasn't femme enough for her.

Of course he didn't tell me all the psychological ramifications at the time—all I knew was that the girlfriend with whom he'd had the best sex of his life (by his own admission) had left him to date other women. I consoled him with a story about a woman I'd known in college who had dated four men in a row who all came out of the closet after breaking up with her. He just looked at me, jaw slack with disbelief.

After a moment, he said, "I'd like to do that again." I assumed he meant dressing as King Louis and Marie Antoinette for Halloween and wondered where we could rent costumes.

"Sure," I said, "that would be fun." The look of shock on his face made me wonder if I'd missed something.

"You're okay with that?" he asked. Of course I was. Halloween was my favorite holiday and I loved period clothes. "You'd have sex with me dressed as Marie Antoinette?" he asked to clarify. Of course I would. Halloween was all about blurring identity, crossing boundaries, seduction and sexuality. At least that's what it was about to me. Being shy, I'd used Halloween to overcome my own inhibitions and dressed as a dominatrix, Catwoman, a naughty Catholic school girl. His wanting to be Marie Antoinette only meant that I wouldn't have to wear the corset and be uncomfortable all night, and that was a blessing.

What neither of us realized at the time is that Halloween is an extraordinary night: one of the few times or places in American culture where crossdressing is acceptable, even encouraged. His expression of interest in dressing as Marie Antoinette was, for him, the equivalent of saying bluntly, "I'm a crossdresser." For me it meant nothing of the kind. That he was hinting at something he needed me to know never occurred to me. I just thought he was playful, and a sure bet as a fun date for Halloween.

I don't remember how he subsequently made it clear to me that his desire to dress as Marie Antoinette was as strong on any given Tuesday as it was the Tuesday before Halloween, but I do know that within those first three weeks, I found myself waiting nervously on the couch to see my brand-new boyfriend dressed as a woman. I rehearsed reaction faces like the ones you use for Christmas presents you don't like. I was determined not to look shocked or appalled. I liked this guy too much to come off as some kind of stick-in-the-mud. I pride myself on my open-mindedness, and nothing—but nothing—was going to get in the way of the relationship that was developing between us.

He emerged as she, tiptoeing in black velvet pumps from the bathroom to the living room where I sat waiting. He hugged the doorway in his black velvet dress, seamed stockings and short, banged, black wig, looking torn between running for his life and facing his fear. He took another step in, but again my memory fails me as to my exact reaction. I ask my husband, who is, as I write this, lying beside me in bed in a silk slip, and he doesn't recall my first words upon seeing him dressed as a woman, either. He does remember that I "looked pleased." I know I smiled—smiled because I was nervous and because, frankly, the sight of a man in a dress is damned comic at first. Socially we're trained to find it funny, from Monty Python's "Lumberjack Song" to

Jack Lemmon and Tony Curtis in *Some Like It Hot*. Open-minded or not, I am still a product of my culture. Maybe because I'm tender-hearted—or maybe because as a writer I'm fond of people's eccentricities—I knew well enough not to laugh. I hugged him instead.

I hugged him just so he would stop trying to read my face so intently. I hid my face from him because I was scared what he might find on it. I was over-whelmed with so many feelings I can't recall feeling any one of them clearly.

I hugged him not only to give myself that precious moment to think, but also for his bravery. He'd come into the room physically shaking, and I could feel his hands still trembling on my back. I hugged him because that is what you do when someone is shaking with fear in front of you. I hugged him because I loved him already, and after seeing how scared he was about how I might react, I knew I loved him even more. I had complained all my adult life about men who couldn't be vulnerable, and this man in a black vel-vet dress had practically torn his skin off so I could see his tender heart beat-ing in his chest. He had laid himself bare. He was the dictionary definition of vulnerable, and I wasn't fool enough to look a gift like that in the mouth.

I found—much to my surprise—that after seeing his face meticulously made-up and framed with a simple wig, I had no further trouble recalling his handsome male face when I wanted to. Even then I remember thinking that was significant. I've since realized it's because I had seen all of him once I had seen his femme self, and that's not a lesson one forgets easily: I remind myself of it every time I wish his crossdressing would just go away.

I MAINTAINED THE accepting and supportive attitude I'd adopted in the beginning for a long time, more than a year. I thought his crossdress-ing was fun, playful, sexy—even subversive. I have always had a taste for adventure. Granted, dating a crossdresser was a little more adventurous than I would have ever predicted. I'd grown bored with more traditional men who could only tell me how pretty my eyes were, and even when I dated more intellectual men I found they were more interesting in think-ing they were educating me than in being my partner. One boyfriend loved that I could be ready to leave my apartment in ten minutes but complained that I never seemed to wear skirts or makeup or high-heeled shoes. Explaining that I devoted my time to more bookish pursuits—as he did—was a moot point. He, like so many other men, thought "looking femi-nine" was a natural state, and had no idea how much time and energy and resources it took to like you've walked out of a magazine. I'd dated artists, activists, and educators—all of whom you'd think would understand how much effort it takes for a woman to look so perfectly put together. These were men who took classes in feminism, after all. No matter how much they respected my mind, they were caught up in the idea that women naturally have cleavage. (They don't, guys.)

Dating a crossdresser—who understood implicitly how long it took to "look like a woman"—was a relief. I love that he knows that time spent poring over fashion magazines was time not used learning HTML. For a while just my appreciation for his understanding made it easy to accept his crossdressing because he was a breath of fresh air after all the deluded men I'd dated. Not only did he understand how long it took to put on your "face," he did mine for me.

Of course I'd also locked myself in by being supportive from the outset. I knew he loved that I could enjoy it, and how could I face up to the fact that I didn't always? I would have felt like a hypocrite. So my twinges of displeasure passed without my saying a word about them, with me barely acknowledging them at all.

I named his femme self "Betty." He has long legs and during our first summer together (probably after he'd tried on one of my bathing suits), I had suggested we recreate that famous Betty Grable pin up. We never did, but somehow "Betty" stuck. We discovered we both liked Betty Page, the 1950s fetish model, and I also learned that "betty" had been slang for girl, like moll. We never thought of Betty as a real name, but more like code: "I think Betty would like to go out this weekend," my husband would tell me on the subway, with no one around us the wiser. All he meant was that he wanted to go out crossdressed, but using "Betty" gave us a way to talk about him being a crossdresser without saying *that word* out loud. When I first went online I found a lot of crossdressers referred to themselves by their femme names, so we used Betty in order to avoid using his real name. Obviously, we still do.

That I chose "Betty" indicates to me now how I thought about his femme self—glamorous and pretty like Betty Grable, fetishy and sexy like Betty Page. How innocent I was. I was willing to indulge his need to dress up because I saw it as a little sexy, a little taboo, and great fun. We went to a T-friendly night at a local club during our first month together. I enjoyed it tremendously. I walked slowly so he could keep up with me in heels he'd only ever worn in his apartment, and simultaneously kept an eye out for any trouble from frat boys or other rabble who might "read" him as a man and decide to harass us. I was delighted to hold open doors and to give directions to the cabbie. I felt so proud when the woman at the door expected me to pay for us both. I was pleased that I had finally found a man who would not only allow me to be chivalrous but who would encourage it, a man who let me flatter and indulge him, and who didn't mind being the center of attention. I have never been very good at being on the receiving end of compliments, mostly because I'm shy and was suspicious of chivalry's implications: can't I open the door and pull out the chair myself? If a man does so, isn't that a suggestion that I'm somehow incapable? If I let him open the door, would he expect me to have sex with him? Like most modern women, I grew up with feminism, and being able to go out with a man who would not only tell me I was beautiful but who could take that burden occasionally off my shoulders was a huge relief. I always envied lesbians for their ability to trade gender roles, but no matter how reasonable it seemed to be a lesbian, I was heterosexual. Dating a transvestite seemed the answer to my own gender issues.

At least, it was, for a while. After that first big night, we were ready for more. Betty and I explored the T-friendly world—from drag and fetish club nights, to crossdressing parties. We found places that provided dressing rooms and makeup application services (although we never used either), and that offered a sense of community.

It was no coincidence that I hit the inevitable crisis right about the time our relationship was becoming very serious. We had been together two years. Two years go by fast, so fast you don't even realize that it's not the first month anymore, that you're not quite as *anything you want honey* as you were once.   Little did I know but he was already planning to ask me to propose and had even told his co-workers.

We decided to venture out into the Real World, to a nearby but unfamiliar restaurant with dim lighting, on a quiet weeknight. It was then and only then that the bubble containing my assumptions and hopes was burst. What I didn't know, and certainly didn't expect, was that my husband's first attempt to "pass" as a real woman would be entirely different from all those times we'd gone to drag shows and alternative clubs. No one at a fetish party cares who wears the high heels, as long as someone does, but being out in public—in the Real World—threw a kind of wrench into our relationship that neither of us could have predicted.

Suddenly it wasn't so cool or exciting to me anymore.   It was terrifying. I ordered all our drinks. I leaned in close because he didn't want to raise his voice. I watched the confident man I had fallen in love with become shy, passive, and quiet. In brief, I saw that "Betty" was nothing like him, that at all the T-friendly nights we'd gone to he'd been himself because it was understood he was a man in a dress. But that night at dinner was the first time I realized how important it was for him to "pass," for others to assume he was a real woman. The implications of his "passing" uncovered fears I had never experienced before. I saw how much he enjoyed it, how excited he was by his success. I was witnessing what's called "gender euphoria," and even though I was familiar with the concept, I wasn't prepared for the reality. I experienced what all crossdressers' wives must confront: a terrible fear that my husband might genuinely want to be a woman.

On the way home I sat sullen in the cab, envisioning my new boyfriend who suddenly didn't jive with the artificial girl sitting by my side. It didn't help to remind myself that they were one and the same person. That handsome man seemed far away and I was terrified that there would come a day that he would be dead and gone and only Betty would remain.

Once we walked in the door of our apartment, he ran off to e-mail our online group with his victory, and I cried in the bath. He was thrilled and I told him I was miserable.

We had a month of long talks during which Betty hid out in the closet with the cobwebs and the shoes we don't wear.

During that difficult time, he proposed and I accepted. Talk about your unusual engagements.

I can say this for sure: it was an important awakening for me. I realized that crossdressing is not just about underground clubs and manicures and fetish clothes. It's not about "subverting gender paradigms" or intentional rebellion. It's about seeing the love of my life suffer. It's about realizing that my feelings matter so much to him that he would be willing to suppress an integral part of his personality just to please me. It's about realizing that I'm with someone who will always feel at least a little constricted by the narrow confines of our society and knowing that my own expectations of a boyfriend or husband are part and parcel of the society that says *No*. It is about having expectations of the man I love that can't possibly be met, and knowing that those very same expectations—whether spoken out loud or not—reinforce the feelings of shame and frustration he has been experiencing all his life.

Sometimes now, he hugs me because I'm the one shaking: scared for our future and scared of the long-awaited creak of that closet door. I'm simultaneously scared of Betty coming out completely *and* of continuing to live with this secret—one of which is inevitable. Sometimes it just feels like he invited me into his closet. He's become inured to his claustrophobia, but I'm not used to it yet and hope I never have to be. Some days wishing his crossdressing would just go away is the only way I can see escaping. I know that's not realistic. I know I'm in it for the long haul, and that it will take much more than crossdressing to estrange me from a man I love so much. But I *do* wish it would go away sometimes. The cost, the confusion, the cultural taboo—all of these add up to a tremendous pain in the ass. I don't like worrying into the night that my marriage might come to an abrupt end if he should discover he is not "just a crossdresser" but transsexual. I dislike keeping secrets from family members or close friends. I resent explaining to aggressive gay men in nightclubs that a man who is wearing a dress is not, by definition, gay. Life with a crossdresser is not easy, and one of the biggest problems is how occupying it is: our conversations, our finances, our plans are all circumscribed by it. It feels sometimes like a runaway train, uncontrollable and potentially destructive. His crossdressing brings up issues I would never otherwise have had to deal with; it creates unpleasant feelings and elicits uneasy conversations.

As we approach our fifth year together, and the writing of this book, I can't say that everything is resolved. In fact, nothing is resolved. In the time we've been together, I have reevaluated and redefined my idea of love so drastically and so often I don't even recognize it anymore. We got married in July 2001—a year after that critical juncture—and argued about crossdressing on our honeymoon. But a year later, for our first anniversary, I gave him a drawing copied from our wedding photo: in it, he's the bride and I don the tux. Being married to a crossdresser has meant giving up certain small things—and being repaid tenfold. It has, most of all, been about stretching myself and my heart to fit around the one I love. It will take, no doubt, more evaluation, more compromise, more discussion, and more growth before I can accept fully and love freely a man who the rest of the world either doesn't understand or rudely rejects.

I have come to understand that most people think crossdressers are freaks because they blur gender lines in a way that makes most of us uncomfortable.

Most people see a man in a dress and see an abomination, a sexual deviant, a pervert. They might—if they like the man or just have an easygoing manner—laugh really hard. If a wife comes home an hour early and finds her husband transformed into a woman, the sight of him might damage her love for her husband so irrevocably that she might refuse to have sex with him ever again. A different wife might seek divorce and use her husband's "sexual deviance" as a crowbar in the courtroom, to separate a father from his children. If his boss found out, the man could be fired from his job—even if he only crossdresses at home. If one of his children discovered his secret, he would worry about the psychological effects it might engender, or worry that the child might tell a friend. If it's the lady across the street, heaven help him: everyone in the neighborhood will know, and he may find himself staying home alone to watch the Super Bowl.

This is less conjecture than it may seem. Every possibility I've presented—including the firing—has happened to a crossdresser, not a hundred years ago or even a decade ago, but in the last five years. In an era when a drag queen like RuPaul gets paid as a spokesperson for makeup, and lesbian mom Rosie O'Donnell can host her own talk show, crossdressers are still rattling the hangers in their collective closet. There is no "movement" to assert their dignity and there's precious little information about them at all. Despite the creative and energetic efforts on the part of the Transgendered Community to assert rights for transsexuals, drag queens, and crossdressers themselves, the average crossdresser still prefers solitude or secret societies that meet behind closed doors and the anonymity of the internet.

Why are crossdressers still in the closet and passing just under the cultural radar? Because they're straight. Because despite their gender dysphoria or fetishistic sexuality, they are still straight men enjoying the privileges of all straight men. As long as no one knows about their stash of corsets and slips, they are average guys with loving girlfriends or wives and good jobs, respected in their communities and successful in their careers. Barbara Ehrenreich described the middle class' "fear of falling" as the anxiety expressed by Americans who worried about losing their privilege. Crossdressers exhibit what I like to call a "fear of freaking." Similar to Ehrenreich's middle class, they stand to lose their privilege if they let the charade slip for an instant.

They are perhaps the last brick in the wall of our cultural construct of masculinity. Women can be aggressive, financially independent, and admired for demonstrating these and other traditionally masculine traits. They wear pants and boots and sometimes even tool belts. It may still be an exception for a woman to run a construction crew or a major corporation, but we do hold up women who do these things as role models for our daughters. We may make jokes about women with mustaches still, but everyone admires Condoleezza Rice. As a feminist I can't possibly say that women have achieved total economic or social equality, but we have made enormous strides in breaking down the cultural ideas of femininity. We can watch a woman don her husband's button-down and not be offended. Her ability to express masculine traits by dressing symbolically in the clothes of the other gender is not considered dysfunctional anymore. In fact, men's clothes aren't even considered masculine anymore, as any girl on a soccer team can tell you.

But we don't send our boys to dance lessons in tutus, do we? Male nurses are still a comic standby. Male beauticians must be gay. We don't encourage boys to apply makeup like Kevyn Aucoin, to cook like Wolfgang Puck, or to design clothes like Gianni Versace. Why? Because the only men who work in traditionally feminine industries are believed to be gay or European (which is, to most Americans, about the same thing). Those jobs are acceptable for gay or effete men, but for straight men the restrictions are still pretty tight. Any single sign of femininity results in relegation to the gay category, and well, we haven't quite given up homophobia as a national pastime, have we? The ironic thing to me is that there is still an association between feminine and homosexual, because I've never met men who are more traditionally masculine than in gay bars. The last time I was at the Roxy, a gay bar in Manhattan, I thought the military was recruiting because of all the cut chests and buzz cuts. But that's what happens when two really important words—gender and sex—get used interchangeably. Because gender is about identity—whether a person is masculine or feminine, no matter if they're male or female, and sex is about biology, chromosomes, and genitalia. A person's sexual orientation— whether they have sex with men or women or both—has little to do with their gender identity. Women have been able to blur gender—by wearing pants and their hair short—without absolutely guaranteeing that they will be assumed to be lesbian. That was not always the case, but it is now. When men blur gender, however, their sexuality is still assumed blurred as well. Even a man who dresses neatly or has fashion sense is jokingly assumed to be a homosexual, and despite the advances of the last thirty years, being a homosexual still means being a freak, an outsider, a person who either doesn't have privilege or who has to earn it. Gay men and lesbian women still have to "prove" themselves in ways straight people do not.

Because most crossdressers are straight men, they're used to the privilege allotted heterosexual men in our culture, which is why your average crossdresser still won't admit to being blurry on gender. If people want to believe that men who wear dresses are faggots or perverts or both, why should the heterosexual crossdresser risk his status in society to tell them otherwise? Why on earth would he throw in his lot with the lot of the freaks and perverts when he doesn't have to? Crossdressing men, with a little discretion and a lot of anxiety, can pass as normal and retain all the privilege of their birthright. They don't have to tell anyone they're wearing lacy panties under their jeans. A dress can be taken off, nail polish removed, pantyhose put back in the drawer. The suit or tool belt or work boots can be worn again on Monday morning. They can put the "man" back on and go about their normal lives. Most of them do, which goes a long way toward explaining why most people think they've never met a crossdresser.

The majority of crossdressers would prefer to keep it that way, having their cake and eating it, too. The problem is, they're miserable. The whole

urge to crossdress, they say, is about putting down the burdens of being masculine in this society, escaping the pressure of being the breadwinner, the
answer man, the decision-maker. Crossdressing is about being able to feel
emotional, to cry, to feel pampered and glamorous and indulged. Most get
to crossdress for an hour here, a weekend there—just enough secret relief
from the stress in order to go on facing life as a man. But by insisting on protecting their privilege as heterosexual men, they deny their possibility as gender dysphoric men—men who would, if they could, find a way to alter our
very definition of masculinity.

I'M WRITING THIS book because many of the crossdressers' wives I've
met are miserable and angry and bitter. Some feel betrayed that they were
told about their husbands' crossdressing years into the marriage. If and
when they do come around to accepting their husbands' peculiarity, they
only tolerate it, and rarely enjoy it. When I first started dating a crossdresser,
I went online. I could research discreetly and I could meet others who were
in my situation. I did. I found websites for and by crossdressers and websites
by and for their partners, and I found support groups for the wives of crossdressers. I found a lot of women who complained, a lot of women who
wanted it all to go away, and a few women who had found ways to cope,
and who generously gave of their time and experience to help others
through. What I didn't find frequently was happiness or contentment. I'm
not saying that life with a crossdresser is easy—it isn't—but I don't see why
it is as traumatic as it is for so many. I wondered if our expectations of masculinity aren't what cause a wife to be abysmally crushed when she sees her
husband in a dress for the first time, and wondered what it would take for
a woman to see her husband in a slip the same way a man can see his wife
in a button-down: as sexy, desirable, and liberated.

In the first group I joined I discovered that my basic tolerance for my husband's crossdressing was not the norm and that other wives who were married to crossdressers treated a new woman on the list who was more
supportive as a bit of a freak herself. I did find my husband's legs pretty in
stockings and was turned on by being able to break a taboo with him. I also
found out rather quickly that saying as much was not acceptable, that I
would only "fit in" with the other wives of crossdressers by being deeply
shocked by the sight of my husband hairless or made-up. My happiness at
having found others in my situation quickly turned to sadness: I was rejected
from that first group for suggesting that women who were at least bi-curious
might have an easier time being married to a crossdresser, and in doing so
didn't realize that I had broken a rule for saying the L word out loud. That

was my first strike. I found another list and got kicked off of it for pointing out that a certain kind of joking among the wives seemed to express a deep anger and disrespect for their crossdressing husbands. That was my second strike. I did discover that most wives harbored three major fears: 1) that their husbands were gay, 2) that loving a man who dressed like a woman would make them lesbians, and 3) that their crossdressing husbands would want, eventually, to become women.

I am the first one to say that women are resourceful, smart, and tolerant— because they usually are all three, and then some—which is why I couldn't figure out why so many of them were so upset about a change of clothes. Women change their clothes depending on the roles they play all the time. They don't dress for a corporate dinner the same way they dress for a child's soccer game. No matter what the range of an individual woman's wardrobe, there *is* range. Women make decisions about comfort and desirability in what clothes they put on every single day. Their inability to see that their husbands' behavior stemmed from similar needs sent me on a sort of mission. I would find out why.

I'm not saying I did. Since I had been kicked out of every group I had found online, I started CDOD in February 2000, an online support group for heterosexual crossdressers and their partners. My main reason, really, was entirely selfish: I wanted people to talk to. I'd been deeply hurt by the rejection from those other groups and felt terribly lonely, despite the fact that most of my friends had known my husband was a crossdresser within the first year we were together. What my friends weren't privy to—and what I couldn't talk to them about—were the specific experiences of a cross-dresser's wife, from the niggling complaints (*I hate it when he doesn't put my makeup back*) to the emotional obstacles (*I resent having to keep this secret from our families*) to the disturbing moments of crisis (*Oh God, how can I be sure he won't want to become a woman?*). In recruiting members, I was very clear that I only sought participants who had reached some basic level of acceptance of crossdressing in their lives. I wanted to connect with peo-ple who could offer advice or just an ear. I needed to seek out women who understood how insulting it could be when your husband, in professing a desire to "feel like a woman," dressed in clothes that to you made him resemble someone you'd call a slut. I wanted to know if other couples brought crossdressing to the bedroom, and how that affected their sex lives. Did other wives question their own sexuality (almost all of them had), and did every other crossdresser seem to masturbate a lot?

Basically, I wanted a community that wouldn't be scared of honesty; that could discuss sex as adults, and that wouldn't reassure me with half-truths.

I sought out couples and individuals who had been inventive about making crossdressing work in their lives.

I found them, and it is my pleasure to introduce them to you in all their inconsistent glory. They have grappled with all the normal problems of relationships—differences in attitudes about money, family, religion, child-raising, and sex—and have also confronted their own notions about gender at the same time. You'll find that they all arrived at happiness by different paths, and that they all started from wildly disparate backgrounds and assumptions. I present them to you because their creativity, commitment, and devotion are inspiring examples for crossdressers and their wives—and indeed, for all couples.

You'll discover that very few of the crossdressers profiled here are completely "out" and that even those who are exercise caution. I have changed some of their names at their request to conceal their identities. It may be obvious that my husband's name—Betty Crow—is his "femme" name, but it's less obvious that mine—Helen Boyd—is a nom de plume. Unfortunately we learned the hard way why most crossdressers and their wives are still in the closet. My husband trusted his ex-girlfriend enough to share his secret with her, and when they broke up—and we began dating—she harassed us and blackmailed us for years on the basis of his being a crossdresser. We

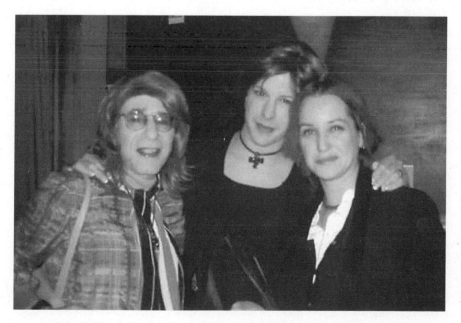

from Right to Left: author Helen Boyd with husband Betty and friend Phylis Anne would love to be brave enough to throw caution to the wind, but it's not yet a realistic option. This book, though, is part of our journey toward coming out completely.

In a culture of proud minorities, it hurts to be misunderstood. Crossdressers are getting lonely in the closet all by themselves, and they express jealousy of others' liberties. They have one hand on the doorknob, and they wait patiently for the world to change enough to accept their peculiarity. They long for freedom and dread the anxiety of being in the closet, living in fear that someone will find out. It is cozy in the closet—but how wonderful it would be to walk in broad daylight down a busy street in a dress! Crossdressers know the first of them to go out there is going to be ridiculed, jeered at, humiliated, or physically attacked. Little by little, though, we will turn the knob and let in the light. No group ever did it all at once. I liken crossdressers of today with the homosexuals of the early 1960s, a time when gay men and women were just beginning to imagine freedom, but hadn't yet found the leaders or the moment to fight for it. Hopefully all liberation movements will continue to gain momentum because of the bravery of the gays and lesbians of half a century ago. Crossdressers—and all those still yearning to live freely as themselves—should acknowledge that debt.

The irony of the crossdresser then is that he is both unknown and invisible in society, and can't become known until he is visible. His wife is even more misunderstood. What kind of woman would stay married to such a deviant? Back in 1976, Deborah Heller Feinbloom, in an otherwise insightful and sympathetic book called *Transvestites and Transsexuals*, mused that women who accepted or encouraged their husbands' crossdressing must either be suppressing lesbianism or suffering from remarkably low self-esteem. Though there may in fact be latent lesbians and women with insecurities among crossdressers' wives, I doubt either of those traits has much to do with why they decide to stay. A woman may just take her marriage vows seriously, or may look past the crossdressing to see that her husband is the same man she always loved. He may have some of those rare qualities that make him a good husband.

Wives are often entirely ignorant of crossdressing when they discover or are told their husbands are crossdressers. Plenty of them laugh the first time they see their husbands dressed because they're culturally conditioned, too: crossdressing has always been a staple of comedy from time immemorial. (I would love for someone to try to find out exactly how many of those guys who dressed "for laughs" were actually crossdressers in private.) Others cry. Crossdressers often express confusion or disappointment at their wives' lack of understanding. The wives almost always admit frustration that their husbands seem obsessed with crossdressing and show little or no desire to control or to suppress it. They also articulate more typical complaints about their husbands: he won't communicate; he can't express his feelings; I ask him questions but he doesn't answer; he gets angry if I suggest counseling. They wonder why, if these men want to be in touch with their feminine side, they don't start by connecting with their own wives. Almost none of the crossdressing literature addresses wives' concerns at all. It is my sincere hope that some wives of crossdressers will find in this book sympathetic voices and examples of women who stayed with crossdressers for reasons far more affirming than Feinbloom's negative assumptions, and that they can find answers to some of the questions that continue to bother them.

The one thing I didn't find when I was the new girlfriend of a crossdresser was a book that had all the basic information I needed: answers to some basic questions, resources, definitions of the TG community, and the experiences of other girlfriends and wives. I did find more online of course, but a lot of that required memberships, or were written from a very slanted perspective. Crossdressers' sites are especially notorious for championing the crossdresser's point of view, and are in fact geared not toward partners but toward other crossdressers. I am not the only wife who has gone online to find information and found instead pictures and pictures and more pictures of crossdressers. I am certain that I am also not the only one to find half-truths, condescending attitudes, and outdated notions of femininity.

I want to provide the guide I didn't find when I wanted one. I have compiled information from private interviews and e-mails, online questionnaires, movies, documentaries, websites, and magazines. I have scoured the entire literature of crossdressing, starting with Magnus Hirschfield's *Transvestites* of 1910, through to Amy Bloom's *Normal* published just last year. I have read books written by Virginia Prince, the founder of Tri-Ess, which is the oldest and largest organization for heterosexual crossdressers in the world. I read books written by Peggy Rudd, the supportive wife of a crossdresser, and books by other crossdressers (Charles Anders, Lacey Leigh, and the author of *Bert & Lori*, to name a few). I have read the books from the medical and psychological and sociological fields (Richard Docter, Margaret Feinbloom, Vern and Bonnie Bullough) and tomes on gender theory either activist in nature (Kate Bornstein, Leslie Feinberg), feminist in nature (Judith Butler), or academic in nature (Marjorie Garber's brilliant *Vested Interests*). I read fiction about crossdressers and transsexuals, like *Trans-sister Radio*, and even snooped around in the pornography catering to crossdressers on sites such as www.fictionmania.com. I went outside crossdressing per se and read books on drag, looked at photographic documents like *Transformations* and *Walk on the Wild Side*. (An annotated list of books appears at the end of this book in Appendix C.) I have corresponded with or spoken to wives of crossdressers, to tranny chasers, crossdressers, drag queens, feminists, boyfriends of drag queens, lesbian couples, transsexual women and their partners, and transgirls, asking them for their unique insight into some aspect of crossdressing men. I have attended support meetings, crossdressing events, drag clubs and performances, and conferences on gender.

I have not, as far as I can tell, left any stone unturned. I have asked questions of myself as a journalist I had not asked myself as the wife of a crossdresser, and surprised myself by seeing things I had not seen before. I have always been an adventurous and curious person with a natural knack for getting people to talk about themselves, but what I sometimes heard or learned upset my pre-existing ideas about gender, sexuality, and identity. Some days I went to sleep wondering if anyone didn't have major questions about these issues, and occasionally made a point of watching sitcoms in order to remind myself that suburban dads on television still make jokes about guys in dresses.

I would like for this to be the kind of book a wife or a girlfriend can read with her crossdressing husband or boyfriend that might lead to a new level of communication between them. I have not filtered this information to be only a positive book about crossdressing, as personally I felt I was handed a great deal of "cheerleading" that was unfair, untrue, and harmful. Life with a crossdresser is not necessarily rosy and I resented efforts by others to tell me it was.

I did try not to emphasize the sadness and adversity, either. By presenting couples who have found either positive ways to "cope" with crossdressing or the ones who have learned to enjoy it as an integrated part of their lives, I want to show—not just others, but myself as well—that there is hope, and more than hope, there is happiness, albeit a deeper, more complicated kind than many expect or can even imagine.

I HAVE COME to the conclusion that some husbands and boyfriends who crossdress are just not good husbands or boyfriends, but it's not because they're crossdressers. Usually they fail to communicate, or lack the sympathy and compassion and patience it takes to help their wives come to terms with their crossdressing. Others have taken the deep urge to crossdress as a motivation, spurring themselves on to greater heights (or is it depths?) of self-discovery and expression. Others still have utilized their desire to be feminine themselves as a way to connect to their wives' lives, to understand the burdens placed upon the women by society and—more often than not—themselves.

The wives I spoke with ranged from unaccepting to being totally gung-ho. Some, like their husbands, explored the questions crossdressing asked of their lives and used the investigation to find new parts of themselves. Others used it to belittle their partners and complain about the unfairness of it all. Still others—and I'd put myself in this third category—utilized some basic personality traits to find a way to understand. Having been something of an academic, a traveler, and a writer, I found my path toward accepting and integrating crossdressing into my life as an individual and as a wife in the writing of this book.

Some crossdressers who read this may decide they are better off in the closet, not telling their wives and opening the biggest can of worms imaginable. Some wives and girlfriends might realize they are not cut out to live with a crossdressing husband, or come to understand that they have been blaming crossdressing for a husband's otherwise bad behavior. Like I said, I have not written a "you can do it" book, but a "you can do it if you work your butt off" book. The level of communication and respect and empathy required of people in a relationship where crossdressing is concerned is intense, and some may not, at this time in their lives, or ever, be ready for it.

That said, I hope, too, that this book might help crossdressers tell their girlfriends about their crossdressing before they propose, or that it might help a man get up the courage to tell his wife after many years of keeping his secret. I have tried to present various types of crossdressers I have discovered, so that a man might more accurately point at a description that is similar to him in order to better inform his wife what she might or might not expect of their relationship. I hope the book can be the kind that one might give to an adult child, a parent, or a friend in order to inform that person of the complexity of a crossdresser's life. Mostly, I hope I have portrayed crossdressers and their partners as their human selves: some of them remarkable, some of them mediocre, but all of them fallible and individual and deserving of love and respect.

CHAPTER 2

Crossdressed Lives

I HAVE SEEN my husband transform himself into a woman many times. Usually he follows a very regular regimen, one formed long before we met but fine-tuned since. He is not easily interrupted while making himself into Betty, and I'm still surprised he picked up the phone when I called that first night to ask him out. First he picks the music he will dress to, starts a bath, and puts on a masque. While the masque dries and the bath fills, he lays all his under-things out on one side of our bed: a pair of off-black pantyhose, cotton thong panties and matching 36B bra, a waist-cinch, control-top panty, shoulder pads, and breast forms. He has his own things now and seldom borrows mine, although we share quite a few pieces—like corsets and hose. He chooses an outfit or two and hangs them on the inside of our open closet door where the cats won't sleep on them and cover them with fur. There is always more than one possibility for shoes, and his selections are placed on the bed as well, heels up. Once he's got the clothes all laid out the bath is ready: he strips off his socks and underwear and throws them unceremoniously onto the bathroom floor, raises the volume on the boom box, and lowers himself into the bath. He washes off the masque and lathers his face with shaving cream. Holding a steam-free mirror with one hand and a Gillette Mach III razor in the other, he shaves his face as he's done nearly every day of his adult life—his beard is light, which is the kind of genetic boon other crossdressers envy. After that he shaves his long legs from ankle to thigh. I love catching him while he's shaving his legs, singing along with Coldplay's music, one long thin leg stretching skyward daubed with shaving cream. He looks perfectly content, as if there is no greater joy than shaving one's legs. I have never felt any joy shaving my legs and in fact usually get mine waxed, but I am not—as I'm reminded frequently—a cross-dresser. I have to shave my legs because I have to, not because I want to, and that makes all the difference in the world. He shaves his underarms, then shaves his face again. He tells me shaving twice is the only way to get the really close shave he needs so his beard shadow won't show through his foundation.

20

While he's drying, he picks out jewelry and starts to think about his makeup. Occasionally he opens Kevyn Aucoin's *Making Faces* for inspiration or to teach himself a new technique, but often he knows what he wants: like me and most women I know, he has his "regular" makeup—the version that's come about over time and repetition, the reliable way he knows looks good. Then it's on with the thong underwear, over which he wears the control top panties, which hold back his bulge. He puts a shoulder pad in each hip for makeshift hips. He sits down to put on pantyhose—he's the only crossdresser I know who prefers them over stockings and garters—and then the bra. He can do the clasp himself. He slips in his breast forms, shakes a little to get them to fall into place, then puts on a corset or waist cinch but more often neither. Sometimes he dresses before he puts on makeup, other times he makes up before he dresses.

As he puts on his makeup, Betty is ascendant: he walks more gracefully, is more precise with his hands—a requirement if you're applying liquid eyeliner—and generally seems lighter, more relaxed. His voice gets a little softer, but no higher in pitch. He may ask my opinion on an outfit or his makeup, but mostly he dresses to suit himself. Sometimes when he is done he is satisfied with how he looks, and other times he changes everything by the time we leave the house (if we're going out at all).

When we're running late he doesn't have time to lay everything out, and the more "out" he's become the less ritualized his procedure: frequently I see him half-dressed scrounging for that other shoe under the bed or checking my drawers for a misplaced pair of underwear. He rarely wears foundation garments now, and when he decides to wear pants he wonders why he bothered shaving his legs at all. As he becomes more comfortable with his femme self, I've noticed he's a little more like a regular woman—cursing at pantyhose that rip, muttering when his mascara dots his upper eyelid, and rejecting those ridiculously high heels for warmer, more comfortable shoes. I wonder if at some point we will meet at a fashion and gender crossroads, with both of us in jeans and oxfords and just enough makeup. Of course, he'll still have to put in his breasts, while I'm stuck with mine.

WHY DO THEY DO IT?

THE MOST COMMON question asked about crossdressers is "Why do they do it?" Like most wives, finding the answer was my most pressing concern, despite my husband's insistence that he had spent at least two decades doing research and hadn't found a definitive answer. He, too, turned to psychology, beginning with Magnus Hirschfield's ground-breaking work *Transvestites*, published in 1910, and to Havelock Ellis' case studies of sexual deviants, all the way through to publications of the late 20th century by Richard Docter, Harry Benjamin, Ray Blanchard, and John Money. He found many theories, sympathetic to outright reactionary, plus everything in between, but never a satisfying answer.

To answer the question "Why crossdress?" one must first ask:

- What is a woman?
- Why do men and women wear different clothes?
- Why is a person's identity so intrinsically connected to his or her clothing?
- Why do gender roles exist at all?

Can you answer any of these questions? I can't. I can provide you with sartorial history, theories of culture and society, and a host of good guesses by psychologists and other "experts," but in the end I can't answer a single one of them in an absolute and definite way.

The best answer is often the simplest, and comes from my husband: "Because I like to be pretty sometimes." Common variations on this explanation include: "It feels good," "It satisfies something in me that nothing else does," and "It makes me feel peaceful." When crossdressers say these things, they are answering more the *how* of it than the *why*— how it affects them and the good feelings it causes. Those good feelings explain—to them—why they do it. Why putting on a woman's clothes feels good in the first place—to some men and not others—is what most of us are trying to figure out.

Perhaps the most important reason crossdressers offer is that, in some sense, they *must*: not must as in eating and breathing, but more like in bathing and sleeping well and getting enough exercise. Crossdressing is not necessary to a person's survival, but it does seem to be necessary to his well-being. Crossdressing is not, as some wives of crossdressers might wish, a selfish whim. Crossdressers as a group do not give it up despite the troubles it can cause in their lives. The phenomenon is stubbornly inexplicable, a cross between a compulsion and a wish. Psychologists over the years have theorized about why.

The study of "deviance" really begins with Richard von Krafft-Ebing's *Psychopathia Sexualis*, published originally in 1887, which presented diagnostic categories for "perversions of the sexual instinct." He did not analyze crossdressing per se, although a few of his case studies included crossdressing. His basic idea was that any sexual perversions were caused by familial influence, and his case studies begin with discussions of the family of origin, listing members who were institutionalized, had legal trouble, schizophrenia, epilepsy, etc. He thought that any sexuality whose purpose was not reproduction "perverted" the natural reason for sex. His crossdressing cases were found in the subcategories of Fetish and Homosexuality.

Not long after Krafft-Ebing comes Magnus Hirschfield, the father of the study of transvestism. He coined the term "transvestite" and wrote the first extensive book on the subject. His theories are constitutional in nature: "He is what he is." There is no other explanation given, and Hirschfield's lack of interest in finding a reason may be related to his own sexuality. He knew he was gay without needing to understand why, and maybe sensed that crossdressers understood their own identity in a similar way. Hirschfield's focus was to provide information to a public and psycho-medical community that was otherwise uneducated about transvestites or unaware of their existence. Transvestites have often been lumped together with homosexuals, fetishists, masochists, and transsexuals. Hirschfield differentiated transvestites from the first three groups, and identified an "asexual" group of transvestites who later researchers would classify "transsexual." Havelock Ellis, a peer of Hirschfield's, thought the term "transvestite" didn't stress fully the gender issues experienced by most transvestites because the term focused too much on the clothing, but he otherwise agreed with Hirschfield's ideas. Unlike Krafft-Ebing, who was openly hostile to all "perversions," Hirschfield was a reformer who worked to de-criminalize crossdressing (and homosexuality), and shared with Ellis a deep interest in studying and understanding the phenomenon, not "curing" it. Reading Hirschfield, especially, is a joy: his work is so free from prejudice and humanistic in spirit, one wonders why, nearly a hundred years later, crossdressing is so misunderstood. It turns out that Hirschfield's Institute for Sexual Science—the first institute of its kind—was destroyed by the Nazis in 1933 and his work thought lost as a result. Hirschfield himself died in exile: he was both Jewish and gay.

Next are the psychosexual ideas about transvestites, which maintain a kind of Freudian party line. Either the transvestite has an absent father from whom he is alienated, and so chooses to make the mother happy by adopting feminine attire, or alternately, the mother is absent and the transvestite son is trying to replace her for the mourning father. A stricter Freudian analysis (psychoanalysis) posits that the transvestite son, in fearing his love for his mother, finds a "safe" way to be close to her by wearing her clothes—

thus allaying his castration anxiety. My favorite Freudian theory is based upon the idea that the young boy, upon seeing some naked female and her "lack" of penis, is so horrified by the idea that he must "create" a phallic woman—that is, in himself, thus reassuring himself that all women have penises under their skirts, and assuaging his castration anxiety. Ah, Freud.

Harry Benjamin is the one who labeled Hirschfield's group of "asexual transvestites" as transsexuals. Benjamin, an endocrinologist, attempted to "cure" transvestites with doses of testosterone (which usually just increased their sex drive but caused no cessation of the crossdressing). Like Hirschfield, he attempted to educate the public. His "Standards of Care" are the rule of thumb in the screening of transsexual people, and their relevance is hotly debated in gender circles, although his contributions are acknowledged.

The "biological determinist" approach evolved from Benjamin's work, arguing that transvestism is caused by hormonal or chromosomal factors. The lure of providing an explanation for crossdressing with the kind of quantifiable evidence biochemistry might yield is great. Biochemical reasons could legitimize crossdressers' behavior in a way nothing else has. That said, it also tempts researchers to find a cure, in that many biochemical imbalances can be "corrected" with contravening chemical cocktails. Because imbalance implies malfunction, some might conclude that malfunction can be fixed. Most crossdressers, however, are not interested in being "corrected" or "fixed" but only accepted. The existence of biological reasons also eliminates other likely influences—like social and cultural factors—entirely.

Sociological and psycho-social theories predominated in the 1950s and 1960s, when behaviorism was the fashion. They were based on the idea that the transvestite had been incorrectly socialized as a child, and that repeated aversion therapy would reverse or correct that early socialization. In the 1960s treatments like electroshock therapy were sometimes prescribed. The transvestite might stop wearing stockings, but his desire to dress didn't decrease. That is, aversion therapy and its ilk only worked on a symptomatic basis, but did nothing to alter the underlying cause, probably because that cause had not—and still has not—been identified.

By the 1970s, sociological models focused more on gender than sex, and the term "gender dysphoria" was created. Gender dysphoria is a basic discomfort with the socially prescribed gender role as determined by the child's genital sex. In a nutshell: a child with a penis is supposed to play with cars, not dolls. Although this term names a phenomenon that motivates crossdressers, it hardly serves as a solution. The next logical question—"What causes gender dysphoria?"—leads us back to square one.

A common belief is that transvestites are severe closet cases, homosexuals who can't act on their desires unless they engage in a heterosexual "masquerade." By wearing the clothing of the opposite sex, crossdressers can attract and have sexual intercourse with men as women. This subterfuge is assumed to alleviate their shame and guilt over being homosexual, at least long enough for them to have sex. Alternately, some argue that the crossdressing is a stepping stone toward "coming out," with the implication being that once the homosexual accepts himself, he will stop crossdressing. Since I've met men who were both homosexual *and* crossdressing from an early age, that seems unlikely.

Virginia (nee Charles) Prince, who has lived full-time as a woman for decades, founded Tri-Ess (The Society for the Second Self, the largest organization of heterosexual crossdressers in America). She started a magazine, *Transvestia*, and wrote books about and for crossdressers in the 1960s. Tri-Ess, with Prince at its helm, gained membership over the years so that by the time the 1980s rolled around, identity politics had emerged and crossdressers started speaking for themselves. The "official" reason given by Prince and other Tri-Ess members is that crossdressers are attempting to express a feminine side of their personality otherwise left unexpressed: their second self. Their urge to crossdress, Prince emphasized, was not erotic, and it did not indicate dysphoria of any kind. It was purely an expression of inherent but repressed femininity, and its expression resulted in happier men who had integrated both their masculine and feminine sides. The cynical observer might ask, if the crossdresser has so fully integrated both sides, why then does he spend so much time looking at lingerie catalogs? Why not express femininity by taking care of children or cleaning the house, instead of devoting endless hours to ritualized crossdressing? Tri-Ess has no answer except to insist on its definition, which must at long last also be taken with a grain of salt, because, as Vern Bullough points out, "those who did not conform were removed from membership." A definition thus acquired is more an enforced opinion than a definition gained from objective analysis.

Where you've ended up is where I ended up, and where my husband before me ended up, which is nowhere certain. There is no single viable explanation, and though some might appeal to reason (more or less), and others seem plausible (more or less), and a few others offer the false hope of a cure (more or less), there is no explanation that holds up under all circumstances. For every attempt at explaining what crossdressing is, there is an exception—often many. I have come to suspect that the attempt to discover the genesis of crossdressing is motivated by the desire to find a cure, and a cure, I assure you, is not forthcoming. Crossdressers—alone and in conjunction with psychologists—have tried it all from purging to repression to electroshock therapy.

Despite the failure to find a cure, we still do not accept crossdressing as a regular behavior. Why? Because transvestism *is* upsetting. Clothes are meant to indicate our biological sex because for some inexplicable reason we need to know if someone is a boy or a girl. Why do we need to know so badly? The easiest answer is that we need to know a person's biological function, whether she or he becomes pregnant or impregnates. If that were the case, we would separate children not at birth but nearer puberty, when a person's sexual function begins. But we separate the boys from the girls at birth, which indicates that gender can't just be about sexual function. We are so insistent upon knowing a child's sex at birth that those born with Intersex conditions—uncertain genitalia or atypical chromosomes— are often surgically altered to look like a boy or a girl, even when the child's biological sex (as determined by their internal organs or chromosomes) is uncertain. Some Intersexed children are made unable to become pregnant or impregnate as a result of these anxiety-driven surgeries, which is strong evidence for gender not being about sexual function at all, but more about the human fixation with dividing us up into one of two gender categories. After all, how offended is a new mother when someone thinks her baby boy is a girl? Very—and she will be doubly sure next time to dress the child in blue. (Interestingly, pink was the choice for baby boys at the turn of the last century, as blue was considered "too feminine" a color, and boys during the same era were often kept in dresses and their hair left to grow long as toddlers.)

Procreation may have something to do with it, but only indirectly in that sexual function determines our gender roles. Because women have babies, they are primarily trained to raise children, and thus their gender role is created: because you are a future woman, you are socialized as a future mother. From girlhood, female children are trained to be nurturing, patient, supportive, and gentle—adept at all the skills they will need to raise children. Boys are future men and fathers, so they are trained to be breadwinners, replete with all the gifts and traits they will need to play their gender role to the best of their ability: competitive, prudent, disciplined, and possessing financial acumen.

It all makes perfect sense except for the simple fact that dads now raise kids, too, and women make money, hold jobs, run businesses. Barely fifty years ago these gender roles were rare exceptions; now they are the norm. Gay male couples adopt and have been proven to raise well-adjusted, well-loved children. There is no "mother" involved in the traditional sense, no woman who plays that role. Maybe both partners "mother" the child in different ways.

Our gender roles are outdated, or at the very least, too rigid. Some women will not have children, others will; some men will become fathers and others won't. Why should a young girl be given a skill set that will in fact disable her from making money? Why teach boys to be aggressive when what they need is tenderness, to take care of a sick child?

Crossdressing, then, shouldn't be upsetting because crossdressers misrepresent gender roles. Lots of things do that now: "Mr. Moms" oppose their traditional gender roles as men, and career women reject their historic gender roles as women. Our lives have changed and most people can acknowledge that it makes sense for the parent who is better at making money to pursue the career. We don't care if that's the man or the woman anymore, as long as someone's paying the bills.

Yet crossdressing still disturbs us, despite our modernized gender roles, so perhaps it's a sexual issue. Certainly a man in a dress sends mixed signals sexually. Is a man in a dress trying to attract another man, or a woman? From a heterosexual context, he could only be using a woman's clothes to signal sexually to another man, as a woman was traditionally considered the "proper" object of a man's desire. That is a heterosexual assumption, however, and we don't live in only a heterosexual society anymore, despite the legal, social, civic, economic, and outright physical attacks on gays and lesbians in America, even in 2004. A woman who dresses sexy may just be signaling to another female, and a handsomely dressed man may be trying to attract other men. So is that man in a dress trying to attract another man, or a woman? You don't know, based on his sex or his presentation. Could be either. Could be both. It could be he's just dressing for his own pleasure and isn't signaling to anyone about his sexual availability at all.

That's not to say we've all caught up with the cultural and social changes of the last fifty years. These changes have been controversial and problematic and not everyone can easily adjust to them. The feminist movement and the changes it brought to our gender roles only date to the 1970s, or—if you want to go back to the Suffragettes—1920. That's still less than a hundred years ago. The shifts in sexual signaling brought by the gay and lesbian movement are even more recent, dating back only to the days of the Stonewall Riots that started on June 27, 1969, or perhaps to Harry Hay's Mattachine Society of the 1950s. These changes are brand new when it comes to cultures, which move about as quickly as icebergs. Our narrow definitions of gender roles may be broadening, but our visceral response to the blurring of those roles is still one of shock or confusion. Our collective consciousness still insists that we differentiate between boys and girls at all times. There are only a few times and places where it's acceptable to blur those lines, such as Halloween or Wigstock and maybe even the occasional political fundraiser. (The former mayor of New York, Rudy Giuliani, got into drag quite a few times during his mayoralty.)

It's as if we are suffering from a cultural hangover from the gender party of the years before. We had unshakeable rules and unbreakable taboos instilled in us from the day we were born and it's hard to get over them. I just learned—from Virginia Prince's 1967 book *The Transvestite and His Wife*—that in the 1960s and 70s women in pants were turned away from restaurants and other public establishments for being improperly dressed. That was a huge surprise to me, since I was born in the early 1970s and grew up with a mom and aunts and female neighbors who all wore pants. It made me wonder: if skirts become acceptable for men to wear, would there still be crossdressers? If men could wear dangly earrings and flowery perfumes, light silk blouses and summer dresses, would crossdressers be able to crossdress? We can't know until men are able to wear all of women's clothes, of course, but my best guess is that crossdressers would still exist. As far as I can tell, men *can* wear frilly things—or they could certainly wear a lot more pretty things than they do now. When I was growing up a man's pierced ear communicated that he was a convict or a homosexual. Now, no one thinks twice about a boy with one or both ears pierced. He can even wear hoops instead of plain studs. Does that mean crossdressers have gone out en masse and gotten their ears pierced? Nope. Plenty do, and others still worry that if they do, someone's going to guess their secret. Ditto with long hair, which so many crossdressers talk about with envy. Do most of them grow their hair long? No. Some do. Some get more unisex cuts that can be styled either way. The vast majority keep their hair short, so as not to raise anyone's suspicions, and wear wigs as their femme selves.

So why is it crossdressers don't take advantage at least of the sartorial freedoms they do have?

Are we back at "why" again?

Crossdressing is not about the earrings or the long hair or the floral patterns. It's not even about high heels (some men wore those in the 1970s) or makeup (some men wore that in the 1980s). Except for the rare crossdresser who can satisfy his needs by wearing an item or two of feminine attire, most crossdressers want to wear women's things as women wear them, and look like women while they do so.

No one knows why.

They don't all do it for a sexual turn-on, though some do. They don't all do it because they are unhappy being men. They don't all do it as a way to release stress. They certainly don't all do it to attract men, or to attract women. Most of them, however, will admit they do it for pleasure of some kind. For some that pleasure is sexual, and for others it is a more tactile pleasure, a sensual appreciation of soft fabrics and fragrances. Others enjoy being able to express part of themselves they feel they can't otherwise express: to be able to cry easily, or giggle, or touch someone to whom they're talking. For every crossdresser there is a different reason to dress, and for each crossdresser there may be a few reasons, but the only true thing I can say is that crossdressers dress for themselves and for the pleasure it brings them.

WHO, WHAT, WHEN, HOW

CROSSDRESSERS COME FROM all walks of life, are all ages and races. There are crossdressers in finance, government, engineering, and other high status jobs. Crossdressers drive trucks, make deliveries, and fix faucets. They act and write. They belong to the Republican and Democratic parties, or vote Independent. They are heterosexual, homosexual, and bisexual. Some are single, while others enjoy long-term marriages or suffer multiple divorces. Many raise children. Some have substance abuse problems, and others have never even taken a drink.

What crossdressers do is a little easier to classify. Most of them share similar "discovery" stories—of the first time they put on an item of feminine clothing and felt that thrill.

There are things children just know without anyone telling them. When a five-year-old boy who finds a pair of his mother's stockings hanging to dry in the bathroom feels a rush of pleasure as he slides them up his pudgy legs, he knows intrinsically not to run into the kitchen to show mom. There are few crossdressers who made that mistake: somehow their childish brains have already filed all the cultural messages about what's okay and what's not, what a boy does and what he doesn't do. Psychologists say children have already learned the difference between boys and girls by age three. Kids know, they file, they separate into the boxes they're given. Pink for girls. Girls wear dresses. Boys don't play with dolls.

Perhaps most crossdressers discover the urge to wear their mom's stockings when they're only five because they're not quite old enough to realize they shouldn't even try them on. After all, kids play dress up all the time, for shows they put on for their friends and parents, for karaoke, for Halloween. All of childhood is about trying new things: a taste of one thing might be the birth of a lifelong love, for lasagna or bubble gum, but a taste of bathroom cleaner lands them in the emergency room. Kids test their boundaries, but when they know they've crossed one, they're smart enough to keep it a secret. So it is for the boy who discovers his love of stockings, who, from the moment he puts them on, knows he will tell no one about it.

The five-year-old sitting on the cold bathroom tile floor in his mother's stockings finds some connection to his own sensuality that he already knows he's not allowed to have. He knows from then on to put on those stockings in the bathroom with the door securely locked. He gets bored with damp panty-hose and wants to try other girls' things, to see if they give him that same excitement, the same rush of pleasure and comfort. He steals from his sister's laundry basket, puts on his mom's slip once the babysitter has fallen asleep, and stares lovingly at his sister's party dress in her little closet with the lamb on the door. He wants and wants and wants these things to be his, to wear them and show everyone how pretty he is, but he doesn't. He remains a boy, and thus the first closet for many crossdressers is in fact the bathroom, or the laundry room, or any room in the house with a door that locks.

Some of them are brave enough to steal an item or two. Most of them just borrow. Colleen, a crossdresser, was so careful about replacing his mother's pantyhose that it was only as an adult that he realized women rarely know how many pairs they have in the drawer.

The laundry basket is a popular place to steal from: items found there are already expected to be missing for a while as they are washed, dried, folded, and put back in the drawer. It's a little like getting a bathroom pass and using it to go wander down the hall to look at that girl in Mrs. Talbot's class, or to see if *this time* the janitor's closet will open. Young crossdressers calculate conscientiously, knowing a sister won't expect her cotton pair with the bunnies on them until at least Tuesday. To forget to return a piece of clothing is the child crossdresser's worst nightmare: When his sister asks, during dinner, "Mom, did you do the laundry yet? Could you pass the butter?" his heart goes into palpitations. He is convinced that everyone at the dinner table knows full well that he is the culprit, that he's hidden the missing item between his mattress and box spring.

Usually Mom's just been late with the laundry.

To keep a secret at such a young age doesn't make the crossdresser unusual. Most kids hide things when they know they've done something wrong. Kids don't confess when they put a whole roll of toilet paper in the toilet, spin rocks in the clothes dryer, or pop the heads off their sister's dolls. But as they get older, at teenage slumber parties or over their first beers, they start comparing notes. Once they reach adulthood, most siblings tattle over Thanksgiving dinner ("You know I never told Mom you were the one who . . ."). Little by little, most people own up to their secret, childhood crimes and so relieve the shame.

Not crossdressers. They may stop popping the heads off their sister's dolls, but they don't stop crossdressing. No one's willing to confess to a "crime" that they're still committing. The five-year-old crossdresser grows into a pre-pubescent boy, and suddenly that thrill he gets from putting on pantyhose might commingle with his first accidental orgasm: the pleasure and sensuality cause an erection, and the taboo is doubled. "Between masturbating and wearing women's clothes I knew I was going to hell," says Colleen, and so did many other crossdressers like him.

Since nothing is more important to a teenager than not being weird, crossdressers dress and jerk-off in private—in their mother's slips or their sister's tights—and meanwhile join the football team and prove themselves star players. They date girls and long to touch the hemlines, finger the earrings, and breathe in the perfume. Some crossdressers avoid girls at this age because they know they risk giving themselves away, but others aggressively pursue girls like most teenaged boys. They are more extraordinarily in love with girls than even your average testosterone-loaded teenaged boy, because their love of girls is more complex: they want to take a girl's clothes off and put them on their own bodies. They want to look *at* them and look *like* them. A crossdresser wants to be near his girl *and* near her things: sitting in her room together he knows she wants him to kiss her, but he's also thinking about all those lovely silky things hanging in the closet. He wants to get into her drawers, all right, but not just the ones her mother warned her about.

My husband challenged his teenaged girlfriends to games of Truth or Dare, hoping like hell it wasn't too obvious that the dares he picked involved putting on lipstick, a necklace, a high-heeled shoe. He found ways to "let" girls put makeup on him, and almost always dressed for Halloween: as a female rock star, a hooker, a flapper, a schoolgirl. (He tells me it largely depended on what clothes were available, that is, available in his girlfriends' or girl friends' wardrobes.) He did whatever he could to get girls or girlfriends to dress him up, even if it meant being blunt. "I bet I could walk in those shoes," he'd say, and the girls would giggle as he put them on and traipsed across the carpet. Other girls would let the subject drop and he wouldn't push it.

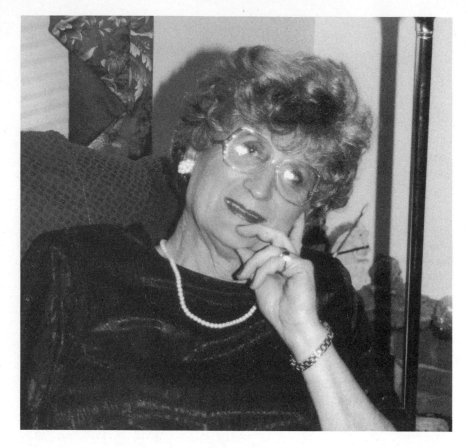

Becky Adams

He was more daring than most. Others never broached the subject with girlfriends and most crossdressers never even tell their wives. They cross-dress in private, and tell no one. They discreetly order everything from panties, stockings, and bras to dresses, shoes, and swimsuits from catalogs. They fight with themselves about their desires yet enjoy themselves when-ever they have a locked door to hide behind. They find racy stories about men who are forced to dress as women for one reason or another, and live lives, as Thoreau put it, "of quiet desperation." They are terrified that some-one will find out.

There are variations of this story, of course. Some put on their first item of female clothing when they're twelve, or fifteen, but rarely are they older than twenty. Kimmi is a definite exception because she started crossdressing only at age thirty-six, and even he can't tell you if his desire was repressed all those years. When Becca was five, he got permission to try on his mother's nylons and wore them right in front of her. He didn't crossdress again until he was a teenager. Crossdressers generally prefer wearing the most intimate of women's clothing, like panties, stockings, and bras, but others are fond of dresses or slips or blouses. Some of them never go out in public en femme, but regularly "underdress"—they wear their feminine dainties under their coveralls or jeans. I am frequently surprised by the feel of a bra strap under my husband's sweater when I kiss him hello and lay my hand on his back. He wears women's panties regularly since lingerie stores like Victoria's Secret make cotton panties in pretty colors. I have to talk him into wearing his male undies, and he puts them on the way straight women put on a lacy negligee for their husbands: to turn me on. He must be coaxed or exceptionally horny, although even he has moments—few and far between—when his male self is "ascendant," as he calls it, and prefers them. No matter how self-accepting a crossdresser becomes, they all still have moments when they wish they weren't crossdressers.

A crossdresser enjoys dressing. It's the popular images and understanding of him that he can't stand and that make him wish he weren't a crossdresser. Transvestites are portrayed in bizarrely bad ways all over the media: in commercials, movies, television shows. The British comedian Eddie Izzard, who is a transvestite himself, makes the perfect distinction: between "weirdo transvestites" and "executive transvestites." He describes a man in the Bronx (one of New York City's five boroughs) who was living in a cave and shooting at geese, and who happened to have several pairs of women's shoes in his cave, which caused the police to decide he was a transvestite. A *weirdo* transvestite, Eddie Izzard argues.

Most of the common portrayals of transvestites are of weirdo transvestites. Frank N. Furter, though well-loved as a cult figure, is a weirdo transvestite. On an episode of *Law & Order: Criminal Investigation,* the detectives note that a man has tweezed his eyebrows. They conclude, as a result, that he is a transvestite, and that being a transvestite, he must also be a masochist. They track down two prostitutes whom he has paid for "forced feminization" scenes, in which they insist he dress as a woman by threatening to punish him in some way. Once he was crossdressed, they explained, they made fun of him until he was in tears, and having reverted to a childish self, he then apologized to his (deceased) mother for something he'd done. It turned out, at the end of the episode, that the man—as a boy—had put ant poison in his mother's lemonade in order to make her get sick and miscarry the baby she was pregnant with. It is only by re-enacting his childhood that he can assuage his guilt. The "forced feminization," one is meant to assume, is what broke his adult ego and allows him to access the guilty child within.*

Weirdo transvestite.

There are tons of other examples. J. Edgar Hoover, for instance. Weirdo transvestite. Robert Durst, a murder suspect, earned headlines like these:

WIGGED-OUT DURST WAS SPOTTED ON LAM IN CALIF.

WHAT A DRAG FOR DURST:

PROBERS SAY THEY FOUND HIS LADY DISGUISES

Weirdo transvestite.

A cop-killer dressed like a woman in order to escape police detection, and his family seemed more embarrassed about his crossdressing than the murder he committed.

Weirdo transvestite.

"Executive transvestites," Eddie Izzard argues, are men like him. Unfortunately he has no other public figures to name, as there is not one other single public figure who is "out," known to be a heterosexual male transvestite. Not one. No wonder then that most crossdressers occasionally wish they weren't crossdressers. The only examples most people see are of the weirdo transvestites, and a crossdresser knows that's what people think of him when he goes out dressed. No wonder a crossdresser's life is steeped in secrecy and shame.

It has been argued that the problems crossdressers suffer are often iatrogenic symptoms, that is, problems caused by the fact that crossdressers have traditionally been diagnosed by the psycho-medical community as "sick." Moser and Kleinplatz argued in their essay, "Transvestic Fetishism: Psychopathology or Iatrogenic Artifact?" that crossdressers are not sick because they are crossdressers, but rather because they are diagnosed as crossdressers—that their "unusual sexual interest" is defined by the medical community as a pathology. They may otherwise be alcoholic, codependent,

---

*This complicated elaboration has nothing whatsoever to do with what most men are looking for when they crave "forced feminization." Indeed, they want a woman to force them to dress as women, under threat of some kind of punishment, but all they are trying to achieve is the ability to be dressed as women without the guilt and shame of wanting to dress like women. By "pretending" that someone else is forcing them to do it, they sidestep the guilt from having such a "deviant" desire, but still get to crossdress.

or even schizophrenic, but they are not those things in higher percentages than are "ordinary" heterosexual men. We have no idea what a "healthy" crossdresser looks like because there are so few in the first place. As generations of gay men and women have found out, it's the closet that's the problem, not the person in it.

LIVES IN THE CLOSET

THE MOST EXTREME manifestation of that embarrassment or shame at being crossdresser is the purge, when a crossdresser gathers up all of his feminine items and dumps them, vowing never to crossdress again. Some do this many times over a lifetime. My husband did it only once—just after he'd been dumped by a girl he liked. It is the moment when the crossdresser symbolically takes his desire to dress as a woman and puts it in the garbage, hoping that doing so will cause him to quit the behavior, too.

It doesn't work. The crossdresser may go for weeks or even months (and in rare cases, years) without crossdressing, but eventually the urge overwhelms him and he buys a pair of panties, or a pair of stockings, or a slip. Soon he finds himself wearing the new item in front of the mirror and shopping for a dress to go with it. Before long, he has replaced everything he owned before. He has wasted time and money, and convinced himself that he is both a crossdresser and a failure for not stopping his crossdressing. It's one thing to live with the guilt and shame of being a crossdresser, but another entirely to suffer the humiliation of realizing that he's incapable of exerting much control over it. When asked what to tell a fellow CD who is about to purge, every crossdresser I asked said "don't bother" in one way or another.

THE PURGE IS one of the few things nearly all crossdressers share. That, and a love of women's clothes, of course. There are other similarities as well. Patterns emerge in the chronology of crossdressed lives. The five-year-old boy putting on his mother's stockings in the bathroom becomes a teenaged boy whose attraction to girls is twofold. It is when that same teenaged boy becomes a man that the decisions he makes about his crossdressing impact his sex life, his social life, and his emotional health. Each decade seems to represent a different kind of struggle for a man who crossdresses, and the decisions he makes during each inform the ones that come after. I have spoken with crossdressers in their twenties to retired men in their seventies, and I'm going to try to describe how a crossdresser's life often progresses.

THE TWENTIES

A lot of crossdressers get married in their twenties hoping that marriage will "cure" them. A very rare few tell their fiancées, but most don't, and before they know it their wives are having babies. Even at this stage, many crossdressers continue to stay silent about their behavior. (Tomye Kelley points out in *Stages of Resolution with Spouses* that many husbands tell their wives "during her pregnancy or at the time that she has just delivered a baby" because they feel "envious of her pregnancy," viewing pregnancy "as the highest form of 'femaleness.' " Kelley mildly asserts that no wife "appreciated such timing." Are you kidding? I'm surprised these husbands don't find their larynxes ripped out.) Married men who stay silent crossdress on business trips, rent hotel rooms in nearby cities, or wait until their wives take the kids to visit Grandma. More than one CD has been "discovered" because his wife came home a few hours early.

The single crossdresser in his twenties dates and crossdresses but rarely mixes the two.

THE THIRTIES

In their thirties, the real dilemmas begin. The crossdresser who has gotten married in his early twenties realizes the behavior isn't going away. The single crossdresser realizes it's not going away. The crossdresser who is in a relationship with a woman he's halfway convinced will be his future wife realizes it's not going away. All three of them panic, to lesser or greater degree. The single CD may purge because he blames his crossdressing for his still being single. The married one may find himself aggressively seeking more opportunities to dress and putting himself at greater risk or discovery; he might also give serious thought to telling his wife. The crossdresser who is dating and heading toward a committed relationship may be so terrified of losing her that he can't imagine telling her, or he makes peace with the fact that if he waited so long for the right girl he has to tell her.

The thirties are a time of upheaval for everyone, not just crossdressers. It's the decade when you've settled down a little about who you are, and look around to see where you are. It's as if thirty is the signpost where you stop worrying about what everyone else thinks of you and start worrying about what *you* think about you. You start looking at the mental lists of what your younger self might have accomplished and begin to realize you had some unrealistic expectations, but you also had great things happen to you that you never expected or planned for. You've probably settled into a career and found a partner and started to wonder what it all means. For the crossdresser it's the same, except he knows that one of his desires—to dress more—has not been met. He wants to start going out en femme. He's been crossdressing secretly in his twenties and not thinking about it otherwise, but at thirty he needs to know why he dresses and whether he could find a way to dress more. A lot of crossdressers start to lose the sexual excitement they got from dressing when they were younger (if they ever had it) and many wonder why they still crossdress if it's not about the turn-on. They look for other explanations. Some of them realize it's about gender, and they might question their masculinity. They might finally acknowledge that they have wondered what it's like to have breasts or to remove all their body hair. They may worry that they are transsexual. Others who have never been "out" wonder what it would be like to pass as a woman in public. Many conflicting feelings come up in the search to figure it all out. Some get so disgusted they purge again, deciding once and for all they're simply not going to do it anymore. That doesn't work because it never works. They are, for the most part, tired of being alone with their secret, and are tired too of feeling "all dressed up with no place to go." They start to experiment and seek options. They find that places host three-day weekends designed for crossdressers, like the En Femme Getaway in Eureka Springs, Arkansas, where they can spend the whole time en femme or they join a support group, or go to a conference focusing on transgender issues.

Pushing themselves to new limits, crossdressers may go out to a T-friendly club, or find a support group, or tell their wives. They often experience what is known as "euphoria" with these victories, an overwhelming sense that they can go anywhere crossdressed. They suddenly want to dress all the time and recapture the feeling again and again. Many do. If they go three days en femme and enjoy it, next time around they want to dress for four days. It is a constant pushing of boundaries—until they get to one and realize it's enough. Ali says he knew he was "just a crossdresser" when he agreed to be in a documentary film about transvestism in his native England: After three days of putting on nylons it was no fun anymore, and he knew he didn't want to crossdress every day. Some crossdressers experiment with their sexuality at this stage for similar reasons and most confirm they're straight—as they thought they were all along. If they can go out and ask questions, they can find answers.

Being the partner of a crossdresser during this time in his life can be especially difficult. There is no certainty, and the crossdresser has not yet figured out what he needs in order to feel satisfied. A couple may make a joint decision that she is okay with him dressing once a week, and he agrees to it, but barely a week later he may realize that's just not enough. She wonders if she missed something, and she did: she missed the sense of urgency and confusion that's going on in his head, and doesn't realize he is at a point where he is entirely unable to make a decision about his crossdressing that will stick for longer than a week. In order to preserve their relationship, a crossdresser will often agree to limits he can't keep, because he's torn between keeping his girlfriend and expressing his femme side. His inability to stick to his promises drives his wife up the wall.

THE FORTIES

A crossdresser in his forties is either one of two types: either he has done all the experimenting he needed to and discovered how often he wants to dress, where, and how; or, he has continued in a state of denial that his crossdressing urge would go away. The crossdresser who has experimented can

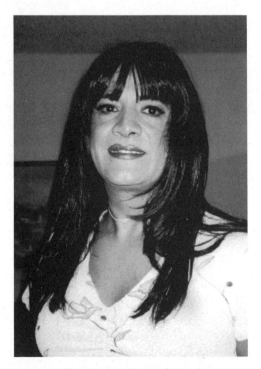

Caroline, a single crossdresser

scttle down a little bit, and because of the general decrease in testosterone, might find less sexual pleasure in dressing if that is what he found in it to begin with. He might realize his crossdressing is an opportunity to access a different, more feminine side of himself. Through support groups, he may want to help other younger crossdressers through their confusion. He is in the enviable position of having answered some questions and put niggling doubts to rest.

The other crossdresser—who has not asked the questions and explored opportunities—is fit to burst at this stage. The combination of a lifetime of repression and loneliness combined with a midlife crisis can cause serious sadness and difficulties in the crossdresser's life. He may blame his cross-dressing for never having been married, or for a failed marriage. He may do reckless things in order to feel feminine, like frequent gay clubs and flirt or date men even if he's been sexually fond of women his whole life. Loneliness and confusion can cause a lot of mischief in a person's life, and the crossdresser is no exception. The non-CD may have an affair or buy a sports car to relieve his midlife crisis, but the closeted crossdresser in his forties has no way out, and is mired in shame and self-doubt. He may find that social drinking has turned ugly, and drinks often by himself, and until he's oblivious. He feels like a failure for not having "conquered" his crossdressing, and heaps blame for his failure on himself as well. Historically, this decade is when late-transitioning TG/TS people realize they are not "just crossdressers," and decide also that it is about time they did something about it.

THE FIFTIES

By his fifties, the closeted crossdresser is ready for a nervous breakdown or worse. He may drink too much, be unpleasant at home, and shut down emotionally. His wife might be the one who sends him to therapy as he becomes increasingly difficult to live with, and depending on the counselor, he may come to realize there is no chance of "curing" himself and reach out for help either by contacting a support group or by telling his wife. He could end up with a therapist who tries to cure him, too. If he does decide to tell his wife, he may do so badly—in anger, or off the cuff, and not be prepared for her feelings because he's not aware of his own. He may find himself divorced for keeping a secret from his wife for several decades, or they may end up in counseling because she is furious, sad, betrayed. His commitment to his wife has probably not changed, and he may have children and grandchildren whom he loves. He faces the prospect of losing it all, and yet many take the risk at this time in their lives. At age fifty, most men know they have to make up their minds: They have reached the age of their maximum earning potential and begin to plan their retirement. They begin to sense their own mortality, especially if they are hearing stories about peers' heart attacks, divorces, early retirements. Many, finally, come out with it: They tell their wives, find the support group, and want to dress all the time. Get out of the way of a crossdresser who has waited all his life for this opportunity! He is euphoria embodied if he finds the support he needs, and by berating himself for not having come to grips with his crossdressing much, much earlier in his life, spurs himself into dressing more often. If he hasn't driven his wife completely nuts yet, he will when he becomes "euphoric."

The crossdressers, who experimented in their thirties and found whatever peace they could with their dressing by their forties, may get to fifty and want to dress more in order to make up for lost time. Those who retire early may want to spend all their time at home en femme. Others discover that the natural decrease in their testosterone has made them a little more "passable" because their skin is softer, and their decreased muscle tone is more pliant for corsets and other body shapers. If they are ever going to, they also may have a bit of money to spend on good cosmetics, breast forms, and body shapers. Many older crossdressers also capitalize on the fact that women above a certain age are not ogled in public; because no one is looking at them too carefully, they pass much more easily in places like malls. Older crossdressers often run their local support group, serving as role models for the younger CDs by sharing practical tips in hair-styling and makeup application. The crossdresser who has found support and is out to his wife may find he is perfectly happy. Some older men are known even to their own grandchildren.

THIS IS ONLY a generalized lifeline, based on the stories I've heard from crossdressers and from their wives. It's hardly the most extreme version— crossdressers consider suicide, end up deeply repressed and thus depressed. Every crossdresser's story is different. Some stay permanently in the closet, others come out in their twenties. Others only start crossdressing at home when they become widowers, others when their wives divorce them. More than one crossdresser has come out as a result of blackmail by an ex-girlfriend or a wife: it's not a good way to come out, but it happens. There are as many life stories as there are crossdressers, but what I have found to be true is that a crossdresser's happiness is largely dependent on his own self-acceptance. How he acquires that—via therapy, a supportive spouse, or membership in an organization of other crossdressers—is up to the individual.

There is a great deal of variety in the community, and despite the narrow definitions inflicted by the psychological community and crossdressing organizations, there are a few distinct "categories" of crossdressers as well. There are as many types as there are crossdressers, and as soon as you try to categorize them, the categories fail. Of course I can't help but try, anyway. My husband and I came up with these categories; we've got crossdresser friends who fit each of the "types," and although I might argue it would be easier to be married to some of these types than others, we imply no judgments whatsoever. There isn't a better or worse kind of crossdresser. That said, even when a crossdresser "fits" one of these categories, he might also fully fit another entirely. He may fit different ones during different times in his life, too.

- The *Straight Drag Queen* dresses to be fabulous, for performance, and is generally over the top. My husband occasionally falls into this category, when we go to themed club events (he does a mean Betty Page) or the like. Donna T of Boulder is a straight drag queen: she dresses and performs as her femme self

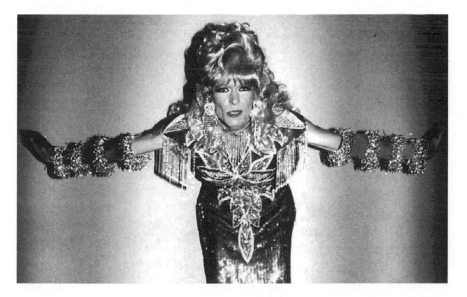

Donna T, a straight drag queen

in order to raise money for Children's Hospitals. She is specifically accepted by the other queens, as a fellow queen. Straight Drag Queens often have a more "regular" crossdressed side as well, because it's difficult to shop in four-inch platform heels and fake eyelashes.

- The *Fetishist* is the type who loves one item of clothing more than any other—like lace panties—and who can dress only in it to feel satisfied. The Fetishist's life is rarely disrupted by his interest, although it can be. The Fetishist is less likely to remove body hair or desire other body modifications for full-fledged crossdressing. When a crossdresser's website is covered with pictures of himself in panties, you can be pretty sure he's the Fetishist type.

- The **Closeted Crossdresser** is exactly that: the crossdresser who doesn't go out at all, and who may not even be out to his own wife. He may attend Tri-Ess meetings and know other "girls" who know him as well, but he's the one who has to dress on-site for the meetings, because he'd never even drive dressed. The closeted CD greatly looks forward to Halloween, as that's the only time he can crossdress in public—and even then will make a point of "not being very good at it" so as not to give himself away.

- The *Transgenderist* has deeper feelings about his gender, and uses crossdressing as a way to express his "inner woman." "She" spends more time en femme than en homme, and might be willing to try hormones for a while, or not. The Transgenderist is not a transsexual woman; "she" can and will dress as a man if the need arises. Virginia Prince, Tri-Ess' cofounder, is a self-described transgenderist, and has been for decades.

- The **Slutty Crossdresser** dresses like a slut and occasionally has a sex life to match. This is the crossdresser who's wearing a dress with a slit to his hip and sitting on a barstool with his legs spread. He makes crass jokes about women, and for him, crossdressing is definitely about his own arousal. He is "a horny guy in a dress." Slutty CDs are usually the ones that most horrify wives at crossdressing events.

- The **Out Crossdresser** goes to work en femme if he wants. His partner knows, his parents know, his grandchildren know. He will appear in documentaries as a crossdresser, has rid himself of shame, guilt, and usually any connection he might have had to the sexual side of crossdressing. He's usually a little bit older. Bobbi Williams, who is also the writer known as George Wilkerson, fits in this category, as do our friends Melissa and Ali.

- The **Classic Transvestite** is the crossdresser who knows he dresses for sexual pleasure, and enjoys the sensual side of crossdressing more than anything else. He may dress fully to go out, or he may not. He is very clear about his sexuality, and can be the most dedicated husband if his wife can even tolerate his crossdressing. Our friend Victoria considers himself a transvestite, and makes no bones that it's about the sensuality for him.

- The **Submissive** or **Sissy Crossdresser**, wants to take orders. Not always sexual, often you can find the Submissive CD in BDSM circles, or mixed in with the fetishists. There are Sissy Maids in particular, who like serving others in full French maid attire. They clean, cook, serve, do the dishes, vacuum—you name it and they'll do it if you ask the right way. They fantasize about "forced feminization" wherein a woman dresses them in women's clothes as punishment for some misdemeanor.

- The **Blend** is exactly that: a crossdresser who fits into more than one of the above categories simultaneously. For instance, a Submissive may also be a Fetishist, and have a thing for shoes, but is entirely in the closet about his desires, and so is a Closeted Crossdresser as well. My husband is a Blend: part Straight Drag Queen, part Transgenderist, and part Out Crossdresser.
  Most crossdressers are Blends.

It's very difficult to talk to a wife of a crossdresser without knowing what kind of crossdresser her husband is, and unfortunately the pervasive definitions are pillar-to-post. On the one hand you've got the crossdressing community, led by Virginia Prince, which has long insisted there is no sexual component to crossdressing. I assume they are willing to put all the crossdressers for whom there is a sexual component into the Fetishist classification and wash their hands of them. I don't think that makes any sense—after all, Magnus Hirschfield would have never identified transvestites as a group if he hadn't been a sexologist in the first place. Denying the sexual aspect is a nice attempt to clean up the images of crossdressers, but the other pervasive definition—which Eddie Izzard so neatly summarized in his routine on the weirdo transvestite—is still the more popular one.

So either a crossdresser is a regular guy who likes to wear dresses sometimes or he's a pervert, a freak, or mentally ill. There must be truth somewhere in the middle, as that's where it usually is. As a culture, however, we admit to no "middle" when it comes to crossdressing. It's either Jerry Springer—or nothing.

I'm not convinced that crossdressing is a perfectly normal thing, but I'm not convinced it isn't, either. I don't really buy the argument that men who crossdress are getting in touch with their "inner woman" because they so rarely have any interest in the actual lives of women. What they are interested in is their own expression of their own version of femininity, which is a whole different thing altogether. What I see and experience and hear about is closer to that idea than any other, that crossdressers are men, with men's notions of what women are, who then choose to express those male-centered ideas about femininity in a very masculine way. They don't help with the laundry or make dinner, they don't train themselves to make more room for others' needs than for their own. They continue to be the same guys they always were, in dresses. They are often selfish in how they pursue their crossdressing, whether by keeping it a secret from their wives or by buying themselves better second wardrobes than their wives' first ones. In a nutshell, they're the same guys all straight women are complaining about, and they are as predictably male about crossdressing as they are about watching football all weekend. (There is nothing more amusing to me than watching my husband, in skirt, heels and hose, shouting at the television when his team misses a pass. I call it "the worst of both worlds.")

I know, too, that it's about sex, and yet it isn't. Too many crossdressers describe deeply gendered feelings about their crossdressing, not so much as a dislike of their own masculinity, but as an expansion of it. Men generally have high sex drives, so it's no surprise that a crossdresser's gender identity gets tied up with his sexuality: For so many men, everything is tied up with their sexuality. That hardly means it's not about their deeper feelings. Men love women because they love sex with them, and they have sex with them because they love them. For the crossdresser, a sexual love of women is deeply tied to his own transgendered feelings; he loves, erotically and romantically and even platonically, that which he cannot be.

But it's also about more than sex, too. So many of them say they want to feel soft, pretty, and gentle. They want to nurture, and to comfort, and to bond. They envy the easy friendships between women, the casual way women touch each other when they talk. Imagine a man gently brushing another man's hair out of his eyes while they're chatting! But women do that kind of thing all the time, even ones who aren't especially feminine. Crossdressers want to talk and laugh, and not have to prove they're so macho.

Our ideas about masculinity leave men little room for their own self-expression. It's been shown again and again that there are no "traits" inherent in either gender, but rather that we all have different aptitudes and proclivities, some of which are encouraged if we are women, discouraged if we are men. Peggy Rudd, another wife of a crossdresser and author of several books about crossdressing, puts "intelligence" in a list of traits traditionally considered masculine. That wasn't, as we now know, because women aren't naturally intelligent—it was because women weren't educated, which makes showing intellectual acuity a little difficult to demonstrate (although so many women did, even at times when women weren't educated).

My best guess is that crossdressing is a reflection of men's needs to experience the whole of themselves, and especially that side of themselves that is denied in a male-dominated society. Men cannot slum by "being women" without the culture having a problem with it, because men are supposed to enjoy the privilege that comes from being on the top of the pile. They are certainly not supposed to reject it. We are all, as a culture, committed to believing that men are in control, because we live in a patriarchal society. We raise them to be the leaders and offer them no other option.

The complications arise because men understand their own "femininity" *as men,* and they know women through their own men's eyes. That may be why some crossdressers portray such a sexualized image of women when they dress as them. It may be why their notions of femininity seem a little absurd and outdated. Men objectify women—meaning, they see them as objects, not people, and what else can we expect when a man tries to replicate something he doesn't understand in the first place?

But the crossdresser, at least, is trying. He may try to emulate women in a particularly thick-headed, masculine way, but he does it out of his love for women—even if that love can only be shown by the short spectrum of emotions men in our society are allowed to express.

*　*　*

KYRIE, A CROSSDRESSER, tries to describe how he feels when he crossdresses:

The thing that immediately comes to me when I am "en femme" is the overall feeling of "well being." It is not something that is very easy to explain. It is both physical and emotional at the same time.

Physically, of course, there are all the sensations that go along with soft, silky clothing next to the body. This is amplified when I am dressed after just having shaved my legs, arms, body, etc. It can sometimes feel like being caressed, or even lightly massaged. The feeling of having a cool breeze beneath my skirt or dress is tantalizing, to say the least. These are physical sensations that are almost impossible to feel while wearing male clothes. They just aren't made from materials or to fit the body in a way that can produce the same tactile response. With a bra and breast forms in place, the center of gravity of the body shifts, and wearing high heels makes it necessary to redefine the way I walk. My steps are shorter and there's that certain "roll" of the hips that nat-

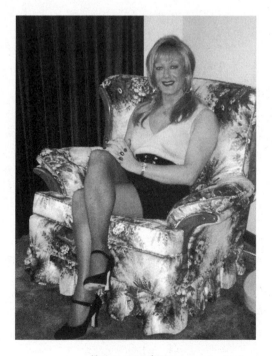

Kyrie, a crossdresser

urally develops. I like wearing a corset also, and apart from the figure is gives me, it also feels nice and supportive for the back. Doing things with long fingernails can be a challenge sometimes, but it causes me to handle things more gently, not that I am a rough and tough person to start with, but there is a definite "thing" that happens with the hands. My ears are pierced and I love that little "tug" and feel of something dangling from them. I used to have my own naturally long hair, but that has long since gone the way of the dinosaurs, so a wig has become necessary. Again, I love the feeling of hair gently caressing my neck and shoulders. It tickles, in a nice way. A hint of perfume adds to the overall "softness" that I feel. I love the feel of garters and stockings (that little tug that lets you know they are there as you walk). I have this little trick I use to create cleavage, and it can be very convincing, so low-cut tops and open-neck blouses are my preference. I am not purposely trying to be provocative, but I do like to see how well the illusion works.

On the emotional side of things, I find that transforming into Kyrie makes me high. I wish I had a better way to explain it, but that's about as close as I can come to anything that I can actually explain. I just feel "good." Aches and pains and stress and worry seem to just melt away, and what's left is just a feeling of well-being! I feel happy and energized. If I stay at home, I will just do simple things (answer e-mails, bake something, iron or maybe watch some TV). If I go out, I get this nervous kind of excitement thing happening. I go shopping or strolling through a mall or even to a movie, and I have this feeling of freedom. I do not have a better word for it. There is also this "naughtiness" about the whole thing. It's kind of like I am out there, looking and acting like a woman, but I know that underneath all the clothes and makeup, I am really a guy. It's like when you are a kid and you are playing "make believe." It's just plain fun. It can be a little unnerving at times, especially if I get read, but that's rare, and as long as nobody bothers me about it, that's okay. I love to dance in girl mode, but I have not done that in a while (apart from Halloween). The club scene is not something I do a lot these days, but that's another story.

The whole process of getting dressed and doing my hair and makeup and catching that glimpse of myself in the mirror afterwards is something that always brings me joy. It's a feeling of getting in touch with something that's important and special to me. Sexually speaking, it is not as much of a "turn on" as when I was younger. I suppose over time,

the fetish part of it has worn off, but I would still love to bring it into the
bedroom sometimes. I find the feeling of silk against silk very arousing.
I have no illusions about who I really am. I know that I am a guy, but
sometimes it just feels nice being a girl for a while. It has been a part of
me all my life, and I suspect it always will be.

Why do men crossdress? Because they can experience sensual pleasure and express it when they're dressed as women in a way they can't when they're men. Because it's playful, a little "naughty," and even a little bit sexy. Because—as they old joke goes—they can.

CHAPTER 3

Crossdressers' Wives, Girlfriends, and Partners

IT IS IRONIC that the most famous crossdresser is Joan of Arc, when she is outnumbered absurdly by men who have worn dresses. Women who crossdress have always been met with greater acceptance than male crossdressers. Marlene Dietrich crossdressed to great effect, and no one laughed when Mary Martin played Peter Pan. There is a long and rich history of women who crossdressed, and Vern and Bonnie Bullough point out in their book *Crossdressing, Sex, and Gender* that stories about women who crossdressed were very popular in the period from 1650 to 1850. These women were often tolerated and even encouraged by their fellow soldiers and sailors. The Bulloughs conclude that the tacit acceptance of FTM crossdressers was based on the understanding that a woman's crossdressing gave her access to a life that she couldn't otherwise have. But why on earth would a man want to emulate a woman? Women have historically been second-class citizens, and a man's desire to dress as a woman indicated that he had to be sick, insane, or at the very least, slumming.

Women do not crossdress the way men do. There are cases of women who dress as men for sensual pleasure, but they are rare. When women do crossdress, they do so in public, in order to "pass" and live as men. They do not put on a button-down shirt and bind their breasts for fun. Some do it because they are transgendered, as a step toward transitioning, or as "drag kings," where the crossdressing is about performance or humor. In the introduction I talked about a woman putting on her husband's button-down, and how we interpret that to mean she misses her husband or boyfriend. Most of the time, we're right. Sure, there are plenty of women who wear men's clothes, but how many straight women dress in men's clothes in order to look like men? Not many. Do any want to pass as men or date women? Not often. (There are exceptions, since there have been cases of FTM transsexuals who after transitioning dated men, but the majority of transitioned or transitioning FTM TSs have relationships with women.) The argument has been made—usually by crossdressers, but also by the psychological community—that women don't crossdress because they don't have to. Woman have greater sartorial freedom, meaning, we can wear what we want. I don't think that is entirely true. Yes, woman can wear jeans and pants, but we are still supposed to wear *women's* jeans and pants. What has happened is that fashions that used to be "for men only" have become acceptable for women—but only in the women's versions. Women's pants, for instance, are usually form-fitting, and so aren't really like men's at all. Ditto for women's jeans and blouses. They are designed for the female form, and often show off a woman's body the same way all women's clothing does. Any woman who wears loose flannel shirts or bulky sweaters in order to diminish her chest is accused of "covering up." I know. I have been shy about my curves for most of my life, and found it easier to get on in the world—in school, at work—by camouflaging my body a little. The less sexual harassment the better, I figured, and removing that threat made me feel more confident. As any woman knows, you can still get a wolf-whistle in sweats and no makeup with your hair pulled back.

Women understand that their clothes have something to do with their sexuality. My sister has worked in banking, a male-dominated industry, for over two decades. She has only recently—after achieving a certain degree of success and power—started wearing more feminine things to work. Before that, she dressed in man-tailored suits that de-emphasized her chest, and hip-long jackets to cover her hips and butt. She dressed, as it were, for work. She was not there to be pretty. She was there to run the place. Only recently have men in male-dominated industries started accepting that women are their peers and bosses. Only now, my sister says, does she feel comfortable dressing in floral silks and brighter colors, because only recently have professional women been allowed to express their femininity in the workplace. They are able to do so because they are finally beginning to be accepted as women. Previously, they de-emphasized their gender in order to be taken seriously.

Women know that women's clothes sexualize the body. They are designed to make the most of curves and cleavage and small ankles. Women's clothes show the female body to its best effect. Different designs highlight different attributes, but in the end, women's clothing—especially evening wear—is about looking attractive, showing off your form, and appealing to men.

This may be why we don't get why on earth our husbands and boyfriends want to wear women's clothes. The example I provided in the introduction—of the man who puts on his wife's slip—is not putting it on because he misses his wife. He puts on a slip because he's missing his own femininity, the part of him that likes pretty things. And that might have something to do with why women have a hard time with men crossdressing.

I have had times when my husband's crossdressing sickens me, baffles me, angers me. I just don't get it. Meredith doesn't, either. She tells me that her husband Victoria claims to be more comfortable in women's clothes: "How can he tell me that? They're not comfortable. I have to wear them. I know they're not comfortable. He's full of it." I can't help but agree. High heels, bras, and pantyhose are *not* comfortable, and the types of lingerie many crossdressers really love—garters, stockings, and corsets—are something close to sartorial torture. What I've learned is that Victoria means he is psychologically comfortable, and that dressing as a woman satisfies him so deeply that the physical discomfort is immaterial. Knowing that still doesn't mean I understand my husband's desire to emulate a woman. But I do know it derives from his admiration of and sexual attraction for women.

The hardest part about trying to accept my husband's love of the feminine was figuring out how I felt about being a woman. I had to come to terms with my own femininity. In my opinion, being a woman is not a walk in the park: shoot, most women can't even take a walk in the park without fear of sexual harassment or attack. We get paid less than we should, are admired primarily for our looks, and are usually assumed to be unintelligent, conniving, or both. So what was it he liked about women? Things I didn't even see as necessarily feminine: my friendships and conversations with other women, the choice to dress up or dress down, soft skin, curves, and the ability to show emotions without criticism. I could cry if I wanted.

I have had to make peace with being a woman in a way I never had to before. My husband has taught me to see my curves as beautiful, when before they only made me feel fat or objectified. He pointed out that I could wear pants or skirts. I had a greater range in how I might present myself: as girly, elegant, butch, or even dowdy. But it was realizing that he has spent a lifetime learning not to cry when he wants to that made me more thankful I was born and raised a woman than anything else. I can't say that I might not have learned these things if I hadn't married a crossdresser, but his love of the feminine has given me the ability to appreciate the good things about being a woman. In return, I think I've given him an education in what real women's lives are like. The conversations we have had about gender help us cross a divide and enriched our ability to communicate. Ultimately this exchange has made our companionship more companionable.

But of course all that goes right out the window when I find out he's lost my favorite lipstick.

*   *   *

ACCORDING TO THE crossdressing community, there are two types of wives: the ones who accept their husbands' crossdressing, and the ones who don't. That is an incredibly facile representation of who we are, and I'm happy to say I'm both types, depending on the day or the week or the moment. I'll bet most wives feel similarly, in that even those of us who are "accepting" have major issues with crossdressing: personal issues, sexual issues, identity issues. Besides, acceptance also exists on a "spectrum." Victoria thinks of his wife, Meredith, as nonaccepting, but Meredith has known about her husband's crossdressing for seven years and she's not going anywhere. In fact, she has been to a Tri-Ess meeting, works with a crossdressing friend of her husband's, and agreed to be interviewed for this book. Is that "not accepting"? I don't think so. She could be more accurately classified as "nonparticipatory," meaning she doesn't buy clothes or jewelry for her husband or chomp at the bit to attend CD social events. Other wives are more decidedly nonaccepting: Dixie's wife has not had sex with her crossdressing husband since he told her he was a crossdresser several years ago. She will not discuss the subject with him, refuses to meet other wives of crossdressers, and has thrown out the literature Dixie provided for her perusal. If there is any "textbook version" of a non-accepting wife, she is it. Then again, she hasn't left him, either. It all depends on how you define "accepting."

In *The Transvestite and His Wife*, a book written by Virginia Prince specifically for married crossdressers, wives are graded like schoolchildren, with "A" wives being the ones who are supportive and participatory, and "F" wives being, well, more like Dixie's wife. I'm not going to reprint these categories on the grounds that the whole exercise is condescending and steeped in male prerogative. Even if it was meant to be funny, it wasn't. Crossdressers often talk about the "spectrum" of transgenderism and seem to forget that their wives are just as varied as they are.

WHEN A WOMAN finds out or is told her husband is a crossdresser, she may:

- Want a divorce
- Tell her husband she never wants to hear another word on the subject
- Tell her husband she never wants to hear another word on the subject but that he can continue doing whatever it was he was doing, provided there is no evidence left in her home

- Accept that he is a crossdresser as long as he understands she doesn't want to see him dressed, see photos of him dressed, or participate in any way. She may acknowledge his need to go to meetings, but insist that he remove any trace of makeup by the time he gets home.
- Accept that he is a crossdresser but insist that he can't do it at home for fear that the children will see him dressed
- Accept that he is a crossdresser but quickly lose interest in having sex with him whether he is dressed en femme for sex or not
- Accept that he is a crossdresser and never want to see him dressed, but go to a meeting or a conference to meet other wives in the same situation
- Accept that he is a crossdresser and secretly try to figure out how to cure him
- Accept that he is a crossdresser and start reading everything she can on the subject—more than the husband himself is usually comfortable with
- Accept that he is a crossdresser and admit she'd like to know more because the idea confuses her
- Fear he's gay
- Fear he wants to be a woman
- Seem to accept his being a crossdresser, yet pick fights about everything else they've ever disagreed about
- Jump for joy because she's secretly wanted a crossdressing husband all her life

That last one is a joke. I've yet to hear of a wife who was happy when she found out. There are women who prefer to date and want to marry crossdressers, and when they find the right guy—and he's a crossdresser—their dreams have come true. The difference is that they have chosen to be with a CD. Most wives do not have a choice, and don't like feeling a loss of control over their own lives. They feel they've been tricked, which leads to feelings of betrayal, broken trust, and sometimes even depression.

Many wives or girlfriends will see themselves in several of these categories, sometimes during different periods of their lives, and other times within minutes on the same day. As wives and girlfriends of CDs, we go through the same kinds of on-again, off-again behavior our husbands do. Crossdressers binge and purge; wives of crossdressers fluctuate between goddesses of acceptance and vixens of vengeance. No matter what a woman's reaction to this news, her emotions will be very strong.

Most women want to love their husbands. Most women are socialized to love men and to make room for their quirks. Doing so when you're married to a crossdresser often means you are challenging yourself beyond your normal limits of love and tolerance, and every time you push your own envelope, a backlash results. I was fine with my husband being a crossdresser until I realized he wanted to "pass" in regular, public places, and then I flipped out. Meredith can stand having a crossdressing husband as long as she isn't asked to participate. Gidget doesn't mind her husband's crossdressing but wish he'd cut his long hair as she feels it "gives him away." Others can stand it as long as their husbands refrain from plucking their eyebrows or shaving their legs; others if they're not asked to take their "wife" to bed. Still others can stand it all as long as there's no flirtation with men. Plenty of wives tell me they could even enjoy it if their husbands' espousal of wanting to "feel like a woman" included cleaning the kitchen once in a while, and others just want their husbands to stay out of the kitchen and leave their own traditional female roles intact. All of the women I have spoken to have different limits, but the one thing that is true of nearly all of them is that they are willing to rise to the challenge because of their love for their husbands, and the value they place on their marriages. Most crossdressers—and most men in general—take a woman's selflessness for granted. Many do not realize how naturally women put their own needs aside for the sake of their husband or family. Pick up one self-help book for women or watch an episode of *Oprah*: Women often have a hard time even identifying their own needs, much less insisting on having them met.

The irony perhaps is that the wives most crossdressers pick are not the best equipped to deal with them. There is a tendency for a certain type of crossdresser to think that if he marries a woman who is conservative, religious, or stern, his wife will keep him from crossdressing. The self-hating reflex steers crossdressers toward women who would never accept them. Regardless, the crossdresser usually begins his own private journey toward self-acceptance. He may do this with the help of other crossdressers, books, or counselors. The only problem is, his wife has never known. She doesn't associate with people like crossdressers, and might think of them as freaks. So when he finally tells her, and asks for acceptance, she is stunned. She never suspected her husband chose her for her conservative qualities. He ends up confused because he wasn't aware of his subconscious hope that she might save him from himself. When their repressive strategies don't work, and they finally seek acceptance, men like this often express confusion as to why their wives can't provide it.

Why can't they? Because they are not the type of people who accept sexual deviance. In fact, his self-hatred indicates that he isn't the type who does, either, but he's got no choice in the matter. Neither does she if she loves her husband. Both of them, as a result, have some attitude readjustment to go through. For him it's private, but still difficult: the only difference between him and his wife is that he has known all along he is and always was "one of those." She resists, because she resists "alternative lifestyles" in general. One shared aspect of their relationship—their traditionalism or conservativism—is no longer shared. He's changed, she hasn't.

There's an old adage that the liberal becomes a conservative when he gets mugged, and the conservative becomes a liberal when she gets arrested. Likewise with being—or being married to—a crossdresser: often an ideological shift takes place in one or both partners once acceptance becomes the goal. However, their community of friends and family are often conservative as well so it is a huge jump for some of these men and their wives to have to re-evaluate their political opinions in the light of their personal realities. The same thing is often true of people who have never had anything to do with a gay person, and whose son or daughter comes out to them. This needed transition is a critical juncture in their lives, and the husband's request that his wife suddenly become more open-minded is resented on her part. Conservative crossdressers sometimes find a way to accept themselves only, which may be why some crossdressers don't understand gays and lesbians or even other transgendered people.

Women who are independent, feel empowered to fulfill their own needs, and demand equality in their relationships are often the best wives for crossdressers. Dr. Roger Peo, who worked in and with the crossdressing community until his death, wrote, "the woman who can best learn to cope . . . is nonjudgmental, has a good self-image, has her own interests and is self-sufficient." She is, in essence, a modern woman, and a feminist (even if she doesn't call herself one). That does not mean she won't have problems with her partner being a crossdresser. She undoubtedly will. She will even share a lot of the same issues a more traditional woman will have.

How well any woman lives with a crossdressing husband and how happy she finds herself in her marriage has a lot to do with other factors: how she is told, when she is told, whether or not she seeks counseling, whether or not her husband is sensitive to her needs, how deeply invested she is in being "normal," and whether or not she can bolster her own self-esteem to the point that her identity is not threatened by her husband's femininity. Her acceptance may have to do with her age, cultural background, or her openness to new things.

*   *   *

THE FACTORS THAT affect a woman's ability to accept a crossdressing partner can be lumped into three big categories: Identity, Trust, and Sexuality.

I. IDENTITY

A WOMAN'S IDENTITY—WHO she is, how she thinks of herself, how she relates to her community, her education, her culture, her political beliefs—are all influential in greater to lesser degrees.

CULTURAL AND POLITICAL IDENTITY

Age can be an important factor, and may dictate how she has responded to the cultural changes that have taken place during her lifetime. Gidget, who is fifty-four years old and the wife of a crossdresser, explains:

> Our age has something to do with our acceptance of this . . . older women are more used to separating the male from the female . . . I think that younger women are more used to accepting that each of us is a shade of the other sex inside . . . I think the fifties had a lot to do with this . . . and then there was the sixties and seventies, that made us "open" our minds up to a lot of differences in people . . . maybe that is good, but some people will see this as a bad thing . . . I myself had to get rid of the fifties mentality to step up into the modern world, and I think that is why it took me so long to accept my husband like this . . . I used to say I was "open-minded" in the sixties and seventies, then when my husband told me about himself, it was the early eighties and I still did not accept him yet . . .

The generational difference cannot be dismissed. There is a different ethic of acceptance now than there was in preceding generations. White people pride themselves on having black friends, and straight people admit to friendships with gay men and lesbians. There is no doubt in my mind that the civil rights movement of both groups greatly contributed to this more public accept-ance, even when it's just tokenism. That said, crossdressers have no civil rights movement to speak of, and are continually failing to engage them-selves in the transgender movement. (More on that in Chapter 8: Gendered Politics.) It's unreasonable to expect, for now at least, anyone boasting that they're married to or know a crossdresser. But the modern acceptance ethic, as I'll call it, may help some wives contend better with being married to a "sexual deviant." The key word is "may."

Emma still has problems, but her sensitivity to prejudice, which resulted from her own life experiences, has helped her accept her husband. She explains:

> I have had several gay friends, black friends, Hispanic friends, Asian friends—all types of people that have one big thing in common, "discrimination." I myself am white but have an Asian look. When I was a child I went to an almost all-white private school and experienced intense discrimination, sometimes violent. So I identify. I think this has helped me adjust to my husband's way of life.

She may not understand crossdressing per se, but that her husband deserves tolerance for being different is something she can relate to, since she's been perceived as "different" herself, and has known others in the same situation. It is obvious from her story that she was looking for a connection, something about her husband's experience as a crossdresser to which she could relate. I think her openness to finding that link accounts for her having found it.

A woman who wants to find a way to understand her husband's crossdressing is sure to find it. If she is generally open-minded, it may be easy for her to handle new ideas and experiences. Attitude is half the battle: a wife who is stuck in her ways and generally resents change is less likely to come to terms with her husband's crossdressing. She may be less likely to participate, as in Meredith's case, or may just take a little longer to get used to it, like Gidget. Dixie describes his unaccepting wife as follows:

> Some of this refusal is nothing more than a built in stubbornness and a refusal to accept the truth—no matter how much it goes against what they think. In my case, my wife has an arsenal of pre-conceived opinions that are used like weapons when the subject comes up and she's in the mood to use them against me to belittle and degrade as she deems necessary at the time. Some of it is due to her upbringing and her determination to hold onto old traditional beliefs that a man in anything other than shirt, pants, jockey shorts, and clunky shoes is an oddity and someone to be leery of.

I can't present his wife's point of view, as she won't discuss crossdressing with anyone, including her husband. There may be other factors that have caused her to shut down so thoroughly, and what those are I couldn't guess.

Open-mindedness isn't a guarantee, however. Liberal women will not necessarily have an easier time with crossdressing since they "accept everything anyway." Once the political becomes personal, all bets are off. I'm a pretty good example. My background is thoroughly pro-Union Democrat, and my personal politics are slightly left of that. My friends are gay, lesbian, African-American, Latin, Asian and "other." I live and work in New York City and it would take work to avoid friendships with nonwhite, non-straight people. I pride myself on being able to accept differences and enjoy diversity because this attitude has enriched my life. I expected my acceptance of my husband's crossdressing to come naturally for me. What I didn't realize was that the acceptance I anticipated feeling would be mediated by my personal expectations of what a husband would be, and how his masculinity would reflect me to the world.

In other words, being friends with Jews and Catholics and Muslims would only make me look open-minded; being married to a crossdresser, on the other hand, might encourage others to make negative assumptions about me. Did something in me attract a feminized male? Was I that stereotype of the castrating female after all? Couldn't I handle "real men"? Wasn't I pretty/sexy/femme enough for a "regular" guy? Maybe I was just a closeted lesbian after all. Maybe, as in Feinbloom's bad guess, I had low enough self-esteem to tolerate just about anything in a romantic partner. Most people would assume all or some of these things are true when they hear I am married to a crossdresser. Ironically, the worst assumptions about crossdressers' wives are made by other crossdressers' wives. Meredith told Victoria after their first Tri-Ess meeting that "of course those women will put up with anything, they can't do any better." Other wives have dismissed my acceptance purely on the grounds that I'm too liberal. Still others have wanted to know why I wasn't obese or unattractive, or have written to me because I didn't look like "all those other wives of crossdressers."

So let's get this straight: crossdressers' wives are not necessarily overweight or suffering from low self-esteem. We are not closet lesbians, although some of us are bisexual, bi-curious, or have had lesbian experiences. We are not desperate, in denial, or submissive to our man's needs. The ones who are accepting do not belong to any one political party or belief. Quite conservative women have wrapped their heads around crossdressing. They have found their way toward acceptance as I have, although we may have taken different paths.

*   *   *

IDENTITY AS WIFE

A woman's identity has traditionally been a reflection of her husband's identity. If he has a good job and makes a lot of money, other women respect her. If her husband is an alcoholic who cheats on her, she is either blamed for his behavior or pitied for her poor choice in a mate. Before women had equal rights, women's reputations were entirely subject to their husbands'. Vern and Bonnie Bullough write on the status of women in the late nineteenth and early twentieth centuries: "A woman's social identity was defined primarily by her marital status; her status, with few exceptions, was entwined with that of her husband, bestowed upon her and not 'earned.' " Despite feminism, a woman's identity is still intensely connected to her husband's, and it is not easy to extricate her from him. To some degree this "merge" is a problem in itself, but when the husband is a crossdresser, the wife's lack of an independent identity becomes incredibly troublesome.

Furthermore, crossdressing is usually a secret. When a husband tells his wife she is basically invited into his closet—one he's become familiar with over the years. She is not used to keeping secrets and is troubled by it, but not because she's a gossip. A woman's honesty in her friendships and family life is often key to her identity. We pride ourselves on openness one day and on the next find ourselves burdened with a secret we can't share with anyone. We feel like liars. I know I have. Elizabeth explains:

> The secrecy bothered me a lot. Could the sister (me) who was known to tell any and all secrets ever keep this one? How could I compartmentalize my life so I did not ever give a hint? Especially to family, those same older sisters who voted me Blabbermouth? So while I agreed with my husband that we should not tell, I certainly struggled with the details of keeping a secret.

For a woman who'd been nicknamed "Blabbermouth" by her sisters, keeping this secret was a challenge to her own identity. Because of her husband's crossdressing, she was no longer the person she had always known herself to be. For women, withholding information is akin to lying. We tell each other everything, and when we can't, friendships feel false. Men—non-CDs and CDs—don't enjoy the same intimacy with their male friends. They often don't understand how difficult it is for a woman to keep something from her best friend or sister. They certainly don't understand that there is a kind of "code of honor" amongst women: by telling each other everything, we watch out for each other. We know our sisters and girlfriends will tell us if we're being treated poorly by our boyfriends or husbands. We find assurances in the fact that someone close to us knows the real deal, and that's how we "check" ourselves. Suddenly, that's all taken away. I had to make it known to all of my close female friends that my husband was a crossdresser before we got married. My sisters knew long before that. They got to ask if I was sure he wasn't gay, if it bothered me, if I felt uncomfortable about it. They also got to hear my answers and know that I was okay. Once that was out of the way, I felt like myself again.

SEXUAL IDENTITY

Another big identity issue involves sexuality. A lot of women are terrified of the implicit lesbianism of making love with their husbands en femme. Even if they feel attracted to the man under the dress, this desire throws them for a loop. Some of them don't like the *idea* of being lesbians. They are not worried about actually being lesbians, especially when they have been married and enjoying sex with their husbands for several decades. Instead, they're scared of feeling like a lesbian. They are terrified that they might find in themselves some genuine arousal when their husbands are dressed. And if they do, they may feel disgusted, scared, or threatened. Feelings like this are not lightly brushed aside. They are very real, and deeply ingrained. Our culture has been homophobic for centuries, so it's no surprise that some women respond this way. The best thing to do, in my opinion, is admit to the feelings and the fear, and to discuss them with a counselor, therapist, or trustworthy friend.

The "fear of being lesbian" is similar to what I called the crossdresser's "fear of freaking" in the introduction. A woman who has always considered herself normal desperately wants to retain that status. I hate to be the bearer of bad news, but a crossdresser is not now in our society considered normal, and his wife of course is guilty by association. That's it, I've said it. But let me reiterate: though being married to a crossdresser puts you way outside the "normal" category, you are, however, still the same *you*. The condolence prize is that people who aren't normal learn not to worry about maintaining normalcy, and they're free to have more fun.

The other really liberating result is the realization that people who aren't normal are often decent, moral, and intelligent. You may find yourself introduced to a whole new world of interesting people who have, in one way or another, dared to be different. They accept themselves as who they are, and are skilled at teaching others how to do the same. The other good news is that you won't have as hard a time accepting your lesbian daughter when she introduces you to her girlfriend for the first time. People will start telling you things they didn't think you could "handle" before. You may realize that nearly everyone has an interesting private side.

What sometimes gets called a "fear of being lesbian" is actually something unrelated to homophobia. What a woman might really be objecting to is actually her feeling that she is competing with her husband for the female role sexually. His sexual identity, even in role-playing, becomes a threat to her own: in her opinion, they can't both be the woman in bed. She may turn off because she feels her sense of self compromised, and feels "forced" into playing a part sexually with which she is not comfortable. She may also be uncomfortable feeling "competitive" at all with someone she needs to trust deeply. A woman needs to feel comfortable with her desire, her sexual role in the relationship, and she needs to feel desirable. Sex with a crossdressing partner can challenge all of these.

Other women may have already asked and answered questions about their sexual orientation that they feel forced to ask again. In my early twenties I was hit on pretty frequently by women, and went through a time when I just didn't feel sure of my sexuality. Many people go through a period where they ask similar questions. What I resented, when faced with my husband's crossdressing, was feeling like I had to open a box I'd already shut years before. Being attracted to my husband when he was en femme didn't make it any easier. I am convinced that when we go to a lesbian bar, the women there think I'm a closet case. I wonder if my friends think the same.

In all three of these situations, the woman's heterosexual identity has been shaken. That's not fun. The crossdresser has had his whole life to wonder if wearing a dress makes him gay, but his wife or girlfriend has to wonder if being with a man who wears a dress makes her a lesbian. Often, she has never before asked herself that question. If he wants to be more the seduced than the seducer, she feels forced to play a role she is unfamiliar with, one that a lot of women are raised to consider "unladylike." Because sex is not something people talk about easily, she cannot separate his crossdressing from her sexual reactions, and the result is that she is terrified, angry, and even disgusted with herself. She comes to the conclusion that it's all the fault of his crossdressing. When she tells her husband she feels like a lesbian, or is in some other way uncomfortable with his crossdressing, he needs to listen and certainly shouldn't dismiss her fears: the feeling of not being heard will only exacerbate her fears.

BEAUTY AND SELF-IMAGE

A woman's looks are—whether she wants them to be or not—an important part of her identity as a woman. How she feels about her appearance and her body constitutes an important aspect of her identity in this culture obsessed with youth, thinness, and beauty. When she finds out her husband is a crossdresser, she has to contend with his ideas of what a beautiful woman is and does, but also with his perceptions of her. So what does it mean to a woman when she thinks her husband looks ridiculous en femme? Alternately, what if her husband looks good dressed and she thinks he looks better than she does? In both cases, she has to face her own self-esteem and body image issues.

Wives are faced with an either/or situation: either her husband challenges her own sense of beauty and she feels his femme self threatens her own femininity, or her husband is the type of guy who is too big or too masculine to ever pass.

The woman with the husband who looks so good "she" passes feels threatened as if another woman were present. The likeliness that he embraces a more exaggerated femininity further undermines the sense of self she has struggled to achieve. All women are aware of the ways in which they fail to embody the feminine ideal: thin women feel their legs are too straight, any woman over a size eight thinks she's too fat. While a woman who dates a non-CD man understands there might be a picture of Christy Turlington in her boyfriend's head, the wife of a CD has to see her husband become that idealized woman right before her very eyes. Years of reassurance from other women ("those skinny girls all do coke/are all bulimic") dissolve in the moment her husband stands before her looking *all that*.

(I can't begin to express my contempt for a fashion industry that upholds a feminine ideal that some men achieve more easily than most women. Read Naomi Wolf's *The Beauty Myth*, please.)

What does a woman in this situation do? I found myself slipping more and more into a masculine role. It was obvious to me I'd been beaten hands down, and never having been one to compete in the beauty pageant of daily life, I threw in the towel. I've done the same thing in the presence of female friends for whom being the prettiest woman in the room is important. I rely instead on being smart or interesting or tough or sexy or funny. My friend Guy calls it "The Rhoda Option": only one girl in a group can be Mary, and the lucky runner-up gets to be Rhoda.

A lesbian couple I know embody this idea perfectly: Sandy is an actual former pageant queen, a charming Southern woman replete with blonde hair and legs up to *here*. Her partner Laura is a comedy sketch writer, wildly acerbic and satisfied to know the beauty queen is with her. I looked to them for some resolution to my problem and then realized, um, they're lesbians. Laura tells me her desire to make love to the beauty queen overcomes her desire to *be* the beauty queen. She likes pretty, feminine girls and makes no bones about it.

Not so for us straight girls dating crossdressers. I do find my husband's femme self attractive sometimes. Unfortunately, though, no matter how beautiful I find him en femme, my desire for "her" does not overwhelm my anger and envy that I'm not prom queen. When I see him dressed up and fitting that magazine model standard better than I can, I become resentful and turned off by "her" beauty. He feels I've rejected his femme self and I'm left with my self-esteem so shot I wouldn't be able to make love to Viggo Mortensen if he knocked on the door at that moment. Like so many wives of crossdressers, I gained weight.

I once beat a boy a year older than me in a race. He'd challenged me and I won. I was told afterwards that I had humiliated him. "You got beat by a girl?" his friends asked. Imagine then what it feels like for a woman to know that her own husband achieves a feminine ideal more completely and more naturally than she ever could. It is humiliating. I have managed to feel comfortable and confident around runway models with PhDs, but I feel entirely defeated that my husband walks in heels more gracefully than I do. Simply put, I've been beaten at my own game, and complaining that I never wanted to play in the first place is just the sour grapes of a sore loser. Women are expected to wear heels naturally, we are all born with graceful arches to our eyebrows and thrive on rabbit diets. Uh-huh. And men never have trouble getting it up. Just as the man who is embarrassed to ask his doctor for Viagra knows, we may recognize these "ideals" as mythologies, but we still internalize them and feel like failures when we don't measure up. (The impact this mythologizing has on men's sexuality is well-documented and addressed in *The New Male Sexuality*, a book I strongly recommend.)

As the grass is always greener, I envy the women whose husbands look like linebackers in dresses. *If only*, I think: my female domain would not feel so usurped. I wouldn't feel the need to look better in a skirt than a guy who is born without that layer of subcutaneous fat.

I know from talking to women whose husbands don't pass that it's not easy for them, either. For starters, *their husbands can be giant women*, and they have to get over the pointing, and stares, giggles and ridicule that are bound to accompany any public appearance by their husbands en femme. That's not to say that they shouldn't go out, because they should. But the wife will have to swallow her own desire to laugh out loud at how her husband looks in sequins because she wants to respect her husband's femme self. When Meredith saw her own husband en femme for the first time at a dinner/dance, she paid him one compliment: "I was relieved to see that you did not look as silly as the rest of them." It takes no rocket scientist to realize that she implicitly said he *did* look silly, but her gentle approach enables him to take the tiny compliment she offered as a sign of progress.

For these women, there is an abyss between their husbands' obvious masculine bodies and manners and their feminine ideal. They don't have the opportunity to see their husbands as attractive women, and the absurdity of it all is something they rarely overcome. "If you're so far away from achieving your goal, why bother?" one wife said. Another wondered if her husband wasn't outright delusional, and whether he is aware of how badly he fails.

He is. The big guys are often painfully aware of that abyss. Without the support of their "sisters" and the mutual admiration system built into the CD support network, these guys might not ever go out. When they do they might laugh about being "guys in dresses" to deflect criticism, but that doesn't keep them from enjoying their femme selves. In fact, the bigger guys often compensate for not passing by dressing more ultra-femme than your average CD. This can lead them to looking more like drag queens, but in their hearts they are crossdressers. Like all crossdressers, their powers of imagination are limitless.

I empathize with them and their attempts to embody that feminine ideal. I feel with them that desire like the moth's for a star.

Why do I envy the wives of those men? If they can get over the embarrassment, they can share with their husbands the feeling of being "imperfect women." Plus, they are reassured by their husbands' undeniably masculine bodies. To put it bluntly, she will always be the prettier woman in the relationship, and she knows the "woman" on her arm is a man.

I don't intend to give anyone the idea that my husband doesn't tell me how beautiful I am. He does, in many ways. I can't ask him to be a little worse at being femme for my sake: that would be unfair. I want him to look as good as he can, to come as close to his feminine best as he can. I already know how acutely he hates his large hands and feet, how deep his need to look like a pretty woman runs. He has to prove to himself and everyone else that he is a woman when he dresses. I sit comfortably on the knowledge that I am one. No one stares at me trying to determine what "gives me away," but that happens to him regularly. A very smartly dressed CD recently came up to us at a dinner party and exclaimed that, though it took her a while, she did finally figure out that it was Betty's hands that gave him away. Can you imagine, as a woman, having another woman approach you and say,

"You're nearly perfect, except for that thick neck/large jaw/*insert physical imperfection here*"? Genetic women may judge other women, but only the really bitchy ones would even dream of voicing their criticisms. But that kind of scrutiny is expected at CD gatherings, and the ones who come closest to passing get it the worst. No one sees it as cruel. In fact, most of the CDs reading this are probably thinking, "He must pass really well if only his hands give him away." Having only one visible masculine trait give you away is considered success.

It is an achievement, I suppose, if your goal is to pass. After the first time or two that he passed, passing became less important to him. My husband's goal is to feel and look as much like a woman as possible when "she" is out, and not to be reminded of anything that reveals his masculinity. He still wants to be treated as a woman even if others are aware he is a man.

Of course we both left feeling that "her" ass-backwards compliment was more an expression of jealousy than anything else. (When we later heard that she was a very expensive prostitute who catered to a very exclusive "straight" male clientele, we realized her attention to detail was professional. We wondered if she was considering him for her "stable" before she found out he was married. *Just great*, I thought, *now I know my husband passes as a high-end call girl, too*. Do the insults never cease?)

SO HOW DOES either type of wife confront the particular dilemma her husband's femme self presents? The wives of the larger crossdressers can bond with their husbands about being imperfect women. It can be a source of companionship. The wife, if she can get past her own embarrassment and suppress her desire to laugh—can become a comforting, encouraging partner who uses her husband's appearance to reassure herself. She can feel more confident supporting him precisely because he doesn't look that good as a woman. When they get dressed together, they can commiserate. Her wish that her butt was smaller is equivalent to her husband's desire that his shoulders were narrower. They can share tips and find each other magazine articles about how to de-emphasize physical "imperfections." Her husband will probably appreciate her empathy as long as she learns not to crow about her biologically-female body. She will appreciate his understanding as long as he doesn't brag about everyone thinking he has great legs. Of course that all depends on the husband's sensitivity and sensibility, too: he needs to let his wife complain and focus on their similarities, instead of harping on his wishes that he was her height or weight or curvy like her. The secret in all relationships is figuring out what you have in common, not emphasizing your differences.

(Have I mentioned recently that the primary responsibility for how well the wife confronts these issues falls on her husband?)

For women like me, who think our husbands look better than we do, our husbands need to do almost the exact opposite of the other type. They need to envy our most beautiful or feminine traits. I never mind my husband telling me how much he wishes he had my curves. The crossdresser can use his skills with makeup to apply hers, and always make time to make them both up before they go out. If she's a woman like me who is more likely to be reading public policy than prêt-à-porter reports, he can read fashion magazines and remember to find clothes that would look good on her, too. He shouldn't need the "coaching" a non-CD mate needs in order to buy his wife clothes. He can, in every way possible, reassure her that her appearance is always every bit as important to him as his own.

Of course it takes a remarkably delicate man to give a woman a skirt that de-emphasizes her butt without insulting her. Praise, praise, and more praise is what's required, and every crossdressing husband who can pass has to remember that his wife is constantly reminded by the media of her every physical shortcoming. Shoot, Marilyn Monroe hated her fat hands, and no one can say she wasn't receiving daily affirmations of her desirability. A man should never point out his wife's problem spots, but should listen to her when she's getting dressed. If she thinks the problem is her short neck and he thinks it's her belly, he damn well better buy her necklaces that lengthen her neck instead of control-top pantyhose. Finally, he shouldn't plan a big night out together when she's got her period because there is nothing that makes a woman feel more gross and unattractive (and no, he shouldn't have to ask when it is: boys can count to twenty-eight, too).

There are, of course, the exceptional women who are very comfortable in their femininity and can go out with their husbands like a couple of chicks on the town. Kathy can do that but she's the first to admit she's an exception. She wanted a crossdressing husband, and her independence and business-savvy never get in the way of her love of velvet and jewelry. She has no gender conflict and her husband, as most CDs who meet them conclude, is one lucky man. They can peruse the fashion magazine racks together, have their slumber parties and make love with him en femme without any repercussions.

II. TRUST

TRUST IS WHAT makes a relationship work, and it's broken in a variety of ways when the husband is a crossdresser. Even when a husband doesn't intend to break a woman's trust, he might; in our case, I felt deceived because although my husband told me he was a crossdresser, it wasn't until years later that he admitted the depth of his transgendered feelings. Like women who have found out about their husbands' affairs, wives of cross-dressers have to find a way to trust their husbands again, after they've harbored a secret for years, sometimes decades. Perhaps the most important factor in whether or not a wife can grow to accept her husband's cross-dressing is how she finds out, and when. Weinberg and Bullough correlate that "the earlier in the marriage the wife learned about her husband's TV, the more positive her attitude was toward this behavior, and the happier she was in her marriage. Women who discovered their husband's cross-dressing well into the marriage typically felt betrayed." A wife's trust in her husband is often destroyed when he tells her the truth after many years of secrecy. She wonders whether she can trust another word he says. Some wives come around to understanding that their husbands didn't tell them because cross-dressing is still culturally unacceptable. They know intrinsically the risks in revealing the truth to others, and are aware that even close friends may respond with revulsion. Often wives become more concerned than their husbands with keeping the crossdressing a secret.

The obvious conclusion is for a crossdresser to tell the woman he loves as soon as possible. Previous to this generation, many in the crossdressing community "understood" why CDs didn't inform their wives. Papers like Weinberg and Bullough's had not yet been published and there was no information available on the topic. Now there is. Plenty of research still needs to be done, of course, but there is no uncertainty about the fact that cross-dressers must tell their partners before any major commitment is made. (There are, of course, exceptions: for example, some men do not discover an urge to crossdress until later in life, well after they are married. One crossdresser I met didn't realize he was a CD until he was a widower.)

Of the wives and girlfriends I surveyed for this book, 15 of 20 rated themselves an 8 (10 being "perfectly accepting"), and—surprise, surprise!—14 of those 15 knew about their partners' crossdressing before making a major commitment (moving in together, sex, marriage, etc). Obviously, wives and girlfriends who are willing to answer a survey about their partner's crossdressing to begin with are more accepting than the average, but the correlation is still apparent.

Sometimes even when a wife is told upfront, or after she has accepted her husband's crossdressing, she finds he is still lying to her about other related issues. A woman who has just been told, for example, might finally make sense of the inconsistencies in their budget due to purchases her husband had hidden. His excuse for failing to paint the bathroom over the weekend she was away suddenly makes sense: he was too busy crossdressing to get the job done. The list goes on and on. Women begin to wonder: If he could lie about something as big as crossdressing, what else has he lied about? Often, plenty. Keeping as big a secret as crossdressing takes work. The crossdresser is so used to lying in order to hide his dressing, his ability to distinguish between truth and lies is compromised. He has told one big lie that must be supported by lots of little ones. Lying becomes an ingrained habit, and one that isn't easy to break—even after he comes clean about his crossdressing. After "Ann" came out to Liz, and Liz accepted his cross-dressing, the lies continued:

- Money for family bills was spent on women's clothes.
- Ann told Liz, when she found a key imprinted "USPS", that USPS was not an acronym for the U.S. Postal System. Liz was offended by the audacity of this whopper.
- After closing the post office box, Ann had the post office in their small town hold the subsequent mail. Ann would pick it up regularly, read it, and throw it away without telling Liz about it. Liz didn't know the post office had agreed to hold the mail, much less that Ann was picking it up. "She" would save select pieces and hide them, too.
- Ann inexplicably hides magazines published by the TG community to which Liz does not object.
- Herbal hormone pills were ordered, received, and hidden, but never mentioned and also never taken. When Liz discovered them, Ann claimed to have forgotten about them altogether.
- Liz insisted no crossdressing sites be accessed from their business computers, and no clothes hidden at their place of business, because Liz did not want Ann outed "by people who would not understand nor try to." Ann continued to do both.
- When expected home for dinner and other family functions, Ann was spending time at work on the computer, and then lied that he was "working" when it fact he was web-surfing, instead.

I don't know what kind of mail Ann was receiving through the post office box, but I understand why Liz would be suspicious. Ann is not atypical. I hear these same kinds of complaints from other crossdressers' partners on a regular basis, and the pattern is the same: the crossdresser persists in lying about things he doesn't need to lie about. His wife is usually frustrated, sad, and disappointed, but more than anything else, she's hurt, confused, and angry. She sees no reason for the continued lies, and tries desperately to convince her husband he can trust her and quit lying. For obvious reasons, she is also deeply suspicious that there is more to the crossdressing than what she has been told.

Husbands don't always realize the impact having kept their crossdressing a secret has had on their marriage. They may think that once the woman knows, she should be appreciative that he has shared the secret. Although some women may be relieved to learn the truth, the doubt that creeps into her mind is almost impossible to prevent. She will wonder all the time what else she doesn't know. It can take years of "good behavior" to convince a woman that her husband has truly stopped lying. His ability to respond to her skepticism with love and reassurance instead of anger will go a long way toward calming her fears.

III. SEX

ACCORDING TO MY findings, almost a third of the crossdressers I surveyed still keep secrets from their partners. They lie most often about their sexuality—sometimes curiosity about having sex with men when en femme, though often with no actual desire to engage in such sex—and purchases. The other two thirds, who are completely honest and open with their partners, are more out than others. To me the obvious conclusion is that the crossdresser who has come out to more than his wife or other crossdressers has had to confront certain issues and, once he makes peace, feels less ashamed and is therefore better equipped to share things with his partner. Most of the CDs who are still keeping secrets do so because they don't think their partners can handle the truth. It's unlikely that a crossdresser is going to tell his wife that he's fantasized about having sex with men if she flips out when she learns the thought has even crossed his mind.

The problems start because crossdressers often tell their partners that they do not dress for sexual pleasure. A wife takes her partner's word for it but then may start to notice that he's not as aroused when he's not wearing panties. She might notice that he seems to be "elsewhere" when they're making love or seems to avoid sex. Or, he may be more passive and not actively seduce her. She starts putting 2 + 2 together, but unfortunately she's already been told—by him or by other crossdressers—that crossdressing has nothing to do with sex. She has a weird feeling it does. She starts to suspect her husband is withholding something and feels distrustful because he can't offer an explanation that makes any sense. The only one that makes sense, she comes to believe, is that the crossdressing is causing their sexual problems. She becomes increasingly uncomfortable with their sex life. Often, they eventually stop having sex altogether.

I've heard or read the same story countless times. A wife or girlfriend writes me an e-mail, talks to other wives and girlfriends, and discovers she's not alone. Lots of wives are coming to the same conclusion: can they all be wrong?

No. They're not all wrong. They're misinformed by their husband's misinformation. There is a history behind the "it's not about sex" myth. In the 1960s, the popular image of crossdressers was that they were either gay or perverted or both. In order to gain respect and public acceptance, crossdressers actively started "cleaning up" that image. In Virginia Prince's *The Transvestite and His Wife*, it is very clear that by the late 1960s crossdressers started emphasizing two things: 1) their heterosexuality, and 2) the concept that crossdressing is about getting in touch with their inner female, and not about sex or arousal or fetishism. Their bid for acceptance was understandable. Their emphasis on being heterosexual was valid, since most of them are straight. Their disclaimer that dressing wasn't about sex, though, was a bent truth. That their primary motivation was to get in touch with an inner female self—the "second self" as Tri-Ess would have it—was only partially true. Many crossdressers do indeed access a more feminine part of themselves when they dress. But the "emphasis" on the one motivation eclipsed the other altogether: not only did they deny it was *entirely* about sex, but they insisted it wasn't about sex at all. Crossdressers reassured themselves that they weren't perverts, and reassured their wives dressing wasn't sexual, and everyone got to feel "normal."

For the record: for many men, there *is* a sexual component to crossdressing. Please notice I did not say for *all* men, or that sex is the *only* motivation. Sexual gratification may not be the main reason CDs do what they do, and it is surely not the only reason, but many (not all) crossdressers experience a confluence of their sexuality and their crossdressing at one time or another in their lives. I'll talk more about this in Sex and Sensibility (Chapter 6) of course, but my point here is that women are not idiots. Once a woman starts to identify problems with their sex life, it won't take long before she sees that her husband doesn't have a "regular" sex drive. She will come to know her husband isn't aggressive and masculine in bed. She will notice her husband spends time online reading erotic stories featuring crossdressing plots, like the ones found at www.fictionmania.com, all of which are user-contributed. Women often know that their husbands are turned on by crossdressing, but they doubt their own intuition and experience because so much of the CD literature denies it.

The result? When a husband denies the arousal aspect, yet spends his time reading stories at www.fictionmania.com and buying lacy panties, his wife knows he's lying, and learns not to trust what he says. A woman cannot understand why a man who says he doesn't crossdress for sexual reasons posts pictures of himself in lingerie online. She can't understand why he feels the need to wax his pubic area if she's the only one who's going to see it. She can't comprehend why he's looking at she-male porn. She doesn't know why he avoids sex. She'd like to know. She needs to know.

I asked a group of accepting wives what questions they would ask their crossdressing partners if they had no choice but to tell the truth. Nearly all of the questions had to deal with sex and fidelity:

- Have you ever had any type of sex with another man, CDer or not, while dressed as a woman?
- What is so private about that e-mail account?
- Which side does he enjoy more? His male persona or feminine?
- Did my lack of libido cause you to turn to dressing?
- If he masturbates when he is dressed while looking at photos of she-males or women in lingerie, and how often he masturbates.
- Is there ever going to be a full-time "us", with both of us happy in our life together?
- I would ask him if he has ever had any affairs he hasn't told me about—and if he was really never attracted to a man—which I think he is truthful about—he has never done these things—but sometimes I wish I could spy on him to be really sure—
- Why the cyber affair?
- I would ask him if he was really at the office until 4 AM (a week straight) four years ago, or in a strip club, etc.
- Exactly what bills do you have, to whom, how much?
- Do you fantasize about men when you are trying to get turned on with me?
- What happened to you to make you like this? (I don't think he knows the answer)
- What do you really think about when we make love? Is it being *with* me, or *being* me??
- Tell me the fantasy you have that you are scared to tell me!

Wives will never understand any of this if crossdressers don't start being honest about their own sexuality. Once he stops lying to himself, he may stop lying to his wife. I believe that most crossdressers are faithful to their wives, and the ones that aren't would be unfaithful regardless of their cross-dressing. Just because a man crossdresses doesn't mean he is gay, but it does have something to do with his sexuality. JoAnn Roberts, one of the founding members of Renaissance and TG Forum, says, "I've always said that my crossdressing says nothing about my sexual orientation but speaks volumes about my sexuality. CDing turns me on and I'm not ashamed of that."

A crossdresser's sexuality is tricky and little understood. Crossdressers often have fantasies of having sex with men while en femme, or they would like to be submissive in some way. He may not desire these things because he's a crossdresser, but I doubt it. If he insists that he doesn't have these desires, or argues that they have nothing to do with him being a cross-dresser, his wife will surely come to distrust what he says. When she finds evidence of these kinds of fantasies, her trust will be broken again. If she already feels betrayed because she didn't know he was a crossdresser in the first place, but decided to learn to trust him again, she will be shattered to learn he has lied about sex, too. On the other hand, his fantasies may be more than she can take. The situation can deteriorate even further if he is unable to admit these things even to himself, or is otherwise unaware of what turns him on. The problem is, a lot of crossdressers don't have these fantasies, and some of the ones who do are so deeply ashamed of them they can't consciously confront them. Unfortunately, there are many wives of crossdressers who assume the worst, when in fact their husbands' sexual tastes are really quite vanilla, and other wives who can't imagine such desires and so can't talk to their husbands about them. In either case, therapy is the only chance they have of sorting it all out.

THE THREE ISSUES that wives have to confront—sex, trust, and identity—often intersect in a variety of challenging ways. When a husband is less than honest about his sexual feelings, his wife may develop suspicions. When she discovers his interest in websites like fictionmania, she will actively begin distrusting him. This may lead to her snooping through his Internet history or eavesdropping on his conversations with friends. These breaches in her own ethics will likely erode or threaten her sense of self. The end result is a very tenuous situation. The crossdressing husband feels doubted and resentful of his lack of privacy. His wife lives in a state of anxiety, fearing that her husband may imminently admit to homosexual feelings. Their relationship is threatened in more ways and on more fronts than most relationships can stand. The only way to resolve these issues—and prevent further deterioration in the relationship—is conversation. A therapist, who can encourage communication, may be the only answer. In most cases, a therapist can prevent this sort of deadlock from developing in the first place.

COUNSELING AND PEER COUNSELING

GIDGET WAS·THE partner who rated herself an 8 on the acceptance scale despite the face that she was informed about her husband's crossdressing after thirty years of marriage. She would say that going to a gender counselor was the key to her success in achieving a high level of acceptance. Counseling is probably the single best thing a crossdresser's partner can do, provided the counselor has some experience with gender issues.

There are many therapists who have no experience or familiarity with crossdressing. I had been seeing a therapist before I met my husband, and when I later told her about his crossdressing, she seemed more interested in his experiences than in mine. She started attributing all of my relationship issues to the crossdressing. I eventually quit. Elizabeth's counselor suggested that Elizabeth's husband's crossdressing be treated as an obsessive-compulsive disorder (which is only useful if the crossdresser also shows indications of being obsessive-compulsive, which is not often the case). Elizabeth discouraged her husband from seeing this therapist.

However, a therapist who is familiar with gender issues or crossdressing specifically can do worlds of good for a relationship. Gidget describes her experience:

> The gender therapist we went to taught us to just listen to each other without comment or criticism . . . he emphasized that it was important that we each express our feelings and emotions and what we were feeling and why . . . so we each took our turn to explain to the other person how we felt . . . my husband told me how it hurt him as he could not change what he was, and felt ashamed he was this way, but felt that he could not stop his behavior . . . I explained how it made me feel "strange" and "unusual" to accept him like this . . . and I also explained my feelings about his long hair and how it embarrassed me to no end, as we both work in a public school system that is very conservative . . . the therapist explained to me that it was important to express my feelings about things, and he should listen without comment or criticism of my feelings . . . and that even though my husband would not cut his hair for me, that at least I did get in my feelings about this.

In order to find a good gender counselor, the couple has to do some research. Doctors may or may not be helpful (mine wasn't). Friends who have been to therapy might be able to offer leads, but a transgender organization (like IFGE, the International Foundation for Gender Education, or www.ifge.org) certainly will. At the very least they may know the names of local transgender groups that would be able to advise further. The internet is also a great resource for essays on how to find a good counselor. If all of this fails, the couple might find a directory through a local gay and lesbian organization, as many gays and lesbians contend with gender issues as well. Couples should ask potential therapists whether they have experience with gender issues and have counseled transgendered people before. Therapists, in fact, should be trained to be able to tell the difference between transsexual people and crossdressers, and may help the average crossdresser realize he is not transsexual. Finding the right person is essential, and couples should even consider commuting some distance to see a counselor trained in gender issues.

Ali, who is a trained therapist in England, explains further:

> I would certainly stress the importance of seeking out a councilor who is familiar with transgender issues. In the majority of cases, therapists have little knowledge of this field. Often, they will end up placing too much emphasis on the crossdressing, etc., and fail to recognise other issues that need to be worked through. In almost all cases, a crossdresser will present issues of guilt, low-self esteem, etc., and these are really the main things that should be dealt with first.
>
> Likewise, when couples come to therapy, I often find, that the problems they have are less to do with cross-dressing, and more to do with trust issues. I often hear wives/partners who have discovered their partners cross dressing after several years saying "I don't actually mind the cross dressing so much. . . . It's the fact that he lied to me for so long that I can't handle." It often emerges that her difficulty in accepting her partner hinges on the fact that in her eyes, her husband is a different man to the one she has previously known. One woman described this feeling to me as like bereavement, after she had discovered her husband's secret after many years of marriage and felt she had to get to know her husband again almost as a complete stranger.
>
> These are just some of the most common issues that are overlooked by many councilors/therapists, so it is worth spending some time finding help from someone who is familiar with transgender issues.

"Peer counseling" is another option. In this form of "therapy," wives of crossdressers meet with each other in a group. They find out that they are not alone and that they share a lot of the same feelings. The bonding and community this kind of conversation can create is hugely beneficial to the wives and girlfriends of crossdressers, especially if their husbands are closeted. The wives finally have somewhere to take their grievances and can share information, approaches, and solutions. Peer counseling groups for crossdressers' wives convene online and in person. Getting support usually depends on where she lives and the quality of her computer access. Unfortunately, how much she may or may not get out of peer counseling often depends on how well she fits into the group.

I love the idea of women's support groups. I'm a feminist, and think that women should have their own spaces. It is important for the wives who are new to the crossdressing community to feel safe. Most of the existing support network caters to the needs of the wife who has just been told or found out. Because she is shattered by the news, and sometimes disgusted and horrified, there is often a high tolerance for anger in these groups. She needs to be able to vent and needs reassurance, because she may be terrified about public exposure, the potential loss of a job, upsetting her children, and about a million other things. A woman who has just been told—or found out—that her husband wears women's clothes is not ready to hear about hormones and bisexual fantasies and—gulp—transitioning, so these topics are discouraged in many support groups which cater to her. Groups that cater to this particular woman can be good "safe spaces" for her to come to terms with her initial shock and sadness and anger.

One of the best of these safe spaces is the Tri-Ess' annual SPICE (Spouses' and Partners' International Conference for Education) conference, whose focus is education for wives and girlfriends only. Crossdressers may attend, but they are not permitted to crossdress at the event. Jane Ellen Fairfax, chair of Tri-Ess, the organization that hosts SPICE, explains:

> Some of the wives who attend SPICE approach the registration desk literally shaking with anxiety and fear. Some have just learned that their husbands are crossdressers. They wonder what it means and where it is going to take them. They come to learn about crossdressing, talk out their issues, develop communication skills, and, with their spouses, define a mutually acceptable comfort zone with crossdressing. Some of those who attend have never seen their husbands crossdressed, and are not yet ready to see men dressed en femme. At SPICE,

they do not have to endure this additional pressure, for no crossdress-
ing is allowed at the conference. This is no great hardship for the hus-
bands, who can attend a transgender conference almost any month of
the year, in addition to dressing up for their local group meetings.
SPICE is the only event in the community that focuses on wives'
needs! Thanks to this conference, couples come away with improved
understanding and renewed relationships. Many of the wives have
become more tolerant or even encouraging. Not only have these
women resolved their problem with seeing their husbands cross-
dressed, many have even begun participating with their husbands. A
small sacrifice for a lot of good!

Last year's program included lectures and discussions on topics like these:

> *Overcoming Fear, Guilt, and Shame—for CDs only*
> *Introduction to Crossdressing—for SO's only*
> *Pros and Cons of Having a CDing Husband—for SO's only*
> *CD's and SO's Bill of Rights*
> *Boundaries*
> *Our Fears and Discomforts*
> *The Kids Bill of Rights*
> *When is She More Than a Guy in a Dress*
> *Hormones NOT!*
> *Safety When Dressed*
> *Addictive Behavior*
> *To Tell or Not To Tell*

SPICE is a good place for a new wife or girlfriend to get the information she needs, meet other women, and to get acquainted with crossdressers as their male selves. SPICE benefits both wives and their crossdressing husbands, and saves marriages, too. However, SPICE only takes place once a year, and requires travel, conference fees, and hotel costs. A woman may not want to wait until next July for help, in which case she usually goes online.

Tri-Ess also runs an online support list called CDSO (CrossDressers' Significant Others), which is run *by* wives of crossdressers and *for* wives of crossdressers. No CDs are on the list, so the women can talk honestly about their fears and anger without feeling pressured to be accepting. This is often the first list women find online and it can be terrifically useful as a "bunny slope" into the community. Elizabeth describes CDSO:

CDSO is an online support community run by volunteers who are them-selves experienced wives of crossdressers. Women stay long enough to feel comfortable, to get their questions answered, to decide whether their relationship is worth saving or not. A few, like me, stay on in hopes we can help the newcomers see that accepting crossdressing is an adjust-ment worth making in a loving relationship and/or because we have no other female friends with whom we want to share this part of our lives. One of the goals of the group is to make it a safe place to vent, cry, laugh, whatever. When your most intimate relationship has become a tightrope walk you need a safety net! Sometimes there's a lot of bitching but recently there's been some wonderful sharing of good times. Bitching is sometimes seen as humorous, letting off steam.

As Elizabeth describes, CDSO can provide a useful forum for the wives of crossdressers. The problem is that CDSO often becomes a huge "bitch" ses-sion, with the moderators silencing women who have anything positive to say. I was kicked off CDSO. I don't remember exactly what it was I said or did to deserve such rejection, but I do remember three incidents: 1) I suggested that being bi-curious might help wives of CDs, 2) I was offended by the cruel "humor" of the women and suggested that they talk about their anger instead of "joking" about it, and 3) I told one woman who sent daily eighteen-page-long e-mail complaints that she should discuss her problems with her husband. Other "accepting" women have had similar problems on CDSO. Kathy is one:

I was nervous that my acceptance and encouragement would scare some women off the list. I eventually got more ballsy with mentioning my thoughts regarding this. See, what bothered me was this scenario: a woman wanted to blame her husband's crossdressing for everything . . . poor handling of family money, spending four hours chatting nonstop and ignoring her, blah blah blah . . . to me it was obvious that this sort of behavior would make even me, Miss Accepting, angry. Not over the CD issue, but misuse of money, lack of attention and such. This is not a "crossdressing" problem. This is a guy being a jerk problem. I think that is the point where I started calling a spade a spade and saying how I felt. Thank goodness when I said, "Hey I went looking for this and this would tick me off. This has nothing to do with dressing like a woman." If you are going to be angry at your husband be angry for the right rea-sons. I also called women to task when they were being unreasonable and had unrealistic expectations of their husbands.

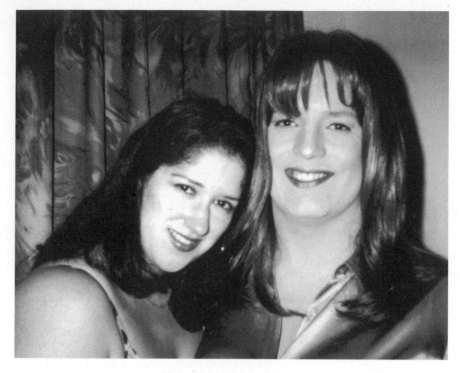

Kathy and her husband, Amanda

Kathy is now moderating a list called CD-WSOS (Crossdressers' Wives and Significant Others Support), which is not associated with Tri-Ess.

I am told CDSO's policies have loosened somewhat since I was a member, but I still get applications for my online group from women who have left CDSO feeling confused and rejected. The list should be moderated by wives with a greater variety of backgrounds, and perhaps involve a professional counselor in order to keep the "bitch fest" to a minimum.

Since Tri-Ess is perhaps the only national organization that specifically provides support for the heterosexual wives of heterosexual crossdressers, the list's culture—of "protecting" women from the supporting wives—is highly problematic, especially as it "advertises" itself (in the description on Tri-Ess' website) as being for all of us. It's not. Just because some of us might not have an issue with crossdressing per se doesn't mean we don't need a community, or support, either. CDSO presents itself as the only "legitimate" game in town, so women who progress past their fears are often forced to rebel against the group in order to acknowledge their growth. When they do, they're asked to leave: so much for acceptance. There is no "intermediate"

list hosted by Tri-Ess, and this leaves women who have reached a certain
level of acceptance without a community of friends or support. Many
women who are being told before marriage do not have the same issues of
betrayal and anger, and as a result are more "accepting" because they were
fully informed. But being accepting doesn't mean that the problems disappear, which I think this book amply demonstrates. I still needed to talk to
other women and I didn't know where to turn once I was rejected from
CDSO.

I started my own list, but most women are not able to commit the time
and effort necessary to do such a thing. As I said, some of the women who
leave (or are rejected by) CDSO show up on my list. Sometimes they show
up on Kathy's list, CD-WSOS. Her list acknowledges that there is more than
one type of wife, just as there are many types of crossdressers.

> As a moderator, our screening process usually involves several e-
> mails where we find out what the status is of their relationship and what
> they would like to gain from joining our group. Women of all ages, all
> backgrounds, all educational levels, all religious beliefs join this list to
> find out the answer to their burning question. Why does my husband
> want to crossdress? Some women are just learning after twenty-five
> years of marriage, some after their second date, some on their honey-
> moon, and some by accident on the computer.
>
> No two women have exactly the same home situation. Every woman
> reacts differently. Some want to actively participate while others have
> strict rules about when and where and how long. Some women have
> allowed "her" into the bedroom while in other homes even kissing
> while crossdressed is strictly forbidden. Some families let their chil-
> dren in on the secret and in other combined families children may learn
> of this through a disgruntled ex-wife.
>
> I have found that women will in some cases cling to their old view
> of their husband. Most want to think this is a midlife crises or phase
> that the man will pass through. In many cases there are other underly-
> ing factors that make women target or come to hate the crossdressing.
> I have often wondered if they would be as angry at a man for spending
> $400 on a custom corset than if it was on football tickets?
>
> Moderating a group of diverse women does come with pitfalls. I
> have been called every name in the book for supporting my husband and
> trying to help wives of crossdressers. I have been called a sicko and sin-
> ner and a messenger of Satan. I have had women ask for information
> on clinics and doctors which use medications or shock therapy to

"cure" their husbands. Women have come to the list as a last resort to save their marriage. They come to find that our list did not hold the secret to stopping their husbands from wearing women's clothing.

I would like to think of the list as being a haven for wives of cross-dressers who feel that they have nowhere else to turn: for the woman in rural Nebraska who catches her husband wearing her pantyhose. She does not have to be alone if she has a modem and a computer. For every man who comes out of the closet to his wife, he in turn puts her in that closet. I just want this list to be the light in there that she can switch on whenever she needs.

Kathy tables at transgender events, posts photos of herself on the internet, and otherwise encourages new wives to enjoy their husbands' crossdressing. She acknowledges that she has always found it sexy, but that doesn't keep her from understanding how painful it can be for a wife when she first finds out. She keeps her light on so others have a guide in the dark. I am tired of strong women like Kathy feeling guilty about their acceptance; we need to celebrate women who provide not only guidance but empathy and experience. They're the future of the community. They are present, political, patient, and painfully rare. Maybe we're just not nurturing this kind of leadership in the CD community, or maybe—just maybe—we're more comfortable staying in the closet.

Moderating my group has been a terrifically satisfying experience. I have learned a great deal, and list members tell me they have benefited as well. But there are quite a few more online support groups for wives now than when I started CDOD. One, TGSO (TransGendered Significant Others), is geared more toward the partners of men who consider themselves transgendered, or who are "more than crossdressers." None of the alternative groups, however, are sponsored by Tri-Ess. Other groups—like Renaissance—provide spousal support but have no online presence, and that's where people are really finding their community these days.

"Support" may not be what the future wives of crossdressers are looking for. They may just be looking for friends, for other women who they can talk to, who know what it's like to be with a crossdresser. They may be looking for community, not help in "coping." Kathy adds:

I was not looking for "help" but just to have others to chit chat with. I can say that in the last two years thankfully I have seen several women join knowing from day one and if not completely accepting, want to be accepting. There is hope I believe. I have gotten to the

point now when I screen women I tell them up front: we don't allow
husband-bashing; be tolerant; listen to those who are accepting. If
your goal is to find ways to make him stop and you have no real want
for acceptance we are not the group for you.

Her last words ring true. The crossdressers may see us as "accepting" or
"unaccepting," but that's a simplistic view. Just as crossdressers have different needs and goals, so do their partners. A wife who is only interested in tol-
erating her husband's dressing is better served where she can bitch with other
women and let off steam. CDSO is perfect for her. But for me, and Kathy, and
Emma, and a whole slew of other women like us, there needs to be other
kinds of support. There will be women who are dating crossdressers who
want to date crossdressers, and who find the idea of a man in a skirt erotic.
There is already an online list for genetic women "admirers" of crossdressers
and t-girls, and as femininity in men becomes more commonplace, more will
join. Women who willingly enter into relationships with CDs in 2004 and
beyond are not going to turn a blind eye to their husbands' feminine sides:
they will encourage their husbands' feminine sides. They may want advice
about strap-ons, T-friendly spas and salons, lesbian erotica, and BDSM information—you name it. They will not feel welcome in the community if they
can't express their true feelings. It wouldn't hurt the SO community to focus
on creativity, positive attitudes, and a willingness to enjoy crossdressing, not
just cope with it. I wouldn't have married my husband if I wanted to "cope."
There's so much more to explore when your husband's a crossdresser, and I'm
not going to sit back and let him have all the fun.

WHY WE STAY

YOU MIGHT THINK a woman who is unsure of her husband's sexuality,
fears he might want to be a woman, and who is forced to confront her own
issues about identity and self-worth and sexuality might make it easy on herself and get out of the relationship altogether. Some do exactly that, and
some even use their husband's crossdressing to blackmail him into paying
more alimony. Others use the crossdressing to get custody of their children.
Still others realize that with their husbands' crossdressing come too many
other bad behaviors, like lying, selfishness, sexual problems, alcoholism or
drug addiction, or a basic unwillingness to compromise or communicate. A
woman who leaves a bad relationship because crossdressing becomes the
final straw is justified. Being married to a crossdresser is not easy, and if the

relationship has other serious flaws, the crossdressing will aggravate them, sometimes to the point of destroying the relationship altogether.

Many more women are proving that marriages with crossdressers can be gratifying. Over time, more women are deciding to stay with transgendered partners. There are a lot of different reasons. The main one is love. Older, more conservative women who already have grandchildren may stay because divorce isn't in their vocabularies. They have spent a lifetime with the man they love, and no dress is going to stop them. They go to counselors and learn again how to talk about their feelings with their husbands. Some couples who have fallen into communicative or sexual ruts have found that crossdressing renewed their relationship significantly. Other women discover sex toys and other ways to "compensate" for their husbands' unusual sexualities. More than one wife or girlfriend has realized that if her husband can come to accept himself, he can leave behind the negative behaviors that make him a difficult partner, and work toward that goal. Many too do the kind of research they can in order to help their husbands reach that goal, even when the husband is unable to take that kind of first step himself.

Here are a few reasons women stay with crossdressers, in their own words:

> **Angela:** *Jerry is good in every single thing in our marriage but the sex so I don't dwell on it because no man is perfect. I could go out and get someone cheap or selfish, who cheats, lies, or has a disease and not telling what all . . . I think I'll just stick with Jerry and the no sex! LOL! Not to say I don't blow up now and then because I do.*

> **Lisa:** *When my spouse and I were having problems I coined a new "mantra" for myself and for conversations with my spouse: The crossdressing IS functional, the manner in which it is handled can be dysfunctional. That helped keep me from blurring the lines because I knew if I ever associated the crossdressing with our problems and developed a problem with the crossdressing our marriage would not survive or would become a bitter unhappy relationship. I wanted our marriage to survive and I wanted it to be happy and fulfilling for both of us.*

> **Emma:** *Most of all I love him so much and he loves me. When things get hard, I try to picture him not in my life and it is not the right picture. Anyway, my acceptance isn't really the problem. When things get hard it is usually about his self-acceptance and his inability to communicate.*

Liz: *Even though it has been hell some of the time from the lying, I'd still marry Ann again. He is usually a wonderful considerate loving man who is a good husband and father. He is the type of man who tries to help others, and is the first one to help carry a package or whatever.*

Elizabeth: *For me, it was more important to see my husband as whole and wholesome than to try to unravel the why. His personality includes this particular manifestation of female. I can't be happy if I insist on seeing him through some theorist's vision of poor personality development. And the chances are he would not be happy with me for doing so. He is not sick to be made well. He is living with a challenging and puzzling variation of gender that is so little understood he has had to find his own way to live well and responsibly without the usual support community can give.*

Gidget: *However, I do love the person underneath the clothing, and that is why I don't leave—after all, he loved me when I was fat, when I was a skinny looking teenager, and he loved me even when I made a lot of fashion mistakes and looked awful—so I love him thru everything—after all, we won't all be able to hold on to "beauty" . . . there will be a time when we will be senior citizens without teeth or hair . . . and there may even be a time when we need a mastectomy—or an operation—let's face it, if you only love the "beautiful" person, there is not much of a relationship there . . .*

There are as many reasons women stay as there are women, but none of us could manage it if we didn't get reassurance that our husbands—the crossdressers themselves—are willing to go out of their way to help us along. The books they offer us, the late-night conversations they engage us in; the handholding and tear-wiping are only the tip of the iceberg. It is as much our love for them as their love for us that makes these marriages work. *Amor vincit omnia*—but only if love is accompanied by compassion, understanding, respect, education, and communication.

CHAPTER 4

Relationships

MY HUSBAND ACCIDENTALLY "outed" himself to my siblings when we were in Vegas for my sister's wedding. A little over a year ago, he couldn't resist trying on a pair of tall, black, women's boots in the Aladdin Mall and Casino, and once the "indoor rainstorm" attraction was over, my siblings came looking for us. My brother's wife walked in and watched as we discussed whether they were snug enough on his ankle. Big oops. We ended up buying the boots and rejoining my siblings outside the store, where my sister-in-law had already filled them in. They obviously expected an explanation.

"I do drag sometimes," my husband said.

My sister-in-law picked up on his nervousness. "Don't worry about it," she clarified, "we knew you two were weird. It's not like this makes you any weirder."

To most people, including my family, crossdressing is weird, and I'd been warming my family up to weird since I was fourteen and dying my hair funny colors and commuting to Manhattan to see bands like Siouxsie and the Banshees. But after I'd kept my natural hair color for a decade, and had started to live a responsible adult life, they were starting to view my teenaged presentation as a "phase." Then I met my future husband, and *they all liked him*. I was about *this close* to winning the "normal" trophy, and *blam!* It was gone: I'm married to a crossdresser, and now I'll never be anything to them but weird.

I could resent my husband for that, but I don't. The real problem is that he effectively decided to out himself to my family without us having talked about it first. That's the kind of decision (or nondecision) a CD can make that makes his wife nuts. Betty already knew of course that I encouraged him to tell others, because I hated feeling like a phony. I still feel dishonest when I visit his family, even though I know they think I'm odd enough already—and they don't even know I'm married to a crossdresser. They do know I love my husband, and that we make each other happy. But being different to begin with didn't save me—or us—from having a lot of arguments about his crossdressing. We fought (and cried, and talked, and fought some more) about every aspect of his crossdressing. The only fight we haven't had is the "Why didn't you tell me sooner?" one, because he told me after we'd been dating a week and a half. We argued about sex because I didn't want to feel like the man in bed, and was tired of him wanting to be seduced. We bickered over clothes because he'd decide to wear clothes I was planning to wear (we're mostly the same size). We skirmished over my makeup being lost or replaced, feuded over how many shoe stores he looked in as we walked down Lexington Avenue, and we disputed whether or not he was being flirtatious—right in front of me—with a gay man. The list goes on.

We have both had moments when we were convinced our relationship was doomed. For most of the time we have been together, I have been the one to seek outside help, from therapists (thank you, Ali), from other crossdressers' girlfriends (thank you, Katie) and from my friends (too numerous to thank here). To give Betty his due, he was working two jobs for most of our first five years together. He didn't have a whole lot of time to explore his gender identity, but he did make time to listen to me, even when it cut into his sleep. I tried to be supportive even during times when I hated his crossdressing. I didn't lay down rules, and he respected me enough to ask if it was okay before he dressed.

On the other hand, his stubborn avoidance of therapy drove me nuts. When I ask him what I did that pissed him off the most, he replied, "The way you belittled me and made me feel like less than a man." *Mea culpa,* he's right: I did do that.

There are periods when we feel like we do nothing but fight. He has sworn off his crossdressing numerous times in our relationship to call a truce, but whether he's doing it or not, we still fight about it. I feel like he's giving me a guilt trip when he says he will take a "break" from dressing because I don't like becoming the reason for his repression. There are other times when the irony of our relationship brings us closer together: he's a crossdresser, and I'm a bit of a tomboy, and the last thing I wanted in life was a husband who wanted to talk about fashion. I wanted a husband who could talk about foreign policy. Then again, he wanted a wife who could talk about foreign policy *and* fashion, so we both got a little of what we wanted, at least when it came to conversation. I know there are days he still wishes I liked shoes the way most women do, but I don't, and there are days I wish he wasn't a crossdresser, but he is. Such is marriage.

*   *   *

THERE'S A BUD LIGHT commercial in which a woman calls her boyfriend at work and entices him with promises of a French maid's outfit, a blonde wig, and a six-pack of Bud Light. The boyfriend is obviously excited by the idea. The next shot is the woman, in a French maid's outfit and blonde wig. The doorbell rings and the camera pans the room as it follows her to the door, passing, of course, a six-pack of Bud Light on the table. She answers the door to find her boyfriend donning a French maid's outfit, and blonde wig—with a six-pack in hand. He greets her, looks over his own outfit, tries to stutter something about how he "thought she meant," and she abruptly slams the door in his face.

That's pretty much what most crossdressers experience from wives and girlfriends. That slammed door manifests itself in as many ways as there are crossdressers. They expect rejection, which is probably the single biggest reason crossdressers don't tell their girlfriends and wives at all (that along with the hope that marriage will "cure" their urge to crossdress). Surprisingly, more and more girlfriends and wives are accepting their partners' crossdressing. This may be because crossdressers are learning from others' mistakes. Articles and chapters on "How to Tell Your Wife" or "How Not to Tell Your Wife" appear regularly in Tri-Ess publications and in books by crossdressers. Here are some basic guidelines I've culled:

- Don't tell your wife when she's expecting or delivering your child.
- Don't tell her by getting dressed en femme and waiting for her in your living room while she's out doing the grocery shopping.
- Don't tell her by leaving massive amounts of literature about crossdressing around the house.
- Don't tell her after you've just watched a crossdressing nut announce to his wife on "Jerry Springer" that he's been having an affair for the previous six months—with a man.
- Don't tell her by suggesting you'd look better in her new red dress than she does.
- Don't tell her by planning a "surprise" visit to a Tri-Ess meeting.
- Don't take her to a drag club and say "I always wanted to do that."

These sound ridiculous, but plenty of crossdressers have thought these approaches seemed like good ideas. They were terrible ideas. A crossdresser has to use his brains and his heart when considering how and when to tell his wife or girlfriend. If he doesn't trust his own judgment, he should read JoAnn Roberts' *Coping with Crossdressing,* which offers the best practical advice about how to bring up the subject, what kind of information to have on hand, and what kind of responses one might expect. (It does fall a little short in discussing the partners' responses and the logic or emotions undergirding those responses.) One of the things crossdressers forget most often is that they have had their whole lives to try to sort out what crossdressing means to them. They have "known" a crossdresser all their lives, yet still experience shame and confusion. Most women do not know crossdressers. And even those who have been exposed to members of other "sexual minorities"— Angela, for instance, works as a beautician and has known gay men all her adult life—will have a very different response to the news of her husband's crossdressing than to finding out one of her coworkers does drag. The cross-dresser has to keep in mind that, at the very least, the news will be a surprise. Most wives fail to see the "signs," although afterwards, with 20/20 hindsight, many wonder how they couldn't have.

How could a wife be unaware of her husband's crossdressing? Because most CDs do some kind of "compensating" for their inner femininity, and have trained themselves in order to "pass" as regular men in society.

Some crossdressers do "out" themselves. Many a wife has found lingerie that is not hers and has assumed that her husband was having an affair. Worse yet, many make peace with their "discovery." When she finds out there is no "other woman"—or rather that her own husband is "the other woman"—she suffers not just the shock and confusion felt by all cross-dressers' wives, but also criticizes herself for having looked the other way. She might believe she has compromised herself, her marriage, and her integrity in doing so, and feels like a fool. The woman who simply didn't suspect feels like a fool, too. She has to rebuild her self-esteem even while she is trying to figure out how her life is going to change based on her newfound knowledge.

Crossdressers who decide to tell their partners have usually achieved some level of peace with themselves and their crossdressing. Dixie's description of his wife's feelings indicates a lot about how the crossdresser himself may be feeling when he finally tells his wife:

> Her lack of acceptance (and there is little or no communication about it any more since she has just about refused to talk about it) doesn't have any effect on my acceptance of myself. I've determined that I am, always have been, and always will be a crossdresser. And like I've told so many others—I'm at peace with myself about that. I know it's not going to change and to be perfectly honest about it I don't want it to. Once one has experienced the delightful world of femininity, it's not

something that you want to just ignore or cast aside. Besides, I've got enough sense to know that even if I could let it go, it would most definitely change my personality and (not trying to sound vain here) I like my personality and it seems that most everyone else I meet does also. There are imbedded feminine components in any crossdresser's personality and if these could be removed, the results would most definitely make a negative difference.

You can feel the defensiveness in his words, the smell of battle, as it were. He knows what he wants, he knows who he is, and he knows his wife doesn't like it. The problem is, he's determined to convince her to feel the same way about his crossdressing, but for her it's a threat which is going to challenge everything she thinks about herself and her life. She is terrified. She is furious.

If a wife is willing to try, what does she do? How does her husband help her begin the long road toward acceptance? A wife may find solace in books or seek help in the SO community. But the key to it all is her husband's ability to listen—even to things he doesn't want to hear. The crossdresser has to be able to hear his wife out, and listen without interrupting. Her job is to be honest with herself, and to communicate her true feelings to her husband. She has to invest some time and energy into thinking deeply about her own feelings and forming opinions so she can share them with him. A lot of couples, like Gidget and her husband, have to learn how to communicate with each other again after the husband comes out as a crossdresser. Relationship problems often cause a breakdown in communication skills, and if my relationship is any judge, it's harder to repair the lines of communication than to keep them open in the first place. If you don't use it, you lose it, and a relationship cannot exist without good communication.

The newly informed wife of a crossdresser will likely go through stages. Accepting an inevitable fact is like facing death: you have no choice, but it takes some work to get there. Psychiatrist Elizabeth Kübler-Ross' five stages of grief provide a template for the phases through which a wife will pass when she hears her husband's news.

1) First she may *deny* it. She may point out how masculine he is and otherwise refuse to see the truth. During this stage she won't want to read or hear anything about his crossdressing. Some women stop here and are unwilling to proceed.

2) When the truth finally comes clear, and she realizes there is no way to avoid it, she may become *resentful and angry*. She feels as if she can't trust her husband anymore, that her sense of him and their partnership is lost. She

feels everything sliding out from under her. As Elizabeth, the wife of a cross-dresser, put it, "When your most intimate relationship has become a tightrope walk you need a safety net!" During this stage she might find a group of other wives and a place to release her anger. She will need to vent with her husband, but, as Gidget points out, the real trick for her and her husband was learning how to communicate without judgment or critique. This is often difficult for the crossdresser, because he may be experiencing the same defensiveness described by Dixie. It's likely that he will want to refute every objection his wife raises (bolstered of course by all the research he's done on the Internet and elsewhere). This tactic is not helpful. The wife needs to be able to communicate how she feels without ending up in an argument. Often she feels betrayed again because she took the time to listen to her husband, and he refuses to listen to her. She may say unpleasant things and pose challenging, confrontational questions. She may remind him of everything he has ever done wrong. She may be angry, sarcastic, or belittling. I know I have been.

Betty often tries to talk me out of my anger, when all I really want to do is scream for a while. Having him listen and tell me he's sorry when I'm done is usually more useful than his attempts to convince me that I shouldn't be angry.

3) Interestingly, the next stage is *bargaining*. In my opinion, this is where most wives stop in the acceptance process. In the crossdressing community it's called laying down "boundaries." The wives make deals with their husbands: "If you don't dress at home," or "As long as I never see it." It strikes me that this approach is misguided. They set "boundaries" instead of establishing higher standards and expecting their husbands to meet them. JoAnn Roberts, a crossdresser, points out that a crossdresser who spends time dressing is "no different from the guy who plops in front of the television on Sundays to watch all the ball games." I agree entirely: men can be selfish and inconsiderate, or maybe they just have a deep need for that kind of "downtime." The women who are married to the guys who watch football all day complain about their husbands' behavior but also take care of the kids and make dinner and otherwise give their husbands implicit permission. Maybe they should stop getting their husbands the chips, instead, or expect them to cook dinner and bathe the kids when their wives sit down to watch *ER*.

A crossdresser's wife may opt for insisting that her husband can't shave his legs or pierce his ears. She may benefit more from expecting and encouraging him to communicate his own needs and listen to hers. That doesn't mean they can't set mutual "boundaries" if that works for them, but a lot of women are very uncomfortable laying down rules: it feels too much like parenting instead of partnership. Crossdressers themselves are often so appreciative that the women in their lives tolerate their dressing that they follow the rules. A rather sexist and unbalanced arrangement is the result: The man wants to crossdress but his wife will tell him how, when, and where he can, which leaves him free to blame her if he doesn't get to dress as frequently as he'd like. To me this is not a healthy or preferable outcome for either partner.

Women already tend to compensate for the fact that many men aren't good at communicating their feelings, are uncomfortable showing affection, and often come up short on selflessness and nurturing. Must we also be responsible for their crossdressing and control where, when and how much they do it? And take on the responsibility for the resulting guilt and shame? As far as I can tell, my husband is a grown man, and if he's doing something that makes our relationship uncomfortable, I expect him to notice and fix it. Our responsibility, as women, is not to disrespect our partners' need to dress. Respect is our only responsibility, and it's quite enough to figure out how to achieve that. We've got to work on our own issues of self-esteem and body image and sexuality, and our plates are too full to "police" their behavior as well. Maybe it's because we're so busy resolving their issues for them that we never get to our own.

I'm not saying that guys who didn't tell their wives for twenty-five years don't deserve the extreme reactions they get. They do. It's a horrible thing for a man to lie to his wife about anything for that long, and to lie about such an important part of himself is even worse. But making bargains is not a lasting solution, although it can be a good way to establish a temporary truce, so both husband and wife can catch their breath. They're going to need it.

4) The fourth stage is *depression*. Realization finally sets in, and she feels powerless, victimized, and betrayed. She doesn't have the energy to get up in the morning, and her interest in sex may disappear. If she is already mildly depressive, as so many women are, she may need to talk to a professional if she hasn't already.

I'd argue, too, that this isn't a good time for her to start learning more about crossdressing. She may seek out the sad stories in the crossdressing community, which aren't hard to find, and become even more depressed. The crossdressing husband often "catches" his wife's sadness. He may go through the depression with her, and the feelings of confidence that spurred him to tell his wife disappear.

5) The last stage is *acceptance*. Every woman's acceptance is different, but at last she now knows her husband is a crossdresser, and they can begin

making decisions about their life together. She may want a divorce, even after working through all these stages. She may be able to tolerate it as long as she's not asked to participate. She may develop sophisticated coping strategies or embrace her husband's crossdressing.

It's important to note that these five stages could take any length of time. Some women settle into the bargaining stage permanently, and others get stuck elsewhere. A wife may be angry for years before she moves to the bargaining stage. A girlfriend may only be depressed for a weekend, but on Monday may realize she does want to be in the relationship. Every woman's experience is different. Once a woman reaches acceptance, the couple has a whole new journey to embark upon. Myriad mutual decisions will need to be worked out, such as whom they tell about his crossdressing, whether or not they take it to the bedroom, whether or not they'll be "out," and whether or not they share clothes.

I have not found a terrific number of women at any of the events I have been to, and I think that's because most women never hit the acceptance stage. I am not sure how otherwise to account for the fact that crossdressers get together once a month at Tri-Ess meetings and other support groups and their wives simply don't come. Some do. Another reason might be their desire for privacy. The "girls" often take group pictures at these events, and they are of course in disguise just by being their femme selves. Wives don't have such a luxury. We come as ourselves. We might be recognized in group photos by friends, work associates, or family members who happen to see a picture online. Maybe we feel too vulnerable at these gatherings. Maybe the guys should spring for a second wig? It may also just be that there are so few other wives at these events, so there's no one for us to talk to.

At the CDM meeting one of the ladies gave us a tip: If anyone we knew ever saw us walking down the street together and Betty was en femme, I should stop and talk to the person while Betty just kept walking. That way, the acquaintance would not guess that Betty was my husband. We thanked her for the clever suggestion, but explained we'd be more likely to just say "hi" to the person we knew. We explained, too, that we are out to most of our friends, and those who don't know the whole story usually know that Betty occasionally "does drag." That's the advantage of being an actor *and* a crossdresser. Actors are supposed to be a little eccentric. A construction worker can't casually tell his friends he does drag on the weekends.

Most wives also practice caution due to the risk of job loss. Peter Oiler, a twenty-year employee of Winn-Dixie, was fired for crossdressing on his own time. Winn-Dixie even won the appeal. Denise, "Melissa's" girlfriend, used to accompany her crossdressed partner to the local Enormo-Mart.

However, once she started working in "Melissa's" school district, she panicked when they ran into a coworker of hers in aisle three. She wasn't ashamed of her boyfriend but experienced a very real concern for her career. Many wives are in similar situations: they can't risk being recognized with their crossdressed husbands if they work with children, live in conservative neighborhoods, or work for conservative companies.

Once the crossdresser comes out to his wife, the decisions about how he dresses and when and where need to be mutual. She needs to feel safe and know that he is, too. They both need to consider real risks to their safety and reputation and livelihood, especially when there are children involved. In order to do that, they must be equals dealing with their crossdressing together. Compromises must be made. Both partners should treat the other with the kind of respect they expect for themselves. I know I want a relationship based on equality and trust. Since I don't expect my husband to tell me what I can or can't wear for a three-day weekend or a night out, I don't expect to tell him what he can or cannot wear. If I want to tell him he can't shave his legs, then I have to be ready to live with the fact that he wants me to shave mine daily because he doesn't like them hairy or stubbly. To me, that's only fair.

I do expect my husband to figure out when I'm in the mood for his guy self. If all I've been talking about is what a rock star he's been looking like, he should grab the hint and keep out of his lingerie. Ditto for verbal

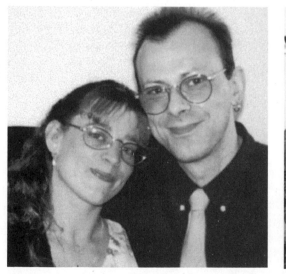

Sue and Adrian, in male mode

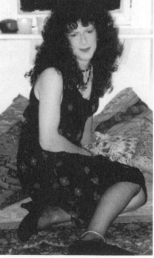

Adrian, en femme, as Ali

appreciations of his stubble, big hands, or broad shoulders. I have been boy crazy all my life and that has not changed for a second. I will always prefer my husband in boxer briefs with a little bit of stubble on his jawbone. But do I love seeing the happiness and peace in him when he's got one leg in the air and a razor in his hand in the bath? Absolutely. He exudes playfulness and sensuality when he's surrounded by bubbles or silk or velvet. When I see him shaving his legs, he can sense what I'm feeling if he bothers to notice. There are times I just roll my eyes or smile and laugh at what a girl he is. Other times I might stop to kiss him or ask if I can help. Still other times I look in and tell him I'll be in the other room. He's not a fool: he knows the difference. He knows my tone of voice. He should know by now that the only time he has to ask if it's okay he gets en femme is when I can't manage even a smile for him.

THE COUPLES

THERE ARE A lot of different types of couples in the crossdressing community. Some are conservative, others eccentric or liberal. It depends on how they function as a couple, what lives they lead as individuals, and what values they hold. They have come to accept crossdressing in their lives in varied ways and to varied degrees. They represent certain paths that can be taken, but couples can find their own. It's only when both partners establish what their own responsibilities are within the relationship that they can really achieve acceptance. Here are six couples I've gotten to know in the time I've been running my online group and how they've worked crossdressing into their lives. Some of them even manage to share the fun of it.

ALI & SUE—HEALERS

Ali *(crossdresser)* is a Reiki master, trained therapist, and Ninjitsu black belt from the southwest of England. He told his partner Sue that he was a transvestite about a month into their dating. She accepted it and took him shopping. They never married and currently live separately, but are romantic partners and raise their son together.

Sue *(genetic woman)* is a thirty-three-year-old second Degree Reiki practitioner and mother from the Southwest of England who provides professional home help to the elderly. She has been with Ali for ten years. She had no knowledge about tranvestism other than from limited media and television coverage, but that didn't keep her from accepting it. They have both always been very eager to help each other in any way possible.

Ali/Adrian and Sue are English, and Ali has often said that might account for their comfort discussing sexuality in general; European culture is often more open about such things. I think it's who they are as people that made it work. These two are kind-hearted, gentle people; they strive with everything they've got to reach a higher consciousness. Their professions indicate their need to help others, and they do. Ali has long been the "ear" of our mailing list, the one person who knows the right thing to say in a difficult situation. Their ease with each other is obvious. They smile at each other and touch frequently, wait for the other to finish speaking, hold hands.

One of the stories Ali and Sue told us was of the time Ali thought "she" needed to know whether being a crossdresser really did mean "she" was gay. Since he'd heard the implications all his life, he needed to explore. Ali told Sue his intentions, and Sue understood. She didn't want a partner who was uncertain of his own sexuality. Although I can't imagine she had an easy time on the evening Ali went out with a man, she managed. Ali got his answer: he liked women. When he got home, they went for a walk and talked. The "space" Sue was able to give Ali blows my mind. I don't think there's a sedative strong enough to keep me calm if my boyfriend were out trying to figure out if he was gay. But Ali and Sue—with their devotion and expansive spirits—have achieved a level of acceptance others only dream of.

In Their Own Words:

Ali: *It is a medical fact that no matter which born gender we are, attributes of both exist in us all. Every man on this earth has a certain proportion of female hormones in his body and vice versa. This is true also on the psychological level too. The functions of the female brain are entirely different to that of a man. Women in fact have activity on both hemispheres of the brain, whereas most men have activity on the right side only. This is not true in all cases though. Some men to a greater or lesser degree have dual hemispheric activity similar to that of women. No links with cross-dressing have yet been proven but many theories as to the why of gender related conditions have been centred on this.*

The Taoist theory of Yin and Yang tells us this also. Everything in the universe has a diametric opposite. Night and day, up and down, hot and cold, etc. but in practice the opposite extremes do not exist. All things exist somewhere in between.

Hot, for example, can always get hotter. There is no point at which we can point that says "that is HOT."

The same can be said for people. No man or woman is 100 percent male or female, no matter how much they like to think they are. We are in reality all individuals somewhere within the sphere.

It seems ridiculous when all the above is considered, that we still have to regard the male and female of the species as two entirely separate classes. Why is it necessary to do so?

It frustrates me that there are so many times when filling out forms or similar things where I have to state if I am Male or Female.

It seemed once I accepted myself as an individual, rather than labeling myself as a Man, or a man pretending to be a woman, I found a lot of the guilt problems disappeared.

It may not work for everyone—but it has worked for me!

Sue: *He told me within a month of our relationship starting. Well in truth you could say I guessed, because of some of the things he had said to me that were so unlike the sort of things one would usually expect a partner to say. Things such as "I bet it feels great to wear that skirt" or "how does it feel to shave your legs and then put a pair of tights on." In the end I just looked at him and said "if you really want to know, there's my wardrobe, knock yourself out." He was amazed to say the least, but after double checking that I meant what I said there was no holding him back. We had great fun that night and have been ever since.*

Finding out so early in our relationship definitely made all the difference. Had I found out years later, it would have been much harder. For me I feel that we started out the way we have continued, with total honesty. That is very important to me.

Ali and I joined the Beaumont Society (a support group for crossdressers in England) which was a great help to us both. Unfortunately there weren't many wives that attended. To be quite honest I didn't really seek support as I didn't have a problem with it. I have tried to do my bit to help others with this. For instance, Ali and I have done several television shows on the subject. We also did a documentary on our relationship and how my partner's crossdressing fits into our lives. It was called Adrian, Sue, and Ali Too. I have also talked to the wives of other crossdressers that were having problems coming to terms with this.

When we decided to go on television we told our friends and families who on the whole were very supportive. Although it's not the first thing we tell anyone we don't

*hide it from anyone including our son. Our belief is that if people can see we don't
have a problem with it then they are less likely to. If they do, hopefully our honesty
will make them feel able to ask any questions which may help them to a better understanding and acceptance.*

*As I said, due to the interviews we had done the decision was sort of made for us.
Ali's family were fine. I know for a fact his mum is very proud of him and even car-
ries a photo of Ali in her purse. My mum was great. She was even in the documentary we did. Unfortunately my dad has big problems with it, to the point that he now
refuses to see my partner and finds it difficult to see me. The rest of my family seem
okay with it but don't really talk about it.*

*Knowing about his cross-dressing has only enhanced our relationship and con-
firmed my own belief that you can't love half a person: you either love all of them or
none of them. You may not like it all but that still makes that person who they are
so you have to like everything even if just a little. I feel so privileged to have been
given the chance to know and love this very special person that I can't imagine how
my life would have been if we had never met (probably quite boring).*

HEATHER & MINNA—CONSERVATIVE ALTERNATIVES

Minna *(genetic woman)* is in her late thirties, mother of two, married to
Heather. She was introduced to crossdressing and BDSM by her husband
after they had been friends for three years but before their friendship blos-
somed into a romance—and after it became apparent that her first marriage
had failed. She didn't immediately accept crossdressing, but found her own
path through the BDSM community. She was raised Catholic, is now Wiccan
and politically moderate.

Heather *(crossdresser)* is a thirty-five-year old, married father of two and
a fourteen-year combat arms veteran of the U.S. Army. Politically he is reg-
istered as and generally votes Republican. He is married to Minna and told
her about his crossdressing and his interest in BDSM before their first night
together. He falls somewhere beyond the textbook definition of crossdresser,
but short of transsexual. He lives and works as a man, but is more comfortable when crossdressed and could happily live as a woman.

Heather and Minna are not a stereotypical couple in any community. He is
a military man, and she is a curvaceous woman with more confidence than
a busload of cheerleaders. They are parents and live in a conservative neigh-

borhood but they refuse to sacrifice their individuality. Their children—
Minna's from her previous marriage—do not know about Heather's crossdressing. Minna's ex-husband is not likely to understand. Heather's military
peers do not know either, as crossdressing is considered a mental illness by
the U.S. Military, and therefore grounds for medical discharge. Their conservative social set, however, has not stopped them from finding other
BDSM practitioners and making new friends, whom they have educated
about crossdressing. Minna has also found herself educating military peers
of Heather's on the Wiccan faith. They are both happily highly sexed.

Although Heather told Minna about his TG nature before they were intimate, it took Minna seven years before she could participate in any way.
Minna found it was through her experiences as a dominant woman, or dominatrix, within the BDSM community that shed light on her husband's needs.
She worked with many submissive men and saw that Heather's desires were
not as unusual as she originally thought. She is continually amazed that
Heather is dominant "herself" when en femme and is only submissive when
taking on his male role.

In Their Own Words:

Minna: *I wish you could walk a mile in my shoes. See what I see the way I see it. See
what I know and experience it. Taste what I taste and see how I enjoy it. My life is
not the same as yours. My husband is a crossdresser. I am a dominatrix. I am a
mother, a wife, a lover and a sadist. I am Republican. I am Wiccan. I am not the
average person and thank the Goddess I am not.*

*You walk by me every day and do not know any of this. I don't stand out in a
crowd. Well, yes, I suppose my bright red hair does and the way I walk does, but I
don't look threatening. I look like an average woman with two kids.*

*You do not know what my double life entails. The frustration of not being able
to let my husband walk out of our house dressed because we are a military family on a military post and that's grounds for him being discharged from the service to his country that he loves. My kids can't know about dad because my son is
from a previous marriage and my ex-husband would take him from me in an
instant if he knew.*

*I worry every time my husband goes out dressed without me that he will be hurt.
It's why I usually don't allow it. Not because I don't trust him, but because I don't
trust you. I hear what others think about crossdressing and I really want to take
interviewers like Jerry Springer out back and get a switch. The average crossdresser*

is not the one you see on TV talk shows. They are normal men and women who have a need to dress in the clothing of another gender.

My husband is not a child molester, a rapist, or some sick perverse serial killer. He isn't morally loose and sleeping around with everyone and everything. He is a man whose internal gender does not match his external gender totally. That is the definition of a transsexual, but he doesn't want to be a woman full time either. It's more complex than him just wanting to be a woman; he wants to be a man, too. It's not some sexual fetish either; he doesn't need to dress in order to get sexually aroused.

I wish you could walk a mile in my shoes. In my friends' shoes. In my husband's shoes. See what we go through every day.

Maybe you'd be a bit more tolerant of those different than yourself.

Heather: When I told Minna about my crossdressing and interest with BDSM it was done for several reasons, not least of which was to make sure She* knew up front. My primary reason however, was to make sure I didn't end up falling in love with a woman whom I couldn't be myself around. If She hadn't been accepting, the simple answer is I wouldn't have continued to develop a relationship with Her. When it became obvious that She could handle part of my oddities with the potential to eventually accept all of them, I made a decision that "a bird in the hand is worth two in the bush"; especially since there was the possibility the second bird might end up in my hand too (and it did seven years later).

That it was important that I inform Her is certain. That I was fortunate to know myself well enough to know I needed an accepting woman from the start is probably more of a testament to my parents' skills at raising a self-aware child than to any wisdom of my own. That it was the only policy that makes sense (though not the only one that will work) seems to have been answered by the number of years of successful marriage Mistress and I have shared without treading the terrible "discovery" pitfalls so many crossdressers go through with their spouses.

I have a Mistress who not only accepts, but also encourages and even brags about my crossdressing (within the BDSM and TG communities). She will not only let me dress around Her, but will even make love to me when I am dressed. I know it doesn't turn Her on when I dress, but it doesn't turn Her off, either. Would I like it to be a turn on to Her? Certainly! Is it reasonable for me to demand it be? Definitely not. I know lots of CD/TV/TS/TG people who would give their left arm to even have a shot at a woman as accepting as my Mistress is. I count myself as exceedingly lucky, and make sure She knows I think that way.

---

*A note on Heather's text: in BDSM culture, a submissive shows respect for his Dom/me by capitalizing references to him/her.

KATHY & AMANDA—GIRLFRIENDS

Kathy (*genetic woman*) has been married to her husband Amanda since 1999. She owns and runs her own business. They live in Ontario and are active in the transgender community there, tabling at GLBT events. Kathy is one of the only wives who was actively seeking a crossdressing husband when she found him, via a personal ad online.

Amanda (*crossdresser*) works for a large company in the automotive industry. He is slightly older than Kathy, but not by much, and was going "out and about" as a crossdresser before they met. It was in fact his website—which of course featured pictures of him en femme—that caught Kathy's eye. An Internet romance was born, and Kathy eventually moved from her native Texas to Canada to start their married life together.

Kathy and Amanda are a special case, and they know it. Amanda spent the time and energy figuring out where "she" was on the TG spectrum, so that by the time he and Kathy met, he had answered all those tricky questions. From the beginning, Kathy knew what she wanted, and Amanda knew who he was. For that reason, they got to avoid many of the arguments other couples experience.

They run information booths on crossdressing and transgenderism at gay and lesbian events, but that doesn't mean they are entirely out. They practice discretion by limiting their CD outings to Toronto—the closest major city to the suburb they live in. Amanda has been going out crossdressed since 1996, and despite the fact that he works at a major employer in the region, "she" never encountered a coworker in public who has recognized "her" en femme, except for a gay man at a local gay bar who of course understood the need for secrecy. Kathy and Amanda believe that if people cannot accept crossdressing, they are not people worth having in your life to begin with. They have structured their lives around being open-minded, and are drawn to others who share the same philosophy. However, they do what they can to educate those who are less understanding.

In Their Own Words:

Kathy: *I am the wife of a crossdresser. My husband Amanda and I met on the Internet in January of 1999. Unlike other wives I knew he was a crossdresser from the moment I laid eyes on him.*

I had been recently divorced and was about to enter a new chapter in my life. I have always had an underlying interest in feminine men since a very early age. Growing up I knew I was heterosexual but had little idea that men who dressed as women would be interested in females. After my divorce I decided to learn more about crossdressers. Who they were, what they did, and mostly if there was a possibility this sort of life was for me.

Being a female who is open to dating crossdressers is like throwing a steak in a pit full of starving lions. Going to transgender friendly bars seemed a good place to start my journey. I had offers left and right but found mostly that many of these men had little in common with me other than my interest in their crossdressing. I also found many crossdressers to be very confused men who were still battling guilt and shame. Many were uncertain as to whether they would ever consider SRS or experiment with hormones once with an accepting girlfriend. I also learned that for some their sexual orientation shifted and changed with the clothes that they wore. Don't even get me started on the rampant alcoholism and drug abuse I saw first hand in this community.

This left me scared and also worried if I was getting myself into something I would later regret. At this time I still had this idea that with the "right" crossdresser I would find the perfect combination of best girlfriend and loving husband in one person. The bar scene left me a bit jaded and I began to rely on the net for potential men to meet, from a safer distance. Scoping websites became my dating service.

That was when I came across Amanda Bowers' website. I sent a simple e-mail saying who I was and that I found his website to be really nice and wondered if he would like to get to know me better. Two weeks of e-mail led to one very long phone conversation. Two months of phoning each other led to him flying down to meet me in my hometown.

Meeting Amanda as a male was even better than I had hoped. He was confident in his gender and sexuality and thankfully had a firm grip on what he wanted in the future. We both would be making huge compromises to make this relationship work so being painfully honest was extremely important. Tough subjects beyond mere crossdressing had to be talked about at length. Money, careers, religion, sex, politics, and what we wanted from each other had to be out in the open.

In August 1999 we were married and I relocated 1,700 miles to live as his wife. Crossdressing has been a source of fun and enjoyment for us. There are very few boundaries we have.

At first I feared that same fear all wives do. Will he eventually take my acceptance as "anything goes" and take his crossdressing to different levels? My friends who knew of our secret life worried what would happen if we have children. I also have worried "what will the neighbors think" as well. As we enter into our fourth year of marriage I feel more secure than ever before of who he is and who "she" is in our life.

As for being "that" woman, I have had women/men/couples come up to me in restaurants, clubs, and stores, and ask "Who is that person you are with?" I find they do this when I am on my way to the bathroom or we are not standing next to each other. When I say "That is my spouse," they look shocked, then ask if "he" already had a sex change, or what. They want to know what's going on. I tell them he is a crossdresser and this is just a fun thing we do and that he has no intention of having a sex change. I find people look at me funny afterwards more than they do Amanda. I usually don't say anything to Amanda as I don't want him to think this bothers me in any real way. Sometimes I wish people would just mind their business but on the other hand if I can educate one person that we are not all wackos, then I am happy.

The more I am married to this man the more I realize what a man he really is. The dream of having a heterosexual male crossdresser with a female mind/heart/soul is pretty much gone. Although my husband is a loving partner he is not a woman in mind or thought. There is a sensitive side to his personality and certainly a less macho attitude than most males, but by no means is he a woman in any way to me.

His crossdressing I believe is more recreation and comfort than transgenderism and certainly transsexualism. There are times I wish he was more feminine in thought or action but then I chastise myself for thinking that way. Would I truly want him to be further down the other end of the scale and then have to deal with all the other things that seem to come with being of that mind frame?

Right now I know that I am one of the lucky ones. I don't fear for the future like I used to and time has only confirmed the promises he made, to stay just a cross-dresser. Choosing this life is something I do not regret and truth be told, I would probably choose it again if I had to start over.

Amanda: *I'd been single all my life until Kathy came along. I'd had a few relation-ships in the past, but nothing that lasted longer than a month or so and nothing too serious. I had a girlfriend in high school, but refused to get too close to her. I never told her about my crossdressing and didn't want to burden anyone I dated with such a thing. Since at the time I had no idea how it fit into my life, I couldn't ask her to try and fit it into her life. It took me about ten years to come to grips with it and quit asking "Why"?*

I was really surprised when I received Kathy's e-mail. At that point in my life I had given up on ever finding a life partner. I was expecting to spend the rest of my life alone. Her e-mail was short but she said upfront what she wanted from a rela-tionship. I was in agreement with her expectations and we continued our relationship through e-mail, then phone, and eventually meeting a couple of months later. Six months after the first e-mail we were married.

We pretty much always go out together. I don't think I've gone out without her.

On the other hand, she has gone out several times to visit with other CDs when I had to work. We go out to everyday events like movies and shopping or dinner and also to CD exclusive events.

I'm out, I guess. My mother knows and is supportive. She's seen me dressed on several occasions and even went out with us for my birthday with me en femme.

It has made things easier to be out. I don't have to worry about keeping everything hidden the way I used to. Now, I don't go exploiting the fact that people know, but I don't really hide it that much either. A lot of it has to do with Kathy, most of her friends know about Amanda either by accident or by being included in the big picture.

On the other hand, most of my friends don't know, but I'm not really that close to any of the guys I know. I have work acquaintances that I socialize with on occasion, but most of the time I prefer to hang around with people that I don't have to hide anything from.

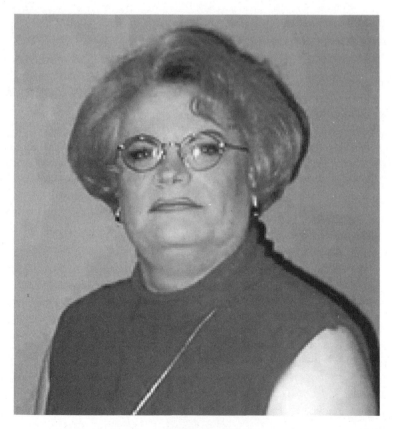

Victoria

I used to feel guilty. "Why me?!" I finally had an epiphany and now know that it's okay to be me. I chatted a lot online, but in the end, it was something that changed inside me. I didn't read anything special or talk to anyone to finally overcome the guilt.

I believe that if you truly love someone, you should tell them about this before you are married. Get it out in the open before there are any strings. I think it's a little easier now being a CD at age fifteen or twenty. The internet has opened up the lines of communication and lets people know that they are not alone.

I'd tell the younger crossdresser: don't be afraid of who you are. It may take some time to accept yourself. Don't do anything crazy until you've figured it out. Lots of people are pushed onto hormones without being ready. Some are never ready and that's okay.

I would not want to be a woman; it's way too hard!

VICTORIA & MEREDITH—PARENTS

Victoria (*transvestite*) has been married to Meredith for twenty-seven years but only told her he is a crossdresser seven years ago. He is a responsible husband and father, has always earned a good income in the tech end of communications. He cares deeply about the happiness of his wife and two adult children. He is out to a degree he never expected to be, and has been in various support groups, including Tri-Ess and CDI. He still hopes his wife will participate more in his dressing, but is satisfied that she tolerates it. He is also a veteran of the Vietnam War. He is in his early fifties, with nearly a full head of hair, on the short side and a little stout.

Meredith (*genetic woman*) is the no-nonsense wife of Victoria. She is also in her early fifties and has an acerbic sense of humor, a professional career, and the usual troubles of a married woman with adult children. She is a thin, impeccably but casually dressed woman whose wit and intelligence light up her eyes.

Victoria and Meredith are in their late middle age, but both of them are youthful and full of life. They have been married twenty-seven years, and the first thing my husband and I were struck by when we met them is how much they love each other. When Meredith rolls her eyes over something Victoria says (like about how corsets are comfortable), she still seems more amused than disgusted, even if she thinks what he's saying is ridiculous. Likewise, Victoria respects his wife deeply, and it was obvious to us that her approval and participation would mean the world to him. He knows she can handle it. He likes her so much he'd have way more fun if she were around. That has begun to happen for them.

Meredith is a traditional woman from a conservative background. She is smart and has had her own career for many years. Living in a suburban community where she is active and respected means she doesn't want to risk losing that "normal" status. As the youngest of six, she has gained approval from older siblings, and "fitting in" was probably an important priority in her life. She has earned her place in society, and is reluctant to risk her standing for the sake of her husband's crossdressing. She likes fitting in and being "one of the girls." Victoria doesn't always seem aware that Meredith is unlikely to give that up for him. His enthusiasm—which comes out whether he's talking about amateur theater or story-telling or corsets—may be what wins his wife over in the end. One of their children does know and has a very hard time accepting crossdressing; the other, who doesn't, still lives with them.

In Their Own Words:

Victoria: *As far as Meredith goes, she has a very structured life and in her mind everything has its place—every piece of furniture, every dish, picture and even the items in any closet. In her house, she puts everything in its place. In all fairness she has found a place for my crossdressing no matter how small a place that is. She said that I speak too much about crossdressing. I now speak very little of it, but it was my intention to let her know of it, in a silly way, to show her it's harmless. Now we both know a number of CDs. But she sees them as people first and CDs second which is how everyone should view CDs. She wants very much to live in a perfect world where everything has its place and no one touches a thing. That will never happen and she is learning to deal with that and all that goes with it, including my CDing. Since I told her about myself, she has come very far in accepting if not completely dealing with it. We have agreed on a number of simple rules both of us can live with, and so there are no surprises: no dressing at home, and no traveling to or from the house dressed.*

As strange as this may seem, but for the both of us, there are a number of CDs in our everyday lives and that's a good thing. I don't think I could have asked for a better understanding short of her wanting me to dress.

Meredith: *Victoria and I have been married for twenty-seven years. When we first got married Victoria took me to a transvestite show and he found it entertaining* *and I found it repulsive. Little did I know that he was trying to tell me that he could relate to these men and would like to be one of them. He hinted at his desire to dress in feminine clothing and I was upset, angry and confused yet I was unwilling to end this relationship. Why? Was it love, my religion or my commitment to a vow? I don't know. I'm sure all of it played a part in my decision to pretend it didn't exist.*

When I was pregnant with my son I found books hidden about crossdressers and transvestites and once again I went into denial and told Victoria I thought it was trash and that I wanted no knowledge of this interest. This was the way of our life until about twenty years later while on vacation he asked me if I loved him. My suspicions were immediately aroused and when I asked questions I learned that while I was away with my children earlier in the summer he had explored this desire to wear women's clothing and through the internet had found a crossdressing group that he felt comfortable with. I had no choice but to deal with the reality of what Victoria wanted. I was hurt, angry, and bitter. Here was a person who I felt betrayed me. I was his wife—loyal, honest, faithful, and always there. How could he do this to me? I certainly didn't deserve to be treated this way. What about my feelings, and what would people say? So many emotions have run through my mind since that summer day. I have wanted to hate him for forcing me to deal with his desire to wear female clothing. It made me question my worth as a female and what did I do that made him want to do this to me? Was he gay? I can't tell you how many times I asked myself that question. Though it all one fact remains—Victoria loves his children and me. His interest in crossdressing is not going away and as long as he doesn't shove it down my throat I can tolerate it. I'll never really like this facet of our relationship but after seven years I can deal with it.

GIDGET & JAYNE—BOOMERS

Jayne *(crossdresser)*, fifty-eight, is a rock'n'roll type who has always been involved in the music industry. He wears his hair long, which drives Gidget a little nuts. They have been married more than thirty years. His crossdressing was the kind of dilemma that eventually brought them closer together. They have one child with special needs.

Gidget *(genetic woman)* is fifty-four years old, and teaches Special Ed. She grew up in a conservative Catholic family and always wore pretty dresses to Church. She thinks her age and conservative background account for her difficulty in accepting her husband's crossdressing, and even now feels a little sad that she didn't get a "normal" adult sexual relationship with her marriage. That said, she loves her husband and has come leaps and bounds toward accepting him for who he is.

Jayne has no wish to go out dressed, for which Gidget is very thankful. Still in all, for her to get used to a man who wanted to be feminine—even at home—was a challenge. It was probably as much of a challenge for Jayne to communicate how deep a part of him crossdressing is. Their relationship reached a standstill when their inability to communicate shut down other parts of their companionship.

Gidget still dislikes Jayne's long hair, but she doesn't talk about him as if he's a petulant child, either. She left CDSO because she disliked the big "bitch" sessions, and was looking for actual help and good advice. Gidget found a gender therapist by calling a local hospital's psychiatric department, and the counselor helped them learn how to communicate again. Within a few months they had become friends again, and learned how to focus on their mutual needs. She came to respect the importance of his crossdressing and he learned to teach her about it and to negotiate.

In Their Own Words:

Gidget: *I think the bottom line is that you must both be in love to come across and meet the other person halfway, as you give up part of what you wanted, for part of him, and he does the same for you. I wasn't the one-hundred-percent accepting person that he wanted, but he loves me and accepted less from me. Also, I did the same for him, as I got myself to take a risk and see and view him as a female. It freaked me out when I first saw it about twenty years ago, but now. . . . It took him being very slow about showing things to me—he first wore a black cotton dress to bed with me, and I imagined this as a black cotton T-shirt and thought "this isn't too bad!!" Then he wore pantyhose, which felt funny to me and I kept getting these lesbian dreams from those things—LOL!!—anyways, it took time . . .*

Pretty soon, he progressed with one more item—I call this "taking baby steps" and that is how I learned to accept everything even now. It had to be done very slowly and at my comfort zone—after all, as I explained to him, he had many years of getting up to this level, and I had no years seeing this kind of thing. He had to go slowly for me to go there with him.

Also, I told him to imagine me without makeup (HORRORS!!!) and with my hair cut in a crew-cut style (I would look awful for sure!!) and then smoking a cigar and wearing a western cowboy look—and then I asked him if he could picture me like that and I told him I needed him to have sex with me like that, what would he think?? He was honest and replied he wouldn't like me that way—so I asked him, "Why not? I'm still the same girl underneath." He used to say to me the same thing—he would always wear his femme outfits and tell me, "Why don't you just love me? I'm still the same guy underneath." Hee-hee—that took care of that!!! He finally saw how I was viewing things—you have to spell it out for them—they think just because they accept themselves dressed as females, that we shouldn't have problems with it, as they see it as no big deal.

However, they do know that MOST women would have problems looking at a man dressed that way—and that is why they hide it from us—they know what the reaction would be.

Another thing, you asked what quality I have that helped me? I have to say, I think having a sense of humor—I laugh at this at times, and he does, too—and we both can feel at ease that way. If you take it too seriously, you get depressed.

Also, he helped me accept him as he was as I could see that he came to bed the first few times looking forlorn and depressed and ashamed very badly—and I felt sorry for him—and knew that he had told me he wanted someone his whole life to accept him as he was, but didn't get it—and I knew he meant it, so I wanted to please him as he was trying to please me by doing things I wanted him to do—such as the dishes, wash the floors, etc.—and that made me want to give up something for him as well.

I know that if he had told me the truth back then, I would have hightailed it out of Dodge for sure—I certainly wasn't raised to have sex with a kink in it—and I associated this as something very forbidden, weird, and bad.

Anyways, my husband and I are very much in love now, we don't fight anymore, and we reconnected to each other in just two months with the marriage counselor— we always were best of friends, but got a little sidetracked, I believe, due to the cross-dressing issues. First of all, I did not understand when I was younger how important this issue was to my husband—and he did not understand that he needed to negotiate and teach me how to tolerate him this way. Now he understands my side, and I understand his, and we respect each other on this issue.)

Jayne: *I told Gidget the night my father died. We were at the hospital. My mother had momentarily lost her mind. I told her "I'm transvestic." "What's that?" she asked. "You mean, you were a woman?" I had been in therapy for about five-six months and was preparing to tell her. I knew by this point that this was not going to go away. I had long thought, "This is stupid. I'm a guy." For a while I even tried to not have sex if I was going to have those thoughts. I was going to "stop thinking" and just stop when I noticed that my thoughts had turned to anything other than what I figured was "real guy" thoughts. I had been tormented with these wishes/ideas/wants to be a girl. My mother had told me since I was very little—*

and till her death—that I should have been a girl. My sister—a tougher model—should have been the boy. After all I had the curly hair, was easily scared, and needed more attention, comfort, and affection. The prevalent view on the cause of this "disorder" at that time was that I was raised that way by my mother and her all-female household. Mother had said that she did not know how to raise boys—having no brothers—and only women present, it would be easier for her if I had been a girl. I have memories of being dressed as a girl—all under five—by my mother and my father—per memory, or false memory—coming in, discovering me dressed, ripping the clothes off and locking me in a clothes closet. The closeting did happen. I to this day have nightmares—not as frequent—of waking in a clothes closet that I can not get out of. I told her after twelve years of marriage. I wanted to tell her many times. I didn't want to lose her. The idea seemed too weird for me to accept—how could I expect her to understand? I didn't want to lose her. I loved her and always will . . .

I did not like to feel that I had hurt her in any way. Early on, I didn't know that I would ever have to tell her, because never having lived before I didn't know that it wouldn't just go away. After all, I'm a guy with women as my object of desire and I now had a woman I loved who loved me. Like a priest who awakes some mornings wondering if there was a God, I wake unaccepting of the notion that this idea of female-interests exists in me. I look to Gidget's love/acceptance of me to calm my own concerns that this weirdness could exist. I am a guy and have always known that I was. But, I'm a guy with these notions that have not gone away—because they are me, too.

Her knowing and "acceptance"—I mean, do even I accept such a nutty notion as a normal looking/acting guy wanting in some way to also be female-like?—has helped beyond words. To put it brief: I was taking tranquilizers for years, largely due to my lack of acceptance of myself and its projection—that others would not accept/love me. Having told her increases my closeness, but—and this will last a while, I'm sure—having been kept in the dark for so long about one thing, she thinks I might be keeping her in the dark about others, such as I'm gay, bi-sexual, or wanting a sex-change, or some other such. None is the case. If there is anything that I am not forthcoming with it is how much money I spend on books and records.

We got real close about two years ago—like when we first fell in love. She's heard it all: no secret purchases (money for books and records is too important to be piddled away on ladies' stuff). No chat rooms, or meetings with gay, bi, transgendered and whatnot individuals. Gidget knows. My friends and family don't. And no one else knows—except you, but you're not real, just virtual.

I have read some of those free stories and bios of like-minded transgendered individuals. The TG stories—fictionmania—are often similar to the fantasies that people my mind during masturbation. Some of the stuff is repulsive. Because I like the feel of women's clothes doesn't mean that everything is acceptable or sexually stimulating to me. I wish we had more sex of any sort together. What is stimulating to me isn't to Gidget, though she can see through the veil that I am me and not another. Most times when we're together crossdressing does not cross my mind. If I'm fully engaged in being with her, there is no psychic space to be in a fantasy mode.

My token feminine component of my presentation is longish hair. Having been a hippyda wanna-be rock'n'roll musician, I have had longish hair for most of the years since the Beatles appeared. I never got into wearing female garments under my clothes. Never went out in public dressed as a woman. Great fantasy, but I'm not passable. If I had a wish I'd like to be more feminine, when in private. And I'd like to be more masculine, in public.

I'm a clinical social worker. Often what I consider as my skills to aid others who hurt is attributable to what I feel are my more feminine characteristics. I'm a feeling person. I've come to learn that I was what they now call a "highly sensitive" temperamental type. This is what my mother misread as feminine. And my pain that I have suffered for living in a society that expects people to fall neatly into one of two boxes—male/female—has aided me in being able to aid others. I don't know if it's my subtle feminine characteristics or my social work training, but these have aided me in being a better dad and a spouse. Gidget may have found that hard to accept initially. Not all that has come of me being transvestic has been negative. Good things can come of things that are initially perceived as bad. Could I still be me without being transvestic?

I'm getting comfortable being this man who secretly dresses partly female (due to laziness, like "Hey, did I get all the mascara off?"). Greater acceptance by the one who knows and still loves me is better than medicine. Love is knowing the other's foibles—knowing them—and still loving.

She has said she probably wouldn't have stayed if she'd known before we got married. She adds that she was so young that it probably would have scared her off. That was what I too had feared. I knew when we met that we were meant to be together. Remember, I knew little and hoped it would just go away. . . . I have never known anyone with the potential for such acceptance as Gidget.

MELISSA & DENISE—GEEKS IN LOVE

Melissa (*crossdresser*) is single and heterosexual. He has been entirely out of the closet for almost five years due to an ex-wife who tried to blackmail him with his crossdressing. He is only slightly active in the transgender community, and lives a mostly quiet life. Professionally, he is an electronic technician. He has two young children by his previous marriage, and thinks of his crossdressing as more of a hobby than a lifestyle. He has no intention of living his entire life en femme, or seeking any kind of SRS.

Denise (*genetic woman*) is a teacher and Melissa's girlfriend. They were friends and dated before they both married other people years ago, and lost touch during their marriages. Later they got reacquainted and became romantically involved again. As a result, Denise knew about Melissa's crossdressing. Her preference is that the male and female sides of Melissa stay separate. Denise is the type of woman who ends up running her son's boy scout troupe, plans the carpool, and brings the cookies and punch to the PTA meetings. She is capable and not easily phased by snafus that would make other people nuts.

Melissa and Denise aren't married, but they have been dating each other exclusively for a few years. Their relationship is most marked by how open and comfortable they both are with being themselves: Melissa as a crossdresser, and Denise as the "take charge" woman she is. They complement each other in remarkable ways, and are both highly intelligent and funny. Interviewing them was like talking with a pair of friends who have known each other for decades. They know each other inside and out and don't keep any secrets from each other. It's clear that they love each other and have fun together—when Denise sets up a joke, Melissa is ready with the punch line, or vice versa. They laugh a lot, which is always a good sign of a healthy relationship.

The secret of their success seems to be the fact that they have known each other a long time, as friends and as lovers. Their earlier platonic friendship provided a strong foundation for their romance.

In Their Own Words:

Melissa: (on going out for the first time en femme) *If you really believe that you are the girl you see in the mirror, then the people around you will believe it too. If you don't, they won't either. Just relax, have faith in yourself, and most of all, enjoy ALL of the sensations. Air on your knees, having someone hold the door for you, the cashier calling you "Ma'am." Its intoxicating, you'll be smiling, life will never be the same for you and you'll want to do it all again. Been there, got the glow, I still get it, five years later, just going to the grocery store. . . .*

(on the femme self and the male self) *I talk about Melissa or John doing something, and it sounds like I'm talking about two different people. Its not that I see myself as*

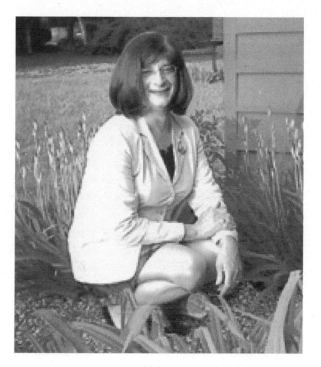

Melissa

two separate entities, its just a convenient way of distinguishing the dressed from the drab. Melissa will go here or do this and John will go there or do that. I find that many people have the idea that we (Melissa and John) exist separately, and react that way. Just another point that needs education. I'm just beyond the point of trying to explain to people that I'm still me when I have a dress on, so I just ignore the misconception, acting like I would normally and letting them figure it out for themselves.

(on getting caught) *The first time I was caught, I was about nineteen (1977). Actually, I wasn't caught dressed, my mother found stockings and heels in my room. I denied the accusations of homosexuality and chalked it all up to "curiosity" and let mom get rid of the things that I "had no use for". Dad made a comment or two about how "maybe we should get you some frilly underwear", which was, of course, embarrassing, demeaning, and laden with the suggestion of homosexuality. Total embarrassment?? You bet!! There was no "talk around town," or anything like that. What did I learn? I learned that I had to be more careful, that I had to hide things a whole lot better, and that what I was doing was supposed to be, well, bad. Funny thing about it is that years later, when my wife was searching for and find-*

ing things (in much the same way Mom did), I once again denied everything. Mostly because, at that time, denial was the only acceptable course, since she would not tolerate my dressing at all, and made that VERY clear. Once again, I learned to be more careful, and to hide better. Now, I put things away when my kids are here, but I refuse to hide.

Denise: *I was dating John and we went to an out of town Halloween party. John dressed as a prostitute and I as his pimp! We stayed overnight and it was that night that I got my first clue about his crossdressing. I was sick with some respiratory ailment and, therefore, not in my correct mind set (partly from medication and the other part due to partying.) So when John, undressing for bed and having removed the outer layers of his costume, stood before me only in his bustier, panties, stocking and garters and asked "what do you think?", I didn't quite know how to respond.*

Now you have to understand that I am a pretty kinky girl going WAY back, so I was not reeling from shock or anything but, rather, I was not really fazed. I think I remember saying that he looked "silly" in the bustier because he didn't have boobs but the rest looked very nice. I remember that I thought he had VERY good looking legs (WAY better than mine). So he came to bed still wearing the stockings. I liked the way the smoothness of the stockings felt and told John that I liked it.

It was from then on that "dressing" became part of our routine in the bedroom, but Melissa was not an entity as of yet . . . that would take years, our break up, his marriage and subsequent divorce to another (whom I have dubbed "the soulless harpy"), and our reuniting to help Melissa "be all she can be." I have helped, I hope, to coach and support Melissa's emergence. I totally accept Melissa, but do have just a few boundaries, which Mel tries to keep in mind. I have to be wary of being in public within the school district that I work. Mel got mad one night at a huge chain store when I practically pushed her into a rack of clothes to hide because I saw a coworker. Yes, I did apologize and we discussed it all afterwards. So Mel is getting to understand that I need to keep Mel in my private life when it comes to my career as a local teacher.

The other issue is that I prefer that John and Melissa remain separate entities. I knew John first and fell in love with him as "John." I have grown to love Mel as well, but I am not interested in the two personalities merging into one. I would rather that John remain John and not have any of Melissa's affectations like jewelry or share the same clothing items. I am not interested in seeing John on hormones or going for the full transition or anything like that, though I have to admit that sometimes I would like nothing better than for Mel to have real boobs at times . . . and so does she.

We are very happy together and I feel like I get to have two lovers for the price of one, so to speak. At holiday time I always remember to gift Melissa as well as for John. I LOVE to shop for her clothes and jewelry and surprise her with what I have found on sale every once in a while. We really do enjoy exchanging roles every now and again. Some days I get to be the girl and some days it's Melissa's turn and I can dig that!

One of the things that became apparent once I met other couples is that there are many different ways to come to terms with crossdressing in a heterosexual relationship. The wife or girlfriend's willingness to accept it may play a part, but it is not the whole story. She may be the type who would prefer to reject such "deviance," but other issues—like religion, or their commitment to a vow, or an understanding that their husbands in turn accept their own quirks—encourage a woman to find her way to acceptance. A wife who is willing to be accepting, however, can't ever become accepting if her crossdressing partner doesn't help her. She may be willing, but he has to find the way.

All of the crossdressers—who dress to varying degrees, are "out" in different ways—were all willing to let their partners figure out how to find acceptance for herself. The one quality they all share is that they trust their partner to figure out for herself what will or won't work for her, and then respect that response. John/Melissa might like to "merge" his personalities more, but he knows Denise doesn't like the idea, and so keeps his femme and male selves separate. All of them have made—and keep—similar commitments to their wives' happiness. Victoria, Jayne, Melissa, Ali, Amanda, and Heather all express deep respect for their wives and mention often how lucky they are to have found any kind of tolerance or acceptance from their partners. They know full well that the odds are against them finding romantic happiness as crossdressers, and when their partners showed any ability to tolerate or accept their behavior, they valued it, and told their wives as much.

One of the things I have found in my own marriage—and not just when it comes to crossdressing—is that taking anything for granted is the first mistake. The other wives and girlfriends—Minna, Gidget, Denise, Sue, Meredith, and Kathy—seem to share that view. We all value the men in our lives, and have found ways to look upon their crossdressing with compassion and respect.

What becomes apparent when talking to these couples is that it's the active participation of both partners that enables them to embrace the husband's crossdressing. Even when the woman is only participating by going to therapy, she is at least acknowledging that his crossdressing is part of their lives, and isn't pretending otherwise. The desire to control the husband's crossdressing causes too much friction between the husband and wife, and if you read these stories carefully, you'll read between the lines that there is not one wife who is trying to control her husband's behavior, and no husband who is trying to control his wife's. Ultimately, the ability to accept a spouse as he or she comes may be the key to crossdressing, as it is with so many issues that come up in relationships.

CHAPTER 5

Slippery Slope?

I GET A kick out of crossdressers. When dressed they're like kids in a candy store: they're having fun. I read somewhere that crossdressers—and other transgendered men—have high IQs. I can't verify that, but I do believe it. I've had crossdressers explain water filtration, telephone communications and computer networks to me. Maybe it's the surprise I enjoy, that under the dress I don't know what kind of person I'm going to find. Some cross-dressers are boring or needy or judgmental, but if you find a crossdresser who can tell a story, you are in for a good tale.

I was a fag hag in my late teens and early 20s. I know the term isn't con-sidered "correct" but the basic gist is that I had a lot of friends who were gay men. I'm a bit of tomboy and a straight woman so I like men and boys instinctually. I think my attraction to gay men as friends is similar to my abil-ity to relate to crossdressers. I feel at odds with my femininity so I can under-stand a man being at odds with his masculinity. I meet crossdressers on the bridge between genders. They get my gender issues in a way most men do not, just as gay men do. Crossdressers—like gay men—have been through a personal trial and have asked difficult questions of themselves. If their lives have been difficult because of their identity, they've usually got the sense of humor to prove it. I admire the courage of people who have to define and respect themselves in a culture that doesn't like them. In a nutshell, I like people who have come up against adversity and won, and who have come away with a surer sense of who they are. They have a special light in their eyes—an inner knowledge that is well-earned. People who know themselves are easier for me to be around. Socrates believed the unexamined life is not worth living, and I agree. Most are never forced to do that examining, but out crossdressers have no choice in the matter.

I can accept the idea that men want to dress as women and want to express their femininity. Their desire to do so doesn't make them any less men in my opinion, just as I don't think of my soccer-playing nieces as masculine because they like to be rough-and-tumble sometimes. For the most part I have found crossdressers to be decent guys who love their wives and Sunday afternoon football. (And when they're jerks they're the same kinds of jerks non-CD men are: selfish, sexist, insensitive, etc.) However, I am often still dismayed that my own husband is a crossdresser. He's the man I love most in the world, and my best friend, but sometimes I can't get to a basic level of acceptance with him that I can manage with perfect strangers. One of the reasons I still find life with a crossdresser frustrating is because there are lingering questions, the biggest of which is whether or not cross-dressing is just a stepping stone to transsexualism.

DOES HE WANT TO BE A WOMAN?

ONE NIGHT I was up late doing research online when I found a Frequently Asked Questions list about crossdressing by a crossdresser named "Diane." I read it, and I was impressed. The FAQ was from 1997. I found Part II of the same FAQ from a year later and read that. A third part was posted the next year. I began to wonder what happened after 1999, and tried to find Diane's homepage in order to locate an index.

While Diane's homepage was loading, I switched to another window and found a different crossdresser's FAQ and started reading the questions: *1) what is crossdressing?, 2) why do people crossdress?, 3) isn't crossdressing a sexual perversion?* I stopped to read the answer. *No, crossdressing isn't a sexual perversion*, the crossdresser argues, *it's about gender.* There's that old half-truth. I proceeded to question 4): *isn't crossdressing just a step to sexual reassignment?* In this case the answer was not just *No*, but a RESOUNDING NO. I skimmed the long paragraph and saw words like "gender" and "transsexuals" and "surgical alterations" and "trapped in the wrong body," in quotes. I made a mental note to read the full answer carefully, but in the meantime went back to see if Diane's homepage had finished loading. It had. The first thing I saw as a photo of Diane herself, in a wedding dress, getting married to a man in 2002.

I didn't have to read the other crossdresser's answer to question #4. I knew, from looking at Diane on her wedding day, fully female, that the correct answer is: sometimes. Anyone who says otherwise is full of it. Charles Anders, in *The Lazy Crossdresser*, relays a "common joke" in the transsexual community: "What's the difference between a cross-dresser and a transsexual?"

The answer? "Two years." He points out that the punch line can be variable. Sometimes it's "one year."

For the wife of a crossdresser this is terrifying news. It's terrifying because even though it only happens sometimes, it does happen. Diane explains:

> *I have been denying my inner self for my entire life, not just the last few years. It's only been in the past few years though that I finally had the courage to face my true self. I am a female and always have been. That has not been easy for me to accept and I feel most can understand why I would not want to the face that truth. Still, no matter how hard it was to confront or how much I denied it, I could not change the facts and trying to do so only made me miserable. When I finally faced the facts and moved forward, my life improved dramatically.*

The newly-married Diane is not the only crossdresser who ever transitioned. One of the couples I interviewed for this book were once "just a crossdresser and his wife." Luke told his girlfriend Katie when they were dating that he sometimes liked to wear women's clothes. Barely three years after getting married, the former "crossdresser" is taking hormones and saving money for various reassignment surgeries.

Katie was the first genetic woman partner of a crossdresser I met online who became a friend. She and I had similar backgrounds and similar attitudes, and we spoke each other's language. We both had weight issues, lived in big cities and grew up working-class. We'd both taken courses in Women's Studies. We saw the world—and crossdressing—through a similar lens. We bounced ideas, fears, and decisions off each other for several years, first by email and then over the phone. Before other friends knew about my husband's crossdressing, she was the only one I could talk to and not feel like I was speaking Greek. In a nutshell, Katie was something like my sister in crossdressing, and we were regularly amazed at the similarity of our lives and our thoughts. Women know how important it is to have a good girl friend. You know that your friend will understand that when you say your boyfriend is a pain in the butt, you still mean you love him. You know too that your friend will know, implicitly, that you are calling her to let off steam—not to hear that you should leave the jerk.

Katie and Luke were married a few months after Betty and I got engaged. We were invited to their "appreciation ceremony" in which Luke was to be the bride. We liked them, and discovered similarities in other aspects of our lives. The four of us talked on the phone together, commiserated about the cost of living, and felt we had forged a friendship within which we could all be fully ourselves. We regretted living on opposite coasts.

I began over time to realize that Luke was tearing out of the closet full speed ahead. Katie supported her husband in his choices, not because she was a fool or a pushover, but because she believed deeply that a relationship based on control is not a relationship worth having. She wanted to be with someone who was fully himself, and if that meant he wanted to go to work crossdressed, she would support him in it. She received the same love and support from him in return. Luke was the best thing that ever happened to her, as she was to him.

I felt challenged by their relationship to be more accepting in mine. While they planned two wedding ceremonies so they could take turns being the bride, and invited all of their friends and family to both ceremonies, my fiancé was in the closet because we'd fought so much about his crossdressing. We were planning only one wedding, and neither set of our parents knew he was a crossdresser. The strides Katie and Luke made in integrating his crossdressing into their relationship always made us both feel a little less competent and accepting. (Telling myself now that it's stupid to compare your relationship to someone else's is useless, hindsight.)

When Betty heard Luke's stories about going to work crossdressed, he wondered how and when he'd be able to do that, if ever. I felt pathetic for feeling like I needed more of a man in my life, especially during our engagement year. Every time we talked to Katie and Luke, Betty and I were left with a sense of "There but for the grace of God, go I." Betty aspired to Luke's level of self-acceptance, but the prospect scared him, too. I was horrified by it.

Luke became a bone of contention. Once Betty told me that he and Luke were talking about hormones in their private email correspondence. I flipped out so completely I had to ask my husband to stop writing to the only other crossdresser with whom he had ever corresponded. In light of the fact that I had encouraged him to talk to another crossdresser in the first place, my reaction seemed especially unfair.

There were periods where Luke and I corresponded more frequently than Katie and I did. I got their mutual news from him instead of her. He would email me reports and it would take days for me to realize I was picking fights with Betty as a result of them. Luke's "crossdressing career" terrified me. I wasn't entirely sure yet that I could live with a crossdresser. I didn't understand how deep my husband's gender conflict went, and we had far more issues than Luke and Katie ever did. I had a lot of fears, and Luke incidentally and accidentally roused them. I was not Katie. As much as I admired her, I was not able at that time to understand or acknowledge my need for control and my resentment at learning that I could only control things so much, for so long. As I saw it, they were already comfortably married and had the luxury of time to examine their gender issues. I was still a bundle of wedding-planning nerves.

I remember Luke telling me "she" had "her" driver's license picture changed to reflect "her" femme self. Luke had legally changed her name to Elle, too. I didn't get it. Why would a crossdresser want a femme I.D.? Katie explained that because Elle presented most of the time as a woman now, it was necessary.

Most of the time? Apparently I had missed a few updates.

Barely one year after their double wedding ceremony, Katie was faced with the prospect of having a woman as her partner.

Elle went on hormones about a year and a half after they'd gotten married. Less than six months after that, she decided she wanted full SRS. Sometime between starting hormones and deciding on surgery, Elle told her wife she was becoming sexually and emotionally interested in dating men. That's when Katie realized her marriage wasn't going to last. She and Elle had done everything they could to make it work. They were in therapy, both individually and together. They worked together and talked together and cried together. They were each the best thing in the other's life, fonts of encouragement and support and friendship and love.

As open-minded as she was, Katie didn't want a female partner. Regardless of her love for Elle, she was heterosexual and missed having a masculine presence in her life. She could deny her heterosexuality about as easily as Elle could forego transition. They were faced with the impossible situation of loving each other deeply, of having worked through all the issues that crossdressing had presented, of having learned to communicate and listen and love each other despite all odds, only to discover that their efforts would not save their relationship.

Katie is my friend. What does a woman do when her friend calls her with a broken heart and a shattered marriage?

A good girl friend blames it all on that asshole man. In this case, I blamed it all on that asshole woman.

It is so much easier to hate the transsexual woman than the genetic woman, isn't it? It's the transsexual woman who is destroying the marriage, right? The evil transsexual lures an unsuspecting woman into her trap and then BLAM, she breaks her heart. That's how it would be portrayed in the movies. But it's not the truth. Elle considered suicide before she could admit she was a woman. She would have done anything she possibly could to be with Katie. She would have tried to live life as a man for her. But Katie isn't the kind of woman who wants a self-repressed, depressed, unhappy person as a partner. She wants a whole partner, someone who is full of love and life and honesty. She could no more ask Elle to be a man for her than Elle could ask Katie to be a man for *her*. They are both women, and straight. They are star-crossed lovers: in love yet unable to be together.

I don't hate or blame Elle anymore. I have too much respect for my friend Katie to do that. I can wish with them that it weren't so, but it is.

Elle has written to me about her electrolysis, her hormones, her planned surgeries. She will suffer a great deal to make her body female. She told me in an email that "MOST of what I'm suffering now would not be necessary if laws allowed the interruption of adolescence with simple pills. We "transsexuals" always knew we wanted those pills as teens." I found myself angry all over again at reading those words. If she knew she was "transsexual" as a teen how could she have gotten married, as a man, to a woman who had already struggled just to accept his crossdressing?

Denial. From *The Columbia Encyclopedia*, Sixth Edition, 2001:

> *In psychology, an ego defense mechanism that operates unconsciously to resolve emotional conflict, and to allay anxiety by refusing to perceive the more unpleasant aspects of external reality. In the psychoanalytic theory of Sigmund Freud, denial is described as a primitive defense mechanism. Most people employ denial at some time in their lives when coping with stressful situations, such as the death of a loved one.*

Elle can look back now and say that she knew as a teenager she was a woman, but that's 20/20 hindsight. Denial, in the Freudian sense, is unconscious, and therefore unknown to the person experiencing it. Elle was not aware of her womanness. She might have had a niggling suspicion, but so do most crossdressers at some point in their lives. Many crossdressers have wondered about hormones or if they'd be happier living as women.

There was no one to blame for Katie's pain, but in my anger and fear that my husband, too, would transition, I blamed Elle. She was the one who had asked my husband when he would start hormones. She was the one who had made me wonder if my husband really was "just a crossdresser." She was the one who had shattered all the peace I had found. She was the first cross-dresser I had ever encountered who transitioned. All the other crossdressers had assured me that never happened.

It has taken the writing of this book for me to realize that Elle did not hurt Katie. Reality hurt them both. I have come to understand that I cannot blame the transitioning woman for "suppressing" her own reality. It is difficult enough to transition without being held responsible for your earlier self-denial. I cannot blame a person who did not know the truth for not making it known.

I do, however, blame the crossdressing community for failing to inform women of the reality that some crossdressers will discover they are transsexual women. It is one thing for an individual crossdresser coming out to his wife after decades of secrecy to assure her he is not transsexual. He will say anything to compensate for the trust he has betrayed. It is an entirely different matter for any crossdresser—as an individual, a representative of an organization, or a recognized figure in the CD community—to tell the girlfriend of a crossdresser not to worry about her husband ever transitioning. A woman must acknowledge the risks if she is to make a lifetime commitment. She cannot make it when no one is telling her the truth. The truth is that there are more than a handful of transitioned transsexual women who once thought of themselves as "just crossdressers," even if that handful is only a small percentage of all CDs.

I didn't know the truth when I became engaged. I still didn't know it a year later when I was married. I was reasonably well-informed about crossdressing; I had contacted support groups and done some research, and I had witnessed the depth of my husband's gender conflict. Nothing I read made me wonder if he might discover he was transsexual at a later date. The fact is, I asked. I read FAQs like the one detailed above. I, like Katie, was reassured continually, by websites and books, that crossdressers are not transsexuals.

Interestingly, while I searched as the wife of a crossdresser, I never came upon the truth: that there is a·possibility *that a crossdresser may eventually want to transition.* Once I started doing the research as a journalist, I did. Perhaps it was a blind eye on my part: the result of my own denial. Maybe the "journalist" title encouraged people to be more honest. It was extraordinary timing that Katie called me with the news about her breakup around the same time as I read *The Lazy Crossdresser* and came across Anders' "two years" joke. Katie tells me that no matter what she had known, she would have married Elle anyway. She wrote these words in the spring of 2003:

> My name is Katie, and I've been married to my partner Elle for about
> 2.5 yrs. When I met "Luke" in Charlottesville in June 1998, "he" confessed to me even before our first date that "I sometimes like to wear
> women's clothes." I had no idea what that meant, and I was a little

apprehensive, but I was already really excited to go out with this sweet,
funny person, so I went anyway.

I had no idea what I was getting myself into. I do not now wish I had
cancelled that first date, although I ask myself that question all the time.
What followed was the most sweet and intimate relationship of my life,
the first time I have felt truly known by another person. Elle and I really
understand each other, which is why throughout our whole relationship
it has been so painful to know there is this issue that gnaws away at us.

Three months after we started dating, "Luke" started crossdressing
more and more, dressing more frequently and more in public. I signed
up for several online support groups for "significant others of hetero-
sexual crossdressers", and I got educated with the terminology and the
issues. I embraced the idea of choosing my love over arbitrary social
rules. After we'd been dating for a year, Luke changed her name to Elle,
and started asking me and everyone else to call her that. By this time Elle
was crossdressing at work, and was out to many friends and family.
Before we got engaged, I asked Elle many times if she was a transsexual.
She promised she would not need to transition. We agreed on a 50/50
rule—a bargain. Elle could crossdress up to 50% of the time, I could
"have" Elle as a man half the time. Not my ideal, but the relationship I
had with Elle was more that I ever expected life with another person
could be. I felt like I could not walk away from it for such a trivial, arti-
ficial social construction as "clothing."

While engaged we were relocated to the West Coast by my job.
I was almost immediately laid off when the dot-com that relocated
us went under, so we lived on Elle's salary and my freelance until
the wedding.

In September 2000 we had two wedding ceremonies, one with Elle
as the bride, one traditional one where I wore the dress. The guest
lists for each were only slightly different. All our parents were at both
ceremonies. We had an amazing three-week honeymoon driving
around Italy.

When we went "home" to California in fall 2000, I got a job, but we
were both laid off within the year, and were to suffer more layoffs and
two unexpected moves to cheaper apartments over the next couple
years. The external stresses of our working lives only bonded us
together. Each time we packed up our books and dismantled yet another
set of IKEA shelving, we felt the only thing stable in our lives was our
marriage.

Throughout this time Elle was crossdressing more and more, usually exclusively for 3-4 months, and then hardly at all for weeks. The 50/50 rule was bending. Each time she stopped crossdressing, I secretly hoped she was getting bored of it. But I was well-read enough on the subject to know that was not likely. Each time she started crossdressing, we had to deal with all the reactions at whatever job she was at. We couldn't help but wonder if she got pushed higher on the layoff short list because she was an inconvenient employee. But then, everyone in Sili Valley is getting laid off, so it's hard to tell.

In fall 2001, after one year of marriage, Elle wrote in tiny writing on a scrap of paper "I am a transsexual woman" and showed it to me. That day she started calling herself a woman, and asked me and everyone else to do the same. I finally hit my limit, and scenes of tears and accusations followed. Finally Elle admitted to me she felt suicidal. We got ourselves into therapy.

Elle began living full-time as a woman. The following spring (2002) she started Hormone Replacement Therapy. One day when we were visiting the Castro in San Francisco, literally standing at the famous intersection of Market and Castro, holding hands, I realized that that tiny corner was the only spot on the planet I could feel comfortable being affectionate with my spouse in public, and even there we got curious glances. It was a cold realization.

We've now been in therapy for a year and a half, going to the same therapist both alone and together. Luckily we live in a great area for transgender resources, and we have a therapist well-versed on the issues. It's been hard. We have been trying to hold on to what we love about each other, without sacrificing our individual identities.

Last fall (2002), Elle and I sat on our couch and I invited her to list for me the surgeries she would like to get. At that point, I stopped fighting for the husband I'd thought I'd had at least a part of.

I've finally come to accept that Elle's womanhood is an intrinsic part of her, and she is not capable of denying it. I used to think if she loved me enough she would sacrifice that part of herself for me. I no longer want to ask her to sacrifice such a deep part of herself for anyone. And I realize that my own attraction to men, and my own heterosexuality, is an equally deep part of myself. And as much as I still love Elle, I can't sacrifice that for her.

It is a deeply lonely and painful thing to live on the fringes of society. And you have to be getting something very deeply affirming to your core *identity to make such a position feel bearable. Elle gets that personal affirmation, but all I feel is our cold spot on the edge. And I've realized I can't do it any more. Elle is going through her first adolescence as a female. She wants to date and explore. She wants to date men. I don't have the strength or will to hold her back.*

As of Thanksgiving, we realized we couldn't picture our marriage in the long-term. We made a plan to continue to live together for another year or two, as time to recover from the instability of the layoffs and moves. Since then we have been living as very cozy roommates. For a couple months it felt comfortable enough, but we are recently realizing we can't live like this much longer.

Last weekend Elle went away to visit a friend. Since we met we've rarely been apart for even a night, but I was surprised by how good it felt to have the apartment to myself. When Elle came back Sunday night we stayed up late crying together. We cry together often these days. We are both sad we can't find a way to make this work.

This week I am not wearing my wedding rings. I have told a few people that Elle will probably be moving out of our apartment soon. We don't know when, probably May or June.

All day long every day I am sad. And scared for the future . . . of being alone, and of how difficult it's going to be financially. And how much I'll miss Elle. But I'm also looking forward to feeling more independent. Transgenderism has been the central issue in my life for 4.5 years, and I'm looking forward to putting it down.

I still do truly love Elle, and I have been closer to her than any other person on the planet. I wish I knew a way we could stay together.

I am, as of this writing, still terrified. I have found other women like Katie, who encouraged and supported their husbands' crossdressing, only to find out they had married women. I am still a little angry at Elle no matter how much I wish I weren't and know I shouldn't be. I am still angry that the partnership that seemed to reflect our own most accurately is now over. I am also angry that my closest friend in the TG community is no longer a part of the TG community. Mostly, I am deeply jealous of Katie: she doesn't have to deal with this shit anymore, and I do.

For the record: crossdressers do occasionally realize they are transsexual women and will need to transition. They will want to get their bodies to look like their internal gender, to have a woman's body in every way they can. Most—though not all—use hormones. Some will seek surgery. The transition process is a difficult time in a transsexual woman's life, when she fully expects to be rejected by everyone she knows. Hormones can cause mood swings, hot flashes, and increased physical sensitivity, all of which are expected but not easy to adjust to. Transitioning is a painful process socially, physically, and emotionally. It is difficult for partners of transsexual women to watch the person they love suffer through electrolysis, worries about passing, family confrontations, job difficulties, and rejection. It is not easy, it is not fun, and it is not a choice. Transsexual women transition because once they have realized the truth about themselves, they must align their public life with their private person, and the best way to do that is for them to bring their bodies into alignment with their female hearts and womanly minds.

As hard as it might be for a crossdresser's wife to believe, there are "genetic women" who willingly enter relationships with transsexual women. Unlike Katie, Kathryn knew her husband Emily would transition from his male body to a female one. "He" was a crossdresser when they met (in an internet chat room for crossdressers), and Kathryn knew about her partner's transition plans before they had made a serious commitment. She says:

> *Before I made a decision as to whether to commit to this relationship, I was fully aware of her plans for hormonal therapy and her desire to live as a woman eventually . . . If I would have objected to the idea, I wouldn't have gotten involved. I am not concerned about SRS, she is adamant she doesn't want it. I have thought about her changing her mind, but I don't worry about it because I tend not to worry about "what ifs."*

Kathryn was in lesbian relationships in her 20s and thinks it is probably easier for bisexual women to be with transsexual partners, but goes on to explain that she doesn't feel like a lesbian in this relationship. She also understands the public might view her that way, but she feels only like herself and doesn't require a label for herself or her partner. She will call her transitioning husband her "wife," and remain a wife herself when Emily begins to live full-time as a woman.

THE TRANSGENDER SPECTRUM

ANYONE WHO HAS even dipped a foot into the transgendered community knows full well that the buzzword is "spectrum." "But considering the spectrum," one crossdresser might say to another, "I'm not putting my wife through that much," or "It was only when I fantasized about having breasts that I realized I was much further along the spectrum than I thought." The "spectrum" (or "continuum") is shorthand for the variation in the trans-gendered community, and encompasses the idea that the crossdresser and the transsexual are differing degrees of one type. The term *gender dysphoria* describes the experience of anyone whose sense of his or her own gender doesn't fit the category he or she was born in. That is, if a baby is born with a penis and insists on playing with dolls, is uncomfortable wearing a boy's clothes, and would prefer to be treated more the way his sister is, he is gen-der dysphoric. His sense of himself is feminine, not masculine. That said, gender dysphoria is only an issue when the difference between the person's internal sense of gender and his or her ability to live in his or her assigned gender role causes problems in the person's life. A man who is thoroughly comfortable with feeling feminine and relating to women is not gender dys-phoric, if he is comfortable not being "one of the guys" and if he is accepted by women as one of their own. Feminine gay men often fall into this cate-gory, and don't feel their feminine identity prevents them from living happy, fulfilling lives. Many may struggle with the issue, but it does not cause them to feel suicidal or present as female. They shop with female friends, gossip with the girls, and present in either a feminine or more gender-neutral way.

Transsexuals experience gender dysphoria in more deep and troubling ways. Evelyn, the author of *Mom, I Want to Be a Girl*, mentions that her youngest child never did very well in school, but that once her child, born a male, admitted to being a girl inside and began planning transition, her grades and study skills improved. This is a simple but basic way in which gender dyphoria can interfere in a person's life. Author Jennifer Finney Boylan, who was once James Boylan, says her gender dysphoria came from a sense that something was wrong. Every day she thought about gender, about her desire to be a girl, until one day she finally realized what she had to do and began to take steps toward transition. Her relief is felt simply by the absence of the question mark that haunted her all her life, and she said recently at a reading in New York City that the big difference now that she has transitioned is that she doesn't have to think about gender anymore.

It could be said, then, that those of us who don't think about whether we're male or female are not gender dysphoric, but that those who do, are. The tomboy who doesn't think there is anything wrong with her boyish behavior and who is encouraged to be the way she is will probably not expe-rience gender dysphoria. The gay man I mentioned above isn't, either. Whether or not a person experiences gender dysphoria may depend greatly on their own upbringing, their own sense of gender roles, and the kind of acceptance or rejection they experience from others.

I tend to think of gender dysphoria as existing on a grid that is defined by two axis lines: one line of *frequency*, the other of *intensity*. That is, the line of frequency would express how often a person thinks of his or her gender, whether or not he or she thinks of it regularly, all the time. Such a person could be described as thinking of gender *chronically*. If the person thinks about gender at different times in their lives, surrounded by times when they don't think of it much, or at all, they could be said to think about gender *episodically*.

The other axis, of intensity, describes the intensity of the person's feelings. If the person's thoughts about their gender dysphoria cause them to consider suicide if they can't fix it, they experience gender dyphoria at a *high intensity*. Someone who daydreams about being the other gender might be considered someone who experiences their gender dysphoria at a *low intensity*.

A person born male who thinks about gender every single day, and often wonders if he would rather be dead than not accepted socially as a woman would be someone who experiences gender dysphoria as chronic, with high intensity. Another person born male who fantasizes about being a woman in the spring, when women start wearing pretty spring dresses, but who never actually buys one of those dresses, would be a person who is gender dysphoric episodically, and with low intensity. These two people are the two extremes of those who experience gender dysphoria, and everyone else falls in between. The first type, who experiences gender dysphoria chronically and at a high intensity, would probably be transsexual, and for the sake of her life and happiness and ability to function, would probably begin to pursue transition. The other type might buy the dress and wear it, and so diminish the desire to be female in some way. That person might be a crossdresser.

The problems arise, of course, because there are an infinite number of possibilities in between these two examples.

Another distinction between gender dysphoric people might be the difference between whether or not the person feels he *is* female, or feminine, or simply *desires* to be. Transsexual women often admit that they had an internal sense that they were girls all during childhood, adolescence, and adulthood—that something wasn't right. On the other hand, the crossdresser might instead have a deep desire to be a girl, but with little sense of himself as actually female. In other words, the self-identity of the transsexual is already female, and she pursues transition in order to make her body and appearance suit the gender that is already present in her head and heart. The crossdresser, on the other hand, may need to express his desire to be a female by crossdressing, but still needs to learn how to be feminine, and remind himself not to think and act in masculine ways.

The way I'm describing it here makes it all seem simple, but that's for the purposes of explanation, only. The reality is, a transsexual woman who does not transition until later in life has spent many decades learning how to live as a man, and may not present as a woman simply as a result of hormones or surgery. It may take some time for her internal sense of femaleness to become apparent after a lifetime of repressing thoughts and feelings that were pushed aside in order to "fit in." No matter how much the transsexual woman has learned to convince others she is a man, internally she is often aware of being female. Likewise, there are crossdressers who express a natural femininity, and can feel fully female when crossdressed, and then revert reasonably easily back to their male selves. They can "put on" their femininity when they put on their dresses, makeup, and wigs, and yet, even so dressed, are fully cognizant of actually being male.

It is because there are so many people who do not fit *exactly* into a type that the concept of a TG spectrum has gained in popularity. However, if we take a look at the history of transgendered science, especially in the field of psychology, we'll find that the idea of transsexual people and crossdressers having something in common is both an old and a new idea.

A HISTORY OF TRANSGENDERED SCIENCE

ONE OF THE things that science does—even the soft sciences, such as psychology—is attempt to classify and categorize. The necessity of defining a phenomenon by drawing parameters around it is part and parcel of the scientific process. New experiments, theories, and evidence are meant to enlarge and change our definitions of the world we live in and how it works. There is theoretical science which posits certain ideas and waits for time and other scientists to prove or disprove a theory. There is empirical science which tries to find evidence that proves or disproves the theory. There is applied science which uses the theory and evidence in order to classify and improve the world as we know it. All three are useful and valid areas of scientific enquiry, and all three are practiced within the field of psychology.

Historically speaking, we tend to have revolutions in science just as we have revolutions in government: someone posits a drastically different theory, counter to the current universally accepted idea, and then the empiricists try to prove or disprove the new theory. (For a remarkable study of how scientific theories are accepted and rejected, read Thomas S. Kuhn's *The Structure of Scientific Revolutions*. It is still the standard text on the subject.)

In the transgendered world, these revolutions have been taking place since Magnus Hirschfield first interviewed his seventeen case studies, who were predominantly males who dressed as women and expressed a desire to be female in some way. The first thing Hirschfield did was eliminate the possibility that these seventeen people fell into any categories that already existed, and one by one, he demonstrated how their behaviors and feelings did not make them classifiable as 1) fetishists, 2) masochists, or 3) homosexual. After that, he knew they needed a new category altogether, and so coined the term "transvestite" (*Trans-* = across, or crossing, and -*vestite* = clothes, or dressing) to describe them, because their one commonality was that they wore women's clothes. Many of them admitted that they became sexually aroused by crossdressing, and so he defined a "transvestite" as a male who is motivated to dress in women's clothes for sexual pleasure. Interestingly, however, his peer and friend Havelock Ellis, also a psychologist, criticized Hirschfield's choice on the grounds that the term emphasized the clothes over the gender issues of the men in question. Ellis' disagreement with Hirschfield's terminology indicated that both men saw transvestites as dressing not only for sexual pleasure but also out of their own sense of gender dypshoria. Ellis suggested and tried to promote the use of the term Eonist instead, after the Chevalier D'Eon, who wore women's clothes, enjoyed sex with women, and retained his primary identity as a male despite long periods during which he presented as a woman (usually to avoid political scandals, as apparently Eon was interested in women who were a little too young.) Eonist, however, never caught on. Ellis' criticism, however, points out that transvestites always had gendered feelings associated with their crossdressing, and the idea that they didn't is a common misunderstanding. Even if Hirschfield failed to highlight that aspect in his choice of terminology, it is clear from his case studies that a number of his subjects, including those who had a history of sexual arousal from crossdressing also had female gender identities from an early age: sexual arousal and gender dypshoria weren't exclusive then, as they don't seem to be now.

His study of the people he called transvestites was, in a certain sense, the first recognition of the transgender spectrum. The men (and one woman) he studied experienced high and low intensity feelings of gender dysphoria, chronic or episodic periods of anguish over their gender, and a few didn't experience sexual arousal as a result of their crossdressing at all. These last few also expressed a more urgent need to be able to live as women. Hirschfield identified this subgroup as "asexual transvestites" whose strong desire to dress and live as women was not sexually motivated.

That he differentiated them from the larger group was essential, because it enabled a later researcher—Harry Benjamin—to continue studying them. Benjamin eventually labeled Hirschfield's subgroup "transsexual." (Benjamin didn't coin the term but did popularize it.) The transsexual case studies were separated from the larger group of transvestites precisely because they were not sexually aroused by their desire to be women. It is important to note here that their lack of sexual arousal as a result of cross-dressing was what caused him to differentiate them from the larger group of transvestites *in the first place,* so it stands to reason that the historic definition of a transsexual came to be that "he" did not experience sexual arousal as a result of "his" gendered feelings.

Hirschfield did his research at a time when surgical and hormonal alterations to the body were not a possibility. Crossdressing as a woman and so passing as female was the only way a transsexual at that time could live as a woman, and Hirschfield, empathetic scientist that he was, often went to the police station with individuals who were miserable living as the wrong gender. He helped them acquire identity cards which indicated their gender as their *chosen* gender, not their anatomical sex, and so, in a sense, helped transsexuals avoid legal entanglements they might have otherwise experienced for "disguising themselves," which—the same as now—caused police some concern for fear the disguise was being utilized to avoid detection of criminal intent or escape from punishment. In a nutshell, he legalized transsexualism for a few individuals, long before there was even a word for it, much less a political identity.

As a result of Hirchfield's and then Benjamin's work, two historic classifications of males who want to dress as women were identified: 1) The transvestite, who wants to dress as a woman because of transgender feelings but for whom dressing creates sexual arousal; and 2) the transsexual, who wants to be a woman, including dress as one, but who does so only because of deeply transgendered feelings with no pattern of sexual arousal as a result of crossdressing.

Benjamin not only helped clarify and define Hirshfield's subgroup of "asexual transvestites" but codified their diagnosis and treatment in what are now called the HBIGDA (Harry Benjamin International Gender Dysphoria Association) Standards of Care. He could recommend that the transsexual person find treatment for his or her gender dysphoria, as medical (surgical and hormonal) options became available in the time between Hirschfield (1910) and Benjamin (1950s and on). In order that a transvestite not mistake his experience as transsexual, Benjamin recommended that anyone pursuing Sexual Reassignment Surgery follow a few guidelines in order to help keep some men from making an irreversible mistake. He also educated other psychologists and the general public about transsexualism, oversaw the major studies of transsexualism for decades, started the IGDA, and promoted the empathetic treatment of transsexual women, especially by emphasizing that their need to transition was not born from a history of eroticized crossdressing. The definition of what transsexualism is seemed clarified and codified as a result of Benjamin's work.

Along comes Virginia Prince, founder of Tri-Ess, who asserts that transvestites are not turned on by dressing in women's clothes. Still Charles at the time, Prince identified as a transvestite, and being one, testified that his own crossdressing was a deep need to express an internal feminine, and was not done for the sake of sexual arousal. Prince thus invalidated the historic definition of "transvestite." Perhaps because Hirschfield's work still stood as the cornerstone, and still seemed to apply to a certain subset of males who crossdressed, Prince coined a new and specific definition for the term "crossdresser" and created a subgroup of males who dress to express their feminine gender identity but who do not wish to live as women (ie, who are not transsexual) but who also do not dress as women for sexual pleasure (ie, not transvestites). The term "crossdresser" never appears in the "deviance" categories set up by the psychological community, but instead, on Prince's insistence, a modified version of "tranvestite" appears in the form of "fetishistic transvestite." This last term describes the crossdresser who not only dresses for sexual arousal, but whose life is disrupted by his desire to crossdress. Neither does the term "transvestite" appear, but the "fetishistic" or deviant tag attaches itself somewhat permanently to "transvestite" in the more general culture, regardless of Prince's efforts.

Because of Prince's explanations of himself and the distinctions he made to both Hirchfield's and Benjamin's work, the psychological community had at that point come to accept three categories of males who dress in women's clothes: the transvestite, the transsexual, and the crossdresser.

Along comes Ray Blanchard, who introduces an entirely new concept to the field of transsexual studies: autogynephilia. Blanchard posits that the autogynephilic, born a male, has a deep desire to be a woman, and to have a woman's body, and that the desire is born from a sexual urge. Quite a few crossdressers—including my husband—have read descriptions of autogynephilia and recognized themselves in it. Some transitioned transsexual women, such as Anne Lawrence, have done the same. Autogynephilia introduces the idea that the transsexual woman can successfully receive treatment despite sexual arousal and/or a history of erotic self-feminization, and that transsexual women who are autogynephilic are no less "legitimate" than their solely gender-driven sisters. Blanchard's concept provides an enlargement, or caveat, upon Benjamin's accepted definition of the symptoms of transsexuals and their treatment. For many transsexual women, autogy-nephilia allows them to admit, finally, that sexual arousal does accompany their gender dypshoria, but that sexual arousal doesn't negate their need to transition.

The definition of "transsexual," so carefully delineated by Benjamin, seems invalidated as a result, because the historic definition no longer describes *all* transsexuals. Blanchard undoes the differentiation Benjamin worked hard to achieve. As a result of Blanchard's work we've got four categories: transves-tites, crossdressers, transsexuals, and autogynephilic transsexuals.

However, autogynephilia is still in its infancy as a concept, and history has not yet proven that it is a valid theory, which brings us to the contro-versy that has been creating havoc in the TG community. Some transsexuals insist that autogynephilia does not exist. Others find the concept liberating, and frees them from the shame of lying about their sexual arousal in order to begin transition.

In other words, we're watching a scientific revolution in the making, and whether or not autogynephilia succeeds in becoming an accepted concept in transgender studies and diagnoses depends greatly on whether or not Blanchard's theoretical idea is defended sufficiently with empirical data.

AUTOGYNEPHILIA AND
THE MAN WHO WOULD BE QUEEN

THE TROUBLE ARISES from a book called *The Man Who Would Be Queen* by Michael Bailey which was published in the spring of 2003. Bailey discusses, in a very broad way, how femininity manifests in gay males and MTF transsexual people. He insists that there are only two types of trans-sexuals. 1) The homosexual or androphilic variety is a person who is born with a male body but is innately feminine and desires sex with men. The androphilic transsexual self-identifies as a heterosexual woman and so opts for transition in order to have sex with men as a woman. Bailey's second group are 2) the autogynephilic transsexuals, who transition out of a deep sexual need to have a female body and are aroused by that female body—or, before transition, are aroused by the idea of having a female body. In his opinion, there is no other possible reason a person born with a male body might transition and live as a woman with a woman's body. Both of his types are motivated to transition out of sexual urges—the first out of an urge to have sex with a man as a woman, and the second from the arousal they experience from having or imagining having a woman's body.

However, Bailey's detractors insist that plenty of people who are born with male bodies desire to transition because of an innate sense of their own femaleness. They have an innate gender identity that is in opposition to their physical body. Historically speaking, the definition of the transsexual group was determined by the fact that some people who dress or desire to be women are not motivated by sexual arousal linked to crossdressing or fantasies of female bodies at all. In fact, evidence of a history of sexual arousal linked to crossdressing could previously prohibit a transsexual woman (a person born in a male body with a female gender identity) from getting the "permission" she needed to transition. The emergence of autogynephilia legitimized transsexual transition for many people who otherwise had to lie about their sexual arousal patterns in their desire to transition. Autogynephilia's acceptance also helped de-stigmatize the sexual feelings of some transsexual women, and helped address the idea that there were equal but different motivations for transitioning. It opened up the idea that because transsexualism is still a phenomenon that is little understood, new advances and understandings could and would broaden its definition so that more people experiencing transgendered feelings could get the help they needed.

But Bailey claims that there are no cases where a person transitions solely because their innate gender identity is opposite their physical sex.

Why is Bailey painting with such a broad brush?

Hirschfeld and Benjamin sub-classified the original group—of males who dress as or want to be women—by their sexual patterns. On the one hand is a group composed of people who were born males and who experience sexual arousal along with their transgendered feelings—transvestites and autogynephilic transsexuals—and on the other is a group of people who were born males who don't experience sexual arousal as a result of crossdressing or other self-eroticized behaviors—transsexual women and crossdressers. The first group, you could argue, have transgendered feelings that are closely linked to sexual arousal. The second group are motivated only by their transgendered feelings. Both types are sexual, but in the first case the sexuality is associated with crossdressing and/or body modification, while the sexuality of the people in the second group focuses instead on making love with partners. Hirschfeld and Benjamin made sexual arousal one of their diagnostic criteria. Their way of distinguishing one subgroup of transgendered people from another has been accepted for several decades.

What Bailey posits in *The Man Who Would Be Queen* is that the second group I described does not exist. He is trying to find empirical evidence for Blanchard's theory. The problem is, he doesn't have much evidence, and he doesn't utilize a control group. He also doesn't seem to consider any evidence that counters Blanchard's theory. As a result, he entirely invalidates the second group's experiences, and insists that if they don't fit into his findings, they don't exist.

I'm reminded of Freud's famous quote that sometimes a cigar is just a cigar. That is, despite Freud's insistence on psychoanalytic truths, sometimes over-interpreting the "evidence" is uncalled for. In a dream a cigar may represent a penis, or it may just be a cigar. I'm also reminded that Hirschfield—who didn't have sophisticated DNA tests and brain-mapping evidence—managed to make an important classification in transgendered lives by listening to people's experiences. He didn't tell them they didn't experience what they experienced. He let them talk, he listened, and *then* he drew his conclusions.

Had Hirschfield done his science the way Bailey did his, we would have never separated transvestites from the massive group of "intermediaries" or "deviants" in the first place. His subgroup of "asexual transvestites" wouldn't have existed for Benjamin to study further, either. If Hirschfield had gone into his research with the idea that all transvestites were homosexual— which was the current prevailing belief—he would have never documented the many existing heterosexual transvestites. His enquiry was open-ended; he was not looking to prove anything except perhaps the existence of his subjects. He sought to validate their feelings and experiences. Bailey, on the other hand, is looking for proof of Blanchard's theory with such blinders on that he is straightjacketing feminine men back into 1950s stereotypes. All feminine men are not homosexual. All homosexual men are not feminine. All feminine men are not transvestites, or transsexuals, or crossdressers, or autogynephilic. All TG people are not motivated by sexual desire. *Sometimes a cigar is just a cigar.*

Up until now, the exact opposite of what Bailey is advancing was believed to be true: that transsexual women are not sexually motivated. Why does he assume the opposite is true when plenty of transsexual women have been saying for years that they are not androphilic and not autogynephilic? That, in fact, sexual arousal has nothing whatsoever to do with their need to transition? They are not self-deluded, or liars, or unaware of their "true" sexual orientation. They are people who know internally that they are female, and their sex drive—and sexual orientation—have little to do with it.

Bailey wants empirical evidence. Right now, the empirical evidence for the existence of transsexual women who are not sexually motivated is based only on their explanations of their experiences. A lack of chromosomal or genetic evidence doesn't mean they don't exist. The possibility that we just haven't found that evidence yet never seems to occur to Bailey, but in the meantime his disrespect toward transsexual women is inexcusable. Trying to prove that there is no sexual motivation is trying to prove a negative, and all that's needed to disprove it is a single erection. However, the erection may not have anything to do with the transgenderedness of the person at all, and the arousal in itself may not having anything whatsoever to do with what actually *causes* transsexuality (whether AG or non-AG), and certainly doesn't disprove the biological theory or prove the psychological theory. Bailey's "evidence" would only stand up in a trial that takes place in a Kafka novel.

My friend Willow, who transitioned a decade ago without the support of her family, is now happily married, and mother to her husband's daughter by a previous marriage. Otherwise she is the same person I knew when she had a male body, except a hell of a lot happier. Some of her family is still estranged, but Willow is a productive and responsible member of society. She so fully identifies as a woman ten years after transitioning that she gives money to organizations like Planned Parenthood and NOW. She is not trans-identified, but lives as a woman. She writes:

> *For me, something was there that shouldn't be. Somewhere, there was an error. I don't think I did it for sexual reasons at all. Hell, right now I am typing to you sitting slouched (a dreadful habit) in a chair wearing a t-shirt, jeans, wool socks, my hair in a ponytail, no makeup, and listening to Eddie Vedder and Pearl Jam sing "Rocking in the Free World." Certainly doesn't seem sexual in my view.*

She may be married to a man now, but her transition was not motivated by her desire to have sex with men. She never identified as a homosexual before she transitioned, and was not markedly effeminate. She does not fit into either of Bailey's categories.

I know a second transsexual woman named Judy who has experienced significant loss as a result of her transition. Estelle, a genetic woman, is her partner. Judy's wife is divorcing her, and although the marriage was in trouble long before she transitioned, it was the final straw. Judy is having a hard time finding a job because she is a woman in her 50s looking for work, and facing the same prejudice other women of her age experience. She is a deeply empathetic and incredibly intelligent person, and went out of her way to make extended family members more comfortable at a required gathering by writing them a letter about her transition beforehand. She had deep feelings about her transsexualism as early as age 30, but couldn't consider transitioning: she was convinced she couldn't do it, had no support system in place, and had two very young children. Seventeen years later, she saw *The*

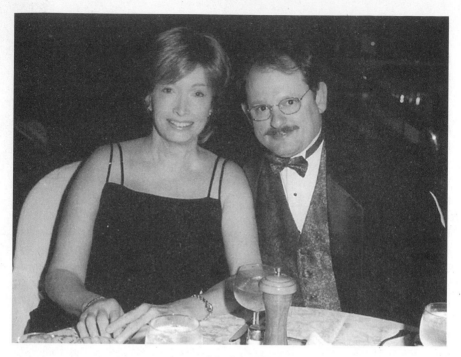

Lynn with husband, Charlie

Crying Game and after a sleepless night made up her mind to transition. Her two children will speak to her by phone but will not interact with her face to face. Her daughter is very angry, and her son actively avoids the issue. She hopes that will change, and has only recently decided that she will stop dressing as a man in order to see them. Her own siblings are supportive, at least. She does not fit into either of Bailey's two categories.

The third transitioned woman I have come to know—in the course of writing this book—is Lynn Conway, who took time to answer countless e-mails I sent her about every single aspect of transsexual women. She responded to every one in depth and with sympathy—sympathy for Katie, sympathy for Judy, and sympathy for me when I expressed concern about my husband's transsexual feelings. She has been, as the English say, an absolute brick. She does not fit into either of Bailey's two categories.

Donna, the fourth transsexual woman I met—also in the course of writing this book—has only recently taken her first step out the door as a woman, but still lives and works publicly as a man because of her ongoing financial and parental responsibilities. She has been taking hormones, going to a gender clinic and examining her options. She used to think perhaps she was simply a crossdresser, until her girlfriend helped her realize that, as she had long suspected, that was not the whole truth. She does not fit into either of Bailey's two categories.

Donna and Judy are both romantically involved with women, and transsexual women who are in lesbian relationships during or after transition do not appear anywhere in Bailey's research, perhaps because he found most of his subjects in gay bars, where it's unlikely anyone would meet a lesbian who was genetically born a woman or not. It could be argued, I suppose, that their lesbian relationships do not eliminate the possibility that they are autogynephilic, but what they tell me does. They are not autogynephilic. Even Donna, who once thought she was a crossdresser, understands that her need to transition came out of a deep sense, present from early childhood, of her own femaleness, not out of a sexual sense of wanting a female body. She says she used to take pictures of herself when she was a crossdresser, but stopped as soon as she began to take hormones and her gender dysphoria began to subside—long before the hormones had any actual physical effect on her libido. Now that she has breasts, what turns her on is her partner's touch. Not herself. Does Bailey think autogynephilia "goes away" once the transsexual transitions? Not according to his book. Does that mean Donna's experience is dismissable? Of course not.

Willow and Lynn Conway are both married to men but never, when their bodies were male, considered themselves homosexual. They are not homosexual now, because they are women who are romantically and sexually involved with men. In their minds, they were always women who desired men. Culturally they might have been seen as homosexual, but internally they knew their desire for men was part of their identity as heterosexual women. During her early twenties, Lynn struggled to fit in as a man, under the threat of being institutionalized, which was a very real possibility for a transsexual woman in the 1960s. The threat of it terrified her into hiding her innate femininity and her womanly sexual responses to men, and out of loneliness and a need for companionship she formed a relationship with a woman. Willow, on the other hand, always felt like a lesbian in her relationships with women, even though her body was male. Bailey would insist on classifying both Lynn and Willow as androphilic, as homosexual transsexuals, but neither of them were men who wanted to have sex with men. Both were women—who happened to have male bodies.

All of these women have expressed to me their deep sense—usually from a young age—that their bodies were wrong. They transitioned—all in different ways and at different times—because transitioning is the only way for a transsexual woman to make her body match her mind and soul. None of them are skittish about sex, and all of them are highly intelligent. Willow was disturbed that someone in one of her support groups—nearly a decade ago—referred to TS women by saying, "well basically we're all homosexuals really." She grew up in a liberal community, and was friendly with many gay men. Why on earth, as she puts it, would she go through all the surgeries and hormone therapy if her motivation was to have sex with men? She could have done that without all the fuss, and embraced a more likely chance of acceptance. For that matter, why would Donna or Judy face being branded lesbians by society if their homophobia is so deep it disables them from having sex with men? That just doesn't make any sense. If they were so severely homophobic, they would have chosen to be with men after transition, in order to avoid being labeled homosexual. Both are content knowing they are publicly identified as lesbians.

It is impossible, still, to say where arousal originates—no one really knows. It could be that the autogynephile's sexual desire for the body she feels she should have is only an expression of her gender dysphoria, and an intense one. Perhaps she is already transgendered and when imagining herself as a sexy woman is exactly like a (genetic) woman who is turned on by the idea of her body being perceived as attractive. Besides, is a transgendered person with a female gender identity who imagines herself as a sexy woman necessarily an autogynephile? Is she an autogynephile if she imagines this once? Ten times? A hundred times? Donna explains:

> No one would suggest that a genetic girl thinks she's a girl because of any sexual motivation; she thinks so because she is one. Isn't it just possible, especially if you accept the possible validity of the biological theory, that a child who's transgendered thinks "she's" a girl just because she really "is" one? And isn't it possible that someone (whether TG or CD) might be happy, and excited, and, yes, aroused at times, by the idea —and for some, ultimately, the reality—one's external form matches one's internal gender identity, without being defined by those feelings as an "autogynephile"(who's just a man interested in having female body parts so he can "play" with them, and for whom this is the "primary" motivation in transitioning)?It's a turn-off when you hate your body, and a turn-on when you imagine you don't. In other words, just because I used to think I was a crossdresser, and, because, yes, there was an erotic element to it, shouldn't necessarily brand me as an autogynephile.

The implication of Bailey's ideas are that many people will "learn" that transsexual women are motivated by their sexuality and nothing more. The response to autogynephilia by some members of the transgendered community doesn't help. Unfortunately they are susceptible to the influence of our puritanical culture the same as the rest of us, and so see the link between sexuality and transsexualism as affirming that they are perverts. Autogynephilia is not perverted: it is a deep sexual motivation, and as such, should be taken seriously.

The other depressing thing about the current autogynephilia debate is that I fear a useful and much-needed concept will be lost as a result. I think autogynephilia is a practical theory for describing the experiences of some transvestites and some transsexuals, and may provide a link that proves, once and for all, that there is in fact a spectrum. It is perhaps one manifestation of transgenderedness, or one "symptom" of it. Perhaps it is not necessarily causal, but symptomatic. The idea that it rules out a pre-existing state of transgenderedness in the individual is ridiculous. Who is to say that the autogynephilic person isn't turned on by the idea of having a woman's body exactly because they are transgendered in the first place? In the case of transvestites, autogynephilia is a useful tool toward understanding the sexual dysfunction many transvestites and crossdressers experience in their romantic relationships with women.

In the crossdressing community, the man who admits he is turned on by his dressing is still considered a pervert. The autogynephilic transsexual will not receive the same sympathy for her transsexualism as the non-autogynephilic transsexual. That's exactly what makes Bailey's book so dangerous: it allows transsexual women to be condemned by our society for having "perverse" sexual arousal patterns.

That some therapists and doctors would consider the autogynephilic's need for transition "less than" any other transsexual's need—exactly because it is sexually motivated—is sad. I understand that there is some need to try to classify transsexuals in order to prevent the wrong people from going through transition, which can result in devastating sadness. But surely doing so shouldn't entail de-legitimizing the experiences of transsexuals who have transitioned and found a great deal more peace. The existence of autogynephilic transsexuals does not disprove the existence of gender-motivated transsexuals. Bailey says it does, and that is where he goes wrong. He also fails to prove that these two motivations—autogynephilia and innate gender identity—can't coexist in the same person.

Despite Bailey's bad science, it may turn out that autogynphelia is a legitimate descriptor of some transgendered experience. If it is—and I do think it is, but not anything near the way Bailey applies it—we are left, in 2004, with Hirchfield's initial case studies. We know his group of seventeen people crossdressed as women: some did so in order to relieve the anxiety caused by gender dysphoria, some just for sexual pleasure, some for both reasons. Some wished to be women 100% of the time, some thought of it chronically, tortured with feeling of being in the wrong body and living the wrong life, and others managed to assuage their anxiety by crossdressing. At the turn of the century, when Hirschfield was doing his work, surgery was not yet a possibility and so, in some sense, the distinctions to be made between these groups not as essential as it may be now. A person born male now has to be very certain of transsexual feelings before getting the radical surgeries and hormonal treatments that will change his life into hers, and it is now—when these surgeries are available—that these categories have failed, coalescing into what is popularly referred to as the TG spectrum.

We are beginning at the beginning, as it were, but at a time when there is more to be undone than the box checked on an identity card.

COMPLICATIONS AND IMPLICATIONS OF THE TG SPECTRUM FOR THE CROSSDRESSER

FOR SOME CROSSDRESSERS' wives, nightmares become reality.

Most crossdressers—by their own admission and insistence—are straight. Many of them are married. The majority of crossdressers, then, have a vested interest in not disclosing the implications of "the spectrum" so as not to freak out wives or potential wives. As it is, many crossdressers do not tell their wives they are crossdressers because they are terrified of rejection, so how on earth can they be expected to tell their wives they may one day find they are transsexual, too? An older crossdresser knows that his wife's two biggest fears will be that he is either gay or will want to be a woman, and he wants to reassure her in every way he can, especially if he has kept his crossdressing a secret for many years.

A younger crossdresser is in a slightly different predicament. In his 20s, he may still think getting married will "cure" his crossdressing, that it is only a sexual fetish. He may know he gets an erection when he puts on a pair of stockings, but not much else. He may have no awareness of his "gender issues." He is not in denial, but is rather ignorant and unwilling to examine the meaning of his crossdressing. He does not know himself that he might be transsexual, so how could he possibly warn someone else?

When today's younger crossdresser meets a woman he loves, he is more likely to tell her he is a crossdresser. My husband told me within the first three weeks we were dating. More and more wives are marrying cross-dressers who tell them long before there is a significant commitment, and those women have an easier time accepting the crossdressing. In fact, they have happier marriages than wives who were not told at the outset. But would these same informed, accepting partners be as willing to marry a crossdresser even if there were only a 1out of 100 chance of him actually being transsexual? If it was 1out of 10? Crossdressers who find supportive or accepting partners have already won the lottery, and they're not fool enough to risk losing it by mentioning an abstract possibility, which is what transsexualism is for most crossdressers in their 20s.

Would an accepting wife withdraw her support if she thought it might lead to her husband's discovery of his transsexualism? Lynn Conway transitioned decades ago, and has seen the patterns of emergence by younger generations of TS women. She explains:

> It's mostly a function of when the transsexual girl gets up the nerve to reach out and try to transition. If she begins transitional efforts in her teens or early twenties, she is unlikely to marry a woman while still a "man." If in her mid-twenties, it's maybe 50-50. If in her late thirties and beyond, even more are married to women. Many pretransition TS women feel profound needs for closeness and companionship, even when all bottled-up by testosterone, and they're easily socially channeled into marrying women. As times are changing, more TS girls are learning that they can find men to love them if they start on transitional efforts early in life. This trend, along with growing recognition that marriage as a man is often a tragic mistake, will likely reduce the numbers who marry women in the future—especially as more TS girls get help at earlier and earlier ages
>
> However, there is a large cohort of TS people who are in the pipeline now who will have to face transition, but who are married now. It's a sad situation for all involved because only about 10% or so of those marriages will survive their transitions.

Katie admits that it was Luke's "profound needs for closeness and companionship" that made him such an attractive partner in the first place. She had found a best friend who was also her lover and husband—every woman's dream. Should she have realized it was too good to be true? Hardly.

The reality is it's probably closer to one in a million crossdressers who realize they're transsexual. Most crossdressers' wives shouldn't worry about their husbands ever wanting to transition, because most of them won't. It's more likely that a woman whose husband has never crossdressed would realize he needs to transition, because his feelings are so deeply repressed he has never even crossdressed. There is no evidence that a woman's support of her husband's crossdressing encourages latent transsexualism. There is also no evidence that her withholding of support can prevent a latent transsexual from self-realization. The one thing that seems to be clear is that a TS woman will realize her innate woman-ness whether she's supported or not. An old friend of mine, Willow, transitioned a decade ago despite hostility on the part of her family. They actively campaigned against her transition by writing letters to her surgeon begging "him" not to go through with it. Her girlfriend at the time left her when she found out Willow was going to transition. In addition, Willow disagreed with a lot of what she heard in TS support groups at the time. She proceeded with her transition anyway. She has been living happily as a woman for a decade regardless of the lack of support from her loved ones.

Certainly the Internet has helped crossdressers educate themselves at a younger age, but the popular mythology is still that crossdressing is only a fetish. It is not only a fetish. Sometimes it is not *even* a fetish, as many crossdressers are not sexually aroused by their crossdressing. If it is not a fetish, what is it? The only answer that makes sense to me is that crossdressers are mildly gender dysphoric. They are on the transgendered spectrum. They do, at some moments in their lives, wonder how life might have been had they been born women. They wonder if hormones and surgery would end their confusion and sadness. (Sometimes they wonder if suicide will, too.) They wonder, in a nutshell, if they are transsexual. Dr. Richard Docter recently gave a seminar on "Crossdressers Coping with Transsexual Feelings" at the 2003 IFGE (International Foundation for Gender Education) Conference. Surely he would not have felt compelled to give such a lecture if there wasn't an audience for it.

The idea that crossdressers and transsexuals experience the same phenomenon but to differing degrees makes life very complicated. The easy (and sometimes illegal) availability of hormones via the internet has prompted some crossdressers to experiment with breast enlargement. They no longer have to visit a gender clinic, even if they should. Because of the proliferation of internet chat rooms and organizations, transsexual people are starting to talk to crossdressers, and vice versa. The crossdresser learns how soft his skin could be if he took hormones, what dosage might encourage breast development, and that Viagra might offset the impact of female hormones on his ability to get an erection. He also learns that his transsexual sisters get taken more seriously than he does.

The TG community, however, is starting to come clean about these issues. In a recent copy of *Girl Talk* magazine, Brianna Austin confesses in a column titled "Truth or Dare" that she was "one of the idiots" who experimented with taking hormones even though she wasn't committed to transitioning, and had not been diagnosed as transsexual. She reiterates the reasoning behind the HBIGDA Standards of Care, noting their stringency but also their intention. Austin also quotes TG musican Lisa Jackson who added, "Taking hormones for the benefit of easier girl maintenance is as absurd as taking heroin to relax." Jane Ellen Fairfax of Tri-Ess, who as his male self is a licensed medical doctor, made a compelling argument against the use of hormones by crossdressers at a recent SPICE conference by delineating the massive health risks the dosages required for feminization of the body can incur: breast cancer (especially if there is any genetic predisposition), risk of liver failure, impotency, stroke, and other risks of high blood pressure, like heart attack. He emphasized, overall, that taking hormones is by no means anything a person should experiment with, and that anyone taking them should be doing so under a doctor's care with twice yearly tests for liver damage and heart disease. He was also very clear that for transsexual people, these risks are necessary to take for their survival and mental health, but for the crossdresser or for the transgendered person with no intention of transitioning, it's reckless and too risky. To boot, he pointed out that the only long-term studies done on hormones are ones involving women taking them as HRT (Hormone Replacement Therapy) for the symptoms of menopause, and those studies too are proving the risks far outweigh the benefits, and should only be used when a woman is experiencing symptoms which greatly disrupt her life or health. Hormone use can also produce permanent body modification that can result, as Fairfax put it, in the person becoming "neither fish nor fowl," meaning that one's body may end up inbetween genders—an unacceptable outcome for the average crossdresser.

The problem is that a lot of crossdressers do have deeply transgendered feelings, and don't know whether or not they are transsexual. A gender therapist should help any individual with such questions, and permanent body alteration should wait until the person is sure transition is their path. This confusion is especially present in younger people, and many are more at risk in making bad decisions as a result of illegal access to these hormones via the Internet. Hormones, in addition, will not help a person figure out whether or not they are transsexual. Tarren, a friend of Brianna Austin's who she quotes, explains: "If you can live a productive life as a man, then you should remain a crossdresser and call it a day . . ." Her comment implies some kind of choice for those whose transgendered feelings are not chronic *and* high intensity, as hers were. She concludes, "If I did have a choice, I would never have never chosen this."

Gidget shares a few thoughts about the TG spectrum that I have seen expressed elsewhere, and more and more frequently:

> *They are looking for answers, and some of them aren't yet sure if they are TG, CD or TS—and they may leap across boundaries for years— some of these people go into TS, and then regret it—and some CDs are unhappy all of their lives as they don't have the gumption to go into being a TS.*
>
> *I started also to realize that maybe we have separated the men into these compartments, but maybe that isn't the way it is—that is, they may all be on the road to TS and, perhaps, the CDers are really TS—but they are frightened off by society's standards, and don't want to lose their wives or their jobs or their families—could this be it??*

I can't answer her question. Perhaps many crossdressers have feelings that are transsexual, but they hold off on transition simply because they realize that the health risks do not outweigh the benefits. Others would like to transition via surgery and hormone use, but pre-existing medical conditions may prevent that. In neither case is the person "frightened by society's standards" but is instead making a rational, informed decision about his life.

WHAT WE DON'T KNOW DOESN'T HAVE TO HURT US

WHEN "CERTIFIED CROSSDRESSERS" like Jamie Fay Fenton opt for transition, I wonder about the advice they've given, just as I wonder about Diane's FAQs, or Elle's insistence that she be able to crossdress at work. I don't blame them. Their previous advice has to be taken with a grain of salt, doesn't it? All three of them were latent transsexuals, not crossdressers, but all three of them gave advice *as* crossdressers. Virginia Prince lives full-time as a woman but insists she is not transsexual. Lynn Conway argues that labels are effectively useless, and one can only identify a person by what they do. If a crossdresser lives fulltime as a woman without surgery and hormones, she is a _____? She may choose to call herself a non-op transsexual or a transgenderist, but does it matter what the term is? She presents and lives as a woman. She should be treated as a woman. End of explanation.

By insisting that there is a box called "crossdresser," we have a tendency to believe that a crossdresser does *this*, experiences *that*, and believes *this other thing*. Crossdressers, some will tell you, *never do that*.

The classifications of the TG community are like the worst language ever invented: there are more exceptions to its grammar than applicable rules. These classifications only cloud the issues, and delude people into thinking that there are strict definitions that hold up under every circumstance. There aren't.

Am I still terrified that Katie and Elle's fate will become my own? You bet I am. I know what transitioning is like, and I wouldn't want to see my worst enemy go through it, much less the person I love most in the world. I do not want to lose the husband I have, the boy I dreamed about meeting since I was a nine year old girl. Who would? The question that plagues me the most these days is whether my encouragement of his gender explorations could open doors to places I do not want to go. My temptation is to stop being so supportive, but I know in my heart that would be a mistake. I, like Katie, want to be with someone who is fully himself, not repressed or denying some major part of his personality. If it turns out that my husband is transsexual, he will become so miserable he will have no choice but to transition regardless of my support of lack thereof. Katie knows Elle held herself back only for the sake of their marriage and that nothing would have stopped Elle from finding her real reflection in the mirror.

What can a wife do? The same thing a wife does when she kisses her husband as they both leave for work: she can value their time together, enjoy their love, and try not to worry about what *could* happen. The only thing she can do is keep herself in the present, and not worry about the "what ifs" as Kathryn points out. Worrying about tomorrow only ruins today. If a couple has achieved some level of acceptance with crossdressing, they have already learned how to communicate and share their fears. The wife can express her fears and the crossdresser can express his. Their mutual expression and shared emotions can bring them closer together and strengthen their bond.

At least that's what I tell myself when I start to freak out. Sometimes it even works. Most crossdressers do not need or want to have surgery or even take hormones. Many are happy just getting a chance to crossdress once or twice a week. I am convinced the difference is in degree. My husband may be gender dysphoric but occasional crossdressing—and being publicly accepted as a crossdresser—may satisfy his desire to be a woman. I worry a great deal about the crossdressers who are uncomfortable being multi-gendered and so think they must be women because they aren't "all man." Kate Bornstein begins her brilliant book *Gender Outlaw* by admitting she became a woman because she knew she wasn't a man. Only now, years after transition, does she think she's not really a woman, either, but something else altogether.

Sometimes I think CDs would rather be "legitimate" like their transsexual sisters. The crossdresser's urge to de-sexualize his condition in order to make it more "acceptable" could lead, I fear, to many crossdressers thinking they need to have gendered reasons for their behavior. They don't. It can be just about sex, and that's okay. It can be about gender, and that's okay too. It's okay to be a feminized man, and it's okay to fetishize women's clothes, and it's okay too to want to feel like a woman. Self-acceptance and self-knowledge are absolutely necessary for the crossdresser, and only a good therapist well-versed in gender can help him find both. But denying that crossdressers do sometimes transition does no one any good. Ignorance of the possibilities allows CDs to convince themselves that they are somehow "separate and apart" from the TG/TS population. Ignorance causes unnecessary heartbreak, and there is enough of that in the TG community without adding to it with our own inability to face the truth. We have to be open to possibilities and honest about how we face them.

The old idea that you could tell if your crossdressing husband would or wouldn't transition based on whether or not he is turned on by his crossdressing is no longer valid. Conversely, a diagnosis of transsexualism cannot be invalidated by a lack of sexual arousal. If in fact autogynephilia is a kind of "unified field theory" of transgenderedness, it still only accounts for one type of transgenderedness. That we don't have empirical evidence for the asexual type of transgenderedness—as exhibited by the crossdresser who presents as a woman for the sake of gender expression and the transsexual woman who is not autogynephilic—only means that we don't have empirical evidence *yet*. We may. We may find that there are two chromosomal variants on the transgendered gene, if there is one, and that one directs a person toward autogynephilia and another to an asexual transgenderedness.

I am, if anyone's not clear on this yet, a transvestite's wife. My husband is not now considering hormones, and as far as he knows, he will not transition. The specter of the possibility—since transsexual women are so often unaware of their feelings—is terrifying to me. I like having a husband, and I don't mind having a girlfriend, but were I to end up in Katie's position—I don't know what I'd do. That said, I don't want anyone to misunderstand me. I don't think my husband discovering he has transsexual feelings is the worst thing that could ever happen. Katie and Elle I'm sure would both admit that their divorce is a far better outcome than Elle's suicide, no matter how painful their separation has been. Transitioning is not easy, but I am sure it is better than the only alternative many transsexual people feel they have.

Estelle dated crossdressers and is now happily living with and loving a woman who transitioned, Judy, and she, having known both crossdressers and transsexual women intimately, sees the difference much the way the child did in the film *Ma Vie en Rose*: that God or Fate sprinkles the transgendered dust on a child when he or she is born, and the amount of dust determines how transgendered the person becomes. It's a fanciful view, perhaps, but *Ma Vie en Rose* is told from the point of view of a child looking for an explanation for herself.

The current research is not dissimilar. Lynn Conway describes it best:

> *Scientific evidence has been growing that somehow certain brain-structures in the hypothalamus (the BSTc region) determine each person's core gender feelings and innate gender identity. These structures are "hard-wired" prenatally in the lower brain centers and central nervous system (CNS) during the early stages of pregnancy, during a hormonally-modulated imprinting process in the central nervous system (CNS).*
>
> *It appears that if those brain and CNS structures are masculinized in early pregnancy by hormones in the fetus, then the child will have male percepts and a male gender identity, independent of whether the genes or genitalia are male. If those structures are not masculinized in early pregnancy, the child will have a female percepts and a female gender identity, again independent of the genes or genitalia. As in the case of intersex infants having ambiguous genitalia, there are undoubtedly many degrees of cross-gendering of brain and CNS structures, so that while some infants are completely cross-gendered others are only partially cross-gendered.*

Instead of God or Fate sprinkling "transgendered" dust, the structures in the brain and central nervous system that control gender are "washed" in hormones that masculinize or feminize those structures. If the child born with a male body has a brain only partially washed with the masculinizing hormones, he will be transgendered. The level or effectiveness of the hormones may determine how transgendered he will be. If those parts are lightly washed by the masculinizing hormones, he may discover later that he is in fact a transsexual woman. If his brain is mostly masculinized, he might grow up to be a crossdresser.

It's a theory and I am not familiar enough with the science to have a strong opinion about it one way or the other. It seems to be based in biological determinism, which is of course the most attractive kind of argument: we have measured the hormones and have proof to show you. Similar studies are beginning to indicate that there may be a chromosomal link. Good science that can prove this theory will help many more transgendered people get the respect they deserve, and prove that crossdressers are on the spectrum along with transsexual people, and are not always transsexuals in denial. Perhaps new studies will prove instead that crossdressers' brains do not show signs of an incomplete masculinization. We can only wait. That's what scientific revolutions are all about. Positing theories is all well and good, but when a researcher is hell-bent on proving something one way or the other instead of keeping an open mind, the result is disastrous. Researchers with open minds, and open ears, are far more capable of finding the empirical evidence that will help us all gain an understanding of transgenderism, and so help our transgendered friends, relatives, and spouses find the kind of affirmation and respect they deserve.

CHAPTER 6

Sex and Sensibility

DO NOT DISTURB, the sign on the door says. As much as I yearn to be able to speak freely of our sex life, I will not. There is still too much stigma attached to a crossdresser's sexuality. I will admit that my husband does experience some of the issues I will discuss in this chapter, but I can only be coy and add: I'm not telling which. Guess all you like but know that most conjectures about how and where and when my husband and I make love have been wrong. Believe what you like. I won't correct you.

IRONIC AS IT may be, the crossdresser's sexuality is his least-explored aspect. It's ironic because everyone thinks he or she knows what turns a transvestite on: he's aroused by wearing women's clothes, right? Well, not exactly. Sometimes. In a way. For some crossdressers, it is that simple. For others, women's clothes have nothing to do with it. So why is it that so many wives of crossdressers find themselves sexually frustrated? Because we don't really know what turns crossdressers on. We assume to know. There are two good reasons why we don't.

The first is that "sexual deviance" has never been taken very seriously. It may be a topic of fascination for some, inspire disgust in others, but only rarely do people—or even sex researchers—remember that a person who is sexually deviant is also still a person, with the same romantic dreams most of us have. The fetishist is as capable of falling in love with another person as he is turned on by high-heeled shoes. The crossdresser, likewise. Since so many crossdressers are not only sexually deviant but heterosexual, they want and need to find happy, fulfilling romantic partnerships with women despite—or maybe because—they are turned on by femininity.

The second reason we don't know what truly arouses crossdressers is because some crossdressers are not turned on by wearing women's clothes, and others are turned on by it but are ashamed to admit it. In a culture that can barely grasp that homosexuality is a naturally occurring phenomenon, how could the average crossdresser expect understanding? He doesn't. He stays in the closet. He does his thing in private, and he talks to no one about it. How much that shame impacts the crossdresser's sexuality is yet to be known. Does repressing or hiding a major sexual turn-on—and so a person's sexual identity—effect his sex drive otherwise? Sometimes, it does. Sometimes it doesn't. Some crossdressers have no trouble being aroused by the sight of a naked woman they find attractive. Others can't perform unless they are seduced, made to feel submissive, or otherwise fantasize about experiencing what they think is a woman's "native" sexuality. Still other put on a pair of panties and are instantly erect; others are turned on by imagining they have breasts, and still others experience all of these forms of arousal.

As with all aspects of a crossdresser, there is no homogeneity. To say "All crossdressers are turned on by _____" is to start a sentence no one can finish.

I do not have a degree in human sexuality, and I have done no empirical studies. I cannot say for sure that crossdressing directly causes the sexual issues faced by crossdressers, but I do know what their wives and girlfriends write to me about. I know how desperate and frustrated they are because many in the community refuse to admit that there is any link between crossdressing and sex. Decades of denial have not helped yield a solution. By shunting off the "fetishistic" types to the *DSM*, the rest of the CD population kept itself out of the Big Book of Psychological Disorders. Crossdressers continue to insist that they are just straight guys whose sexual problems (if they have them) are just the average sexual problems of heterosexual men.

Their wives tell me otherwise. Wives of crossdressers can be brutally honest about their experiences making love with their husbands. I have learned more about crossdressers' sexualities from the genetic women who date them or married them than from the crossdressers themselves. Without their input, I could never have written this chapter.

Maybe it's a remarkable coincidence that so many wives and girlfriends of crossdressers experience husbands with similar sexual problems. I doubt it. I understand men are not willing to stand up and say they have sexual problems. After all, who is? Crossdressers, who are already considered deviant by most of our society, are not going to start a conversation about themselves by pointing out how often they are sexually submissive. They can't tell their wives about their fantasies because a lot of women find men's sexual fantasies threatening to their relationship. They can't confide in other crossdressers because men don't foster intimate friendships. But women do. A woman would ask a complete stranger for advice if she thought he had the answer to her (or her husband's) problems. Sometimes they even ask me.

COMMON MYTHS ABOUT MEN'S SEXUALITY

I THOUGHT I should begin by debunking some basic myths about sexuality. The standard archetype, or "fantasy model" of male sexuality as sex therapist Bernie Zilbergeld calls it, is the very first problem. The myth is that a man has a large penis which is always rock hard for as long as he wants it that way. Many men do not measure up to this ideal. They cannot always get and/or maintain an erection, and that ability can be greatly impacted by their relationship, their health, and their experiences. A man who lacks sexual confidence may have trouble performing because of past difficulties, or because he wants to impress a woman he likes a lot, or because he hasn't gotten enough sleep. If he feels a woman is judging his performance, it may disable him entirely. Some men have major issues with a woman's genitalia, and may be scared to touch/taste/enter her vagina. Others feel guilty about receiving sexual pleasure. Those who have been sexually assaulted may be completely terrified of being touched. Some men prefer a passive role, others like to be punished, and still others are turned off as soon as they develop deep feelings for a woman. Some men require tactile stimulation to get aroused. Men do not have to develop or maintain an erection—or have an orgasm—to have a satisfying sex life, but almost all of them, and all of us, think that they do. One wife told me her husband fathered two children but has never had an erection.

The theme here is that all men are not the same sexually, and that men have deep feelings about sex. They are not all out to "get laid" without concern for the woman or the circumstances. Many men want to feel loved and trusted, and want to love and trust their partners.

None of the above variations is weird, abnormal, or make a man less than a man. The "fantasy model" is ridiculous for most men, but it's even more insane for crossdressing men, who have been told since they were children that the pleasure they have found is perverted. They have hidden a sexual turn-on from everyone in their lives—even their sexual partners—and then wonder why on earth they don't feel like regular men. The answer is that they aren't "regular men," because regular men don't exist. There may be men who are statistically average, but I'm not even sure I can believe statistics when it comes to male sexuality: guys often lie about their sex lives.

The second set of myths revolves around the expected sexual behavior of men and women. A lot of people believe, for example, that men enjoy porn and women don't, which is untrue. Moreover, women are not always sexually passive or submissive, and men are not always dominant, or aggressive. Men do not necessarily prefer casual sex or "getting off" to cuddling, and many women will take an orgasm over a backrub in a heartbeat. That is, most of our cultural stereotypes about sex are untrue, but the ones that are gender-specific are ridiculous. Our sexualities are deeply personal, tied up with issues of self-esteem, morality, religion, body image, and who knows what else. However, no sexual preference or behavior is inherently male or female. Desire is not that simple. There may be behaviors and preferences that are average, but we don't know how many people behave the way they do because of what is expected of them. Orgasm itself used to be a "gendered" aspect of sexuality: fifty years ago, many women considered sex their "wifely duty" and didn't expect pleasure from intercourse. Obviously that has changed, so orgasm is no longer considered only a male sexual behavior.

We are, of course, socialized sexually based on our genders. What I find amazing is how—despite that socialization—a person's unique sexual desires assert themselves regardless. When a person's requirements for arousal are not met, their sexuality may freeze entirely, or go deep into hiding. Men who are not Don Juans—who prefer making love to having sex—often retreat from typical male sex lives (the "notch in the bedpost" variety) and in some cases retreat from sex and relationships altogether. Women, who are supposed to be passive and pliant and wait for a man to make the first move, often get more satisfaction out of asking men out. Luckily there are exceptions to every rule. The sexologists at the turn of the century, who lived in far more sexually repressive times than our own, found plenty of cases of women who preferred to be dominant in bed, and men who preferred a dominant partner. There are plenty of masculine men who love a dominant female partner, and many feminine women who are tigers in the bedroom. Sexual roles have so little to do with gender identity because so often sexuality is a realm to explore those desires that can't be addressed elsewhere. The powerful politician goes to a dominatrix to be ordered around; the shy girl has fantasies of stripping for a roomful of men. Sex is a lot like Halloween: it's where you get to express those sides of yourself you don't show in public.

It makes perfect sense that a crossdresser's feminine leanings are tied up with his sexual urges. A lot of them discovered at a young age—and quite accidentally—that crossdressing brought sexual release. For some of them, orgasm simply brings an end to crossdressing fantasies, and is more a means to an end than pleasure in itself. Crossdressers know they're not supposed to be turned on by putting on pantyhose, but many are. The terrifying thing about desire is that we can't control it: we might all prefer to have "vanilla" tastes, but we don't. There is no shame—or ought not to be—in having an atypical desire.

CROSSDRESSERS' SEXUALITIES

THERE ARE THREE main types of sexual problems crossdressers face: 1) some CDs want to feel like the woman in the bedroom, 2) other CDs are predominantly autoerotic and, 3) still others are nearly asexual. None of these problems is static, and some crossdressers experience all three. Where one begins and another ends is hard to say, but one or more of them will cause significant problems in a crossdresser's relationship with his wife or girlfriend.

I. SUBMISSION AND THE DESIRE TO BE SEDUCED

The first type is the desire to be "the woman" in bed. Some want to be en femme in the bedroom, dressed in a silk slip. Others prefer to be dressed fully as a woman, including fake breasts. Some crossdressers want to be seduced, to be told they are beautiful and attractive. Others would love to feel penetrated, or to feel like they are doing more "giving" than "taking." This desire is not a problem in and of itself but becomes problematic within a heterosexual relationship. Why? Because, as the wives and girl-friends of crossdressers have told me time and again, they married a man and they want a man in bed, and they have very specific ideas about how a man behaves sexually. If they wanted to be with a woman, they'd sleep with women—not men dressed as women. They are straight, not lesbian, and they want to be desired and seduced. What a lot of women don't real-ize is that their sexual socialization included this script: that as women, they are the object of men's desires. Men will want to look at them, court them, pay them compliments, make love to them. A woman's role in this script is to be demure, gentle, and coy: she is to be taken by him. It's a Victorian standard that hails from the era of chivalry, when women, trapped in castle courtyards, waited for their men to come home from killing the dragon. He would prove his valor, and she would swoon. A lot of women think this is just the way sex is supposed to be, that is natural. It's *not* natural. It's a script from a time when women—whose children were princes or peasants, depending on their lineage—had to be controlled sexually. Society had to be sure that a woman's husband was also the father of her children, and so she couldn't have desires of her own. She made love only with her husband because in a patriarchal culture, it is men who count: a father's sons received his land and his titles; a daughter mar-ried someone else's son, who in turn received his father's land and titles.

Understanding where a sexual script like this comes from doesn't mean it's dismissible. It isn't. Women are taught that this is proper and natural for them and that being sexually aggressive isn't ladylike. We have roles to fill as women, and some of those roles are sexual: we have the babies, after all, and in order to become pregnant we have to be desirable, and in order to be desirable we have to be the right kind of woman—and the right kind of woman in Western culture is a submissive one. We can only be faulted for learning our roles too well. In other words, a sexually aggressive woman, who acknowledged and acted on her own desires, might end up giving birth to another man's son, and so sexual aggression in women was discouraged. We were only good "catches" if we weren't interested much in sex, which is why women learned to put on a show about not enjoying sex and being coy and needing to be won over.

What happens when your average woman meets a crossdresser who wants to play the woman's role in the bedroom? Confusion usually occurs, because they both want to play the same part. Authors Clunis and Green, in their book *Lesbian Couples*, recount a joke in the lesbian community: Two women on a date sit on a couch together. The sexual tension is thick. At exactly the same moment, both women throw open their arms and exclaim, "Take me, I'm yours." It's pretty similar to what a crossdresser and his girlfriend often feel like: They're both waiting for someone to step in and start the seducing, but both of them want to be the one who's seduced. Some women can't conceive of being seducers. Wives of crossdressers who are totally incapable of playing this role will have more sexual difficulties than the women who can. Other women enjoy sex enough to play the seducer even though it's not "natural" to them, but end up with a nasty backlash of guilt and shame for having transgressed their "proper" role. I took to doing the seducing pretty easily and even enjoyed it, but a day or so later found myself feeling undesirable and even a little guilty. I felt like a lesbian, or a man. I had broken the rules, and all my internal voices told me I was wrong.

It's not just in the heterosexual community that people believe man = top, woman = bottom. We all do. It causes as much trouble for feminine gay men as it does for feminine straight men. My friend Richard is a feminine, gay man. He grew up learning how to crochet, sew, and knit. He played with Barbies and preferred girls' company to the boys. As an adult, he is a costumer and for a time did drag. In recent years he has opted to "butch up," primarily because his sexual desire is to be "the man," during sex—a dominant top—and his feminine identity misled potential sexual partners. I have always attracted feminine men because I am a bit of a tomboy and otherwise register as a "strong woman," but what a lot of men who liked me didn't realize is that my social (public) identity has nothing whatsoever to do with my sexual identity.

I like to seduce as much as I like being seduced. For women who can't or won't do the seducing, sex with a crossdresser who wants to feel feminine in bed is nearly impossible. Angela explains:

> I know Jerry is the submissive type but I can't get myself to be the "Man" when it comes to sex. I also could not tell him how beautiful he looks . . . I just can't or won't do it.

For me, it was half-possible. I was willing to experiment with reversing roles. I did ask my husband out, and I asked him to come home with me. I wonder sometimes if that didn't give his poor crossdressing heart the wrong idea entirely. I like being able to play both parts, but I hate feeling like I *have* to play only one—the seducer—all the time. In other words, I don't mind being in a "lesbian" relationship, as long as the "woman" in bed knows I like to be seduced, too.

So why do crossdressers often prefer to be seduced? Because they want to feel beautiful. Because they think—just like their wives and girlfriends do—that a woman's role in the bedroom is to be coy and desirable. There is a little bit of the chicken and the egg to this idea, because I'm not sure if the desire to be a woman came first, or if the desire to be desirable came first. Since a lot of men for whom crossdressing isn't a sexual turn-on say that it's all about wanting to feel pretty, my guess is that crossdressers want to be desired, the objects of affection, the seduced, not the seducer. However, they see all of those desires as being proper to a woman, and so they assume—they want to be the woman sexually.

The problem for a lot of crossdressers is that they're really only turned on when they feel feminine. They can achieve this by various means: reading a story about a man being feminized, imagining they are women, or crossdressing. This is another chicken-and-egg type problem, however, because it is unclear whether the crossdressing itself causes the arousal, or if feeling like a woman—which occurs as a result of the crossdressing—causes the arousal. I'm also still not sure where their avoidance of the male sexual role fits into their fantasies of being women.

Autogynephilia

I introduced the concept of autogynephilia in the last chapter in the light of the TG spectrum. How autogynephilia may or may not impact a crossdresser's sexuality is an entirely different issue. The concept in and of itself is useful in understanding some crossdressers' sexualities, especially when their arousal seems somewhat dependent on the fantasy of being a woman. Even then, the crossdresser himself can decide if he is autogynephilic and how autogynephilic he is; that is, he can use the concept as a way of understanding his own sexuality.

Ray Blanchard, a psychologist, "discovered" autogynephilia and Bailey, in *The Man Who Would Be Queen*, paraphrases Blanchard's explanation of what autogynephilia is and why it might happen:

> *Blanchard believes autogynephilia is best conceived as misdirected heterosexuality. These men are heterosexual, but due to an error in the development of normal heterosexual preference, the erotic target (a woman) gets located on the inside (the self) rather than the outside. This is speculative, and what causes the developmental error is anyone's guess.*

I personally don't like the use of the term "error" when it comes to sexuality, and I'd suggest you read the same passage again substituting the word "variation" for "error." The theory seems to describe some crossdressers' sexualities in a nutshell. They always talk about their "inner woman," don't they? And they identify themselves as heterosexual men as well (unlike the TS women Bailey labels autogynephilic, who don't identify as men at all). I'll go Blanchard one step further and posit the idea that the reasons crossdressers locate their erotic target internally is variable: some crossdressers are sexually intimidated by women (and their "inner female" is more forgiving); others were raised with strong emotional ties to women and have a hard time objectifying them, especially in the way men are "supposed to" objectify women sexually, and still others have feminine sensibilities, which were turned inward because they found no expression for that femininity in environments that enforced very traditional gender roles.

The way I see it, most crossdressers are straight men who are socialized to objectify women sexually. Therefore, if they in fact do have an "inner woman" (for whatever reason) they objectify "her," too. Or maybe they objectify their *internal* woman precisely because they are uncomfortable objectifying *real* women. This line of reasoning makes some sense out of the inconsistencies women who date crossdressers become aware of: their guy is considerate, sweet, forgiving, loving, and otherwise enlightened, but when it comes to his own femme self, it's all Victoria's Secret, spike heels, and short skirts. It sure makes the slutty clothes comprehensible, doesn't it? Let me push my point a little further: What if it turns out that the reason crossdressers are so nice and so nonaggressive in bed is *because* they don't objectify real women? What if the reason they don't objectify real women—their wives and girlfriends—is *because* they have an inner woman to objectify? Doesn't it seem likely that they are somehow sidestepping their sexual socialization (that is, to treat women as sexual objects) by being crossdressers? And isn't that rejection of the traditional, sexually predatory male a *good* thing?

My husband was the one who introduced me to the autogynephilia theory because he thought it applied to him. Other crossdressers have seen themselves in the description as well. It sure does explain all those pictures, the endless hours in front of the mirror, and the desire to have breasts. It explains why they want to play the woman in bed, too, because that's what women do in bed. Ironically, the very men who are asking their girlfriends to play the aggressive seducer are the ones who believe most decidedly that "women" should be submissive and seduced.

The big surprise is that I think it's all bizarrely functional. Theoretically it's a useful psychological defense mechanism. Wives and girlfriends of crossdressers know how sweet our guys can be, how gentle, and vulnerable. A lot of them show an uncommon ability to empathize with women. Crossdressers often prefer women's friendships, and admire how women talk to each other, and support each other, though of course once again this is a crossdresser's sentimentalized view of women's friendships. What they don't see is what women go through to achieve the kinds of friendships they describe, the teenaged and young adult years of competition between women. Women nurture their friendships with each other with compliments and honesty, via mutual revelation and trust. Crossdressers don't see, in a nutshell, all the hard work that goes into the deep and lasting friendships women sometimes have, and as with all things feminine, only see the surface level and so sentimentalize it. They also don't see that their own friendships with women are based on the fact that they are men, and that women, in many ways, trust male friends more easily than they do women.

Still, a lot of crossdressers have a deep respect for women, and in some crazy way, it makes perfect sense that they took the crass things they were supposed to think about women and locked them away in their minds. They invent an "inner woman" so they won't treat real women in the objectified way they were raised to. Of course, there are men who desire women and who avoid objectifying them sexually without being autogynephilic. The difference may be that the man who is autogynephilic was born transgendered in some way to begin with.

As compelling as this theory is, questions remain: Did the crossdresser as a young boy sense his own femininity which resulted in his refusal to "buy into" stereotypes of women? Or did he so fear the taboo of treating women like objects that he couldn't later develop even a healthy sexual objectification of them? Likewise, did he admire the women around him to such a degree that he wanted to be one of them? Or, did he recognize that his own desires to be submissive and coy and assume they meant he was feminine? When he first put that stocking on at the age of five, what did that shiver of excitement mean?

My belief is that he felt pretty, plain and simple. But he also knew that boys aren't supposed to be pretty. Psychologists believe that children learn the difference between boys and girls at about the age of three. So the five-year-old crossdresser was aware that feeling pretty meant he was feminine. Since boys can't be feminine, he locked his feminine side up in his head where no one could see "her" but him. When puberty came around, his sexual desires might have overwhelmed him, made him feel dirty or guilty or incompetent—or all three. Maybe he didn't want to take his "filthy" ideas out on girls he actually knew and respected. Maybe instead it was easier to *be* the girl himself, in his own head, and in so doing avoid hurting any real girls with his sexual desires. He masturbated like all boys do, but for some reason—the crossdresser couldn't even let himself imagine doing the things he wanted to do to a real girl. And maybe by being his own girl, he sidestepped all those other scary things about sex: performance anxiety and erectile dysfunction, diseases and pregnancy, and, well, maybe even that "scary" vagina itself. He kept masturbating to the girl in his head, and as a result wasn't forced—like most boys are—to be with real girls. Maybe the CD never gave himself the opportunity to discover that girls aren't so scary after all, that having sex with them isn't harmful or disrespectful because girls like sex, too. Or maybe he discovered the truth too late, when a lifetime of autoeroticism was already such a pleasurable habit that real sex couldn't replace it. Maybe, too, the crossdresser happened to have a low libido, so his urges were never strong enough to force him to seek sex with real women and learn that he could perform after all?

I don't know how many men read stories about boys being turned into girls and masturbate to the idea, or how many put on stockings to do so. I don't know how many feel okay enjoying sex more when they're dressed as women because they don't have to feel like men "taking" pleasure from a woman's body. A lot of the crossdressers who are married to the women who write to me do these things. I don't think it's just a coincidence.

If crossdressing is indeed some kind of functional defense mechanism or survival response to the unpleasant feelings crossdressers have about being men and desiring women, then the *dys*functional part is that he's rendered himself incapable of playing the male role sexually. Then again, some crossdressers are perfectly capable of having sex with a woman without needing to be en femme or needing to feel like a woman. My guess is that these men either have higher libidos, or perhaps have a different variety of feelings about women. Some may feel entitled to desire their wives, but are uncomfortable desiring other women. Regardless of what they actually do, most crossdressers would love to be taken to bed by a woman when they're en femme. Some play the male role, others can't. The wives of the ones who can perform without crossdressing or other autogynephilic props don't have as much of a problem. It's the rest of us who don't know what to do, and unfortunately a lot of women come up with the worst possible solution: they have affairs, and in so doing not only create an atmosphere of distrust, but validate their husband's feelings of not being "man enough." There are surely more creative ways to have a satisfying sex life with the autogynephilic crossdresser.

The Lesbian Model

Let's go back to the two lesbians on the couch both wanting to be taken. In the book *Lesbian Couples*, where that joke is told, the authors Clunis and Green make a couple of useful points for crossdressers and their female partners.

> If one partner is more skilled and comfortable with initiating, she may resent being responsible for taking the lead all the time. It is likely that the high desire partner is also the one who initiates more.
>
> Partners who are less comfortable with initiating may want sex to "just happen." The problem is that for most couples, after the romance and infatuation stage, sex does not just happen. So it is important that couples in long-term relationships talk about their wants and feelings in order to address concerns about unbalanced initiation. . . . **The partner who tends not to take the lead may also need to become more aware of what interferes with her initiating, and what she might do to overcome these hurdles.**

The emphasis is mine. These authors, of course, are talking about two women, and the hurdles they refer to may be associated with the notion that "ladies don't initiate" which I discussed earlier. Maybe some crossdressers can become the kind of "women" who do initiate, by getting those old-fashioned notions of "ladylike" sexuality out of their heads. One of the reasons they're crossdressers in the first place is because they believe at some gut (or psychosexual) level that sex roles are determined by gender. However, my husband and I did watch an amazing porn film made by and for lesbian women called *How to Fuck in High Heels*. Lesbian friends recommended it, in fact. The "star" of the film is a very feminine woman—makeup, high heels, long hair—who wears a strap-on to satisfy her female partners' desires and her own. We both thought it was the hottest thing we had ever seen because the whole idea—of *femme* = *top*—was incredibly sexy. She knew what she wanted and she was getting what she wanted: the ability to please other women. She was a woman with a dick, which is, if we're going to be honest, pretty much what a crossdresser is when he's en femme.

If a woman is willing to go there, she may find that strapping it on is a very powerful aphrodisiac indeed. Many women are astounded by how much it turns them on to be the top, and can really enjoy the role reversal both sexually and emotionally. There is something liberating and empowering in it. It isn't just the wives and girlfriends of crossdressers who are getting hip to strapping it on. Some of the staff of Good Vibrations in San Francisco, one of the new types of sex-positive stores selling sex toys, made a video called *Bend Over Boyfriend* that was so popular they decided to make a sequel: *Bend Over Boyfriend 2*. The men in the video are not cross-dressed (although one appears to be in lingerie). One is a submissive, and others are just men who have discovered what millions of gay men already know: that the prostate is a powerful aid toward sexual fulfillment. In other words, men enjoy being anally penetrated because it feels good, and for many it unlocks the door to multiple orgasms. Tons of crossdressers would love to find a woman willing to strap it on, because some do fantasize about penetration and aren't sexually attracted to men. It can be a powerful and bonding exchange for a heterosexual couple, and *Bend Over Boyfriend* offers all the information you need: how and where to buy a good harness and dildo, the importance of lubricant, and how to have safe anal sex.

Corinne, a dominant woman who has been dating a crossdresser, enjoys playing the dominant role. She likes that she is not the object of desire, and that her role is more about what she does than about what she looks like. She also likes the power implicit in the fact that her partner wants to make himself desirable and attractive for her. She is not the only woman I have spoken with who feels similarly. These are heterosexual women who prefer the dominant or Alpha role. A woman is an Alpha when she "wears the pants" in the relationship. She may be in charge financially, emotionally, and/or sexually. Plenty of women are Alpha without acknowledging it, but a woman like Corinne both accepts and enjoys her dominant role. In the lesbian community, Alpha females are referred to as Butch, and share a lot of similarities with their straight Alpha sisters, although many Alpha females present in a more feminine way than their lesbian counterparts. Sexually speaking, some dominant women dislike penetration, or they find clitoral orgasm as stimulating (which is achieved via careful placement of the dildo's base). Corinne sometimes has a hard time understanding why I am disappointed with my husband's lack of sexual aggression because she is perfectly happy playing only the dominant role.

Despite my willingness to play sexually, the old-fashioned problem remains: I still want to be taken by the handsome, sexy *man* who is my husband. I want him to feel confident enough to be aggressive sexually when he's in boxer shorts. I want him—as Clunis and Green suggest—to figure out what hurdles are in the way of him initiating when he's not dressed en femme. I want him to initiate as a man. Sometimes—if a lot of conditions are met—he can. The more time we've been together, the more he trusts me emotionally and sexually, and that has had a tremendous impact.

One of the key issues to having a good sex life with a crossdresser is accepting him for who he truly is. Donna, a transsexual woman friend, said, "Sometimes, when you learn who you really are (and don't have to depend on clothes or other "props" anymore), things get better, not worse." She had been married to a woman for ten years who rejected her, and although the wife didn't even know about Donna's gender issues, they didn't have sex at all. At the time Donna thought "he" was a crossdresser, but she's since met a woman who not only accepted the crossdressing but realized there was more to it than that, that in fact her new boyfriend felt more like a girlfriend. She encouraged Donna as she started transitioning, and Donna has never been happier. She has also never been more turned on, and enjoys sex more than she ever did, even without dressing, despite the fact that the hormones she is taking—which usually inhibit a male body's sexual desire—make erections rarer. I wonder sometimes if my difficulty with my husband's femme side is why he isn't entirely comfortable with his sexual self yet.

II. FICTIONMANIA SYNDROME AND SEXUAL ADDICTION

The other kind of crossdresser with sexual problems is the oversexed type. A few key habits distinguish the oversexed crossdresser. They tend to spend a lot of time online, either 1) reading erotic or pornographic stories about feminization, forced or otherwise; 2) viewing either boudoir-style or hardcore pornographic photographs of other CDs or MTFs (she-males, TSs, etc); and/or 3) participating either en femme or en homme in chat-room fantasies and flirtations. The oversexed crossdresser may do all of the above with only the intention only of masturbating, but some CDs do "make dates" with interested parties. Either way, their wives and girlfriends are often threatened and infuriated by these activities.

Many crossdressers indulge their erotica habit on the sly. But their wives and girlfriends find ways of checking the computer to see what their husbands have been viewing, either by checking Internet history, or by installing "spy software" that tracks each user's activity, including websites visited, IM (Instant Messaging), chat, e-mail, and even keystrokes. I don't think a relationship where this kind of snooping takes place is healthy. That is not to say that people don't have their reasons, and unfortunately, a lot of men—CDs included—have bad track records. In fact, a crossdresser's wife may be more suspicious, especially if she didn't even know about the crossdressing for many years. The goal should be for the crossdresser to discuss his fantasies and interests with his partner, but some crossdressers admit that some of the thrill is in the possibility of being caught. Many cannot admit their desires even to themselves, and so consistently seek out their turn-ons, have their orgasms, and afterwards resolve to quit their "filthy habit." As in the case of the crossdresser's purge, the resolve eventually weakens and the cycle starts over again.

In their own self-defense, some crossdressers argue that a lot of men have sexual fantasies they can't share with their partners. They may be entirely right statistically, but that doesn't make crossdressers' wives and girlfriends feel any better about it. They still feel that their partners' computer cruising is the same as cheating. Other men who spend enormous time downloading porn that it begins to affect their relationships suffer the same accusations as the crossdresser.

Some of the problem, as I see it, is the huge gap between what men want to do and what they actually do. The evidence seems to support the idea that men, gay and straight, have more interest in casual sex activities then do women, straight or lesbian. The difference between gay and straight men shows up in what they actually do: straight men experience far less casual sex than do gay men. The idea posited is that the pace and type of heterosexual sex is determined by women, since lesbians and straight women have similar patterns of interest in casual sex and fewer experiences of it.

Anthropologist Donald Symons explains in more detail:

> I am suggesting that heterosexual men would be as likely as homosexual men to have sex most often with strangers, to participate in anonymous orgies in public baths, and to stop off in public restrooms for five

*minutes of fellatio on the way home from work if women were inter-
ested in these activities. But women are not interested.*

Women of course have good reasons for not being interested: fear of sexual
violence, a greater risk of catching Sexually Transmitted Diseases, risk of
pregnancy and a "bad reputation" are a few. An argument can be made that
women are not innately "sexually cautious" but forego casual sexual activity due to very real concerns for their health and safety. Some men make similar decisions, but less frequently than do women.

What this means is that many women—and not just the girlfriends of
crossdressers—are living with men who desire kinds of sexual contact
they're not expecting, like oral sex or threesomes. They turn to porn and
masturbation for an outlet, and some, unfortunately, look for sex outside
their monogamous relationships. Women who are with non-CD men know
about their partners' interests, and many accept the porn/autoeroticism outlet as the lesser of two evils.

For crossdressers' partners it's not that simple. The *types* of erotica the
crossdresser is viewing or reading is often more the issue than the behavior
per se. A crossdresser's sexual interests can include a desire for forced feminization, submission, masochism, and sex with men.

One of the most popular "story sites" for crossdressers is *www.fiction-
mania.com*, which features everything from asexual stories about crossdressing to hardcore porn. The crossdresser can search through stories rated
from "G" to "XXX." Here's a list of the keywords to be used to search the
story database at *www.fictionmania.com*:

- Appliances Attached
- Breast Implants
- Chastity Belts
- Diapers or Little Girls
- Hormones
- Petticoats and Crinolines
- School Girl
- Wedding Dress
  or Married

- Autobiographical
- Bridesmaid
- Cheerleader
- Extreme Body Piercing
- Long Fingernails
- Pregnant / Having a Baby
- Use of Sex Toys

- Bondage
- Castration
- Corsets
- Hair or Hair Salon
- Maids or French Maids
- Prom Girl or Fancy Dance
- Very High Heels

Some stories—like the ones by writer/crossdresser Alyssa Davis—are not
erotic at all. They often feature an intrigue—WWII pilot forced to take
refuge in nunnery—where the erotic component is not readily apparent to
the non-CD reader. They are usually marked by extended and highly

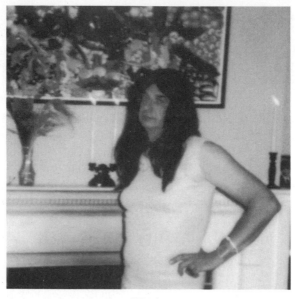

Wendi

detailed descriptions of the clothing and toilette needed to transform the man from male to female, and include excruciating minutiae like the width of the lace trim on any given undergarment. Terrifically boring reading for a non-CD, but terrifically erotic for your average closeted crossdresser.

Interestingly, a lot of the same themes come up no matter how graphic the story. Here's a typical plot one might encounter in crossdressing erotica: A man is feminized (turned into a woman by being dressed and made up as one), often by his wife or girlfriend, in a manner that sometimes suggests punishment. The sadistic wife then forces him into a situation—for example, a double date with two men—in which the crossdresser passes as a female and is expected to give "his" date a blow job. Sometimes the wife or girlfriend witnesses the sex. There are variations on these themes, but not much. Some plots specifically involve magical physical transformation from male to female, and other stories utilize fetishes—bridal gowns, high heels, stockings—as a feature of the story.

My husband's complaint is that the crossdressed male nearly always ends up having sex with a man, which turns him off. My husband had to hope that the story focused more on the crossdresser being feminized by a woman so that he had time to get off before the homosexual aspect of the plot showed up. There are stories at the site in which the crossdresser ends up "lesbian," but not many, although the wife is still the one who "transforms" the crossdresser, by putting female hormones in his cornflakes. Crossdressers are turned on by women and by being turned into women, and so it is almost always a woman's hands that dress and makeup the crossdresser. Only rarely does the crossdresser have sex with the woman, however.

There is one consistent motif: the crossdressed male is forced to give a blow job. The popularity of this scenario is underscored by Kelly's disturbing discovery that her closeted crossdressing boyfriend actually belongs to a Yahoo! group called "Enforced TV Cocksucking." The blow job scenario is probably crossdressers' most popular sexual fantasy after the fantasy of being dressed as a woman. Why does it not surprise me that when a crossdresser—who is socialized as a straight man—fantasizes about being a woman sexually, he envisions himself giving a blow job? This provides further evidence that the crossdresser's "inner female" is painfully loaded with stereotypical male ideas about women, in this case, women's sexual behavior. The idea that your average woman equates "I feel sexy" with "I want to give a blow job" is a remarkably male notion of women's sexuality. That's not to say that women don't find giving a blow job sexy—many do—but many also enjoy multiple orgasms, sensual massage, and receiving cunnilingus. The crossdresser does not choose to express his "internal woman's sexuality" as being multiply orgasmic, but in giving blow jobs. Crossdressers ultimately reveal that their fantasies of women are still based on the fact that they see women through straight men's eyes. That they focus on the one form of women's sexual activity that is primarily about male pleasure is no coincidence.

Responsibility and Sexual Addiction

I don't have an issue with erotica or porn or even men's sexual fantasies. Some days I wish my husband liked erotica more as it might put him "in the mood" more often. There is no shame in a man wanting to give a blow job or wanting to be submissive or even doing these things—as long as he does them safely and without hurting anyone else.

The problem is that many crossdressers cannot bring their femme selves and fantasies into the bedroom because their wives or girlfriends are uncomfortable with them (either due to the perceived lesbianism or for other reasons). Therefore, crossdressers indulge in erotica and fantasy because they are prevented from bringing their strong desires for feminization into their actual sex lives. The crossdresser's decision to indulge in autoeroticism with the aid of erotica is actually a healthy way for him to release these desires, as it avoids the risks of actual sex with another person: STDs, risks to personal safety, blackmail, "outing," and all the other possible consequences of infidelity.

It is one thing for the girlfriend of a crossdresser to be unable to indulge her man's feminine desires in the bedroom. It is her right not to do anything sexual she is uncomfortable doing, no matter what it is. It is another thing entirely for her to ask him to repress those desires entirely. A person can't promise not to have certain sexual fantasies: like dreams, sexual fantasies come unbidden and are uncontrollable. How a person acts upon those desires is the real issue. A crossdresser—or any man in a committed relationship—has a responsibility to prevent his autoerotic pleasure from taking over his life. He has a responsibility to communicate his desires to his partner and not let them interfere with their shared sexual pleasure. If he doesn't enjoy sex unless he is en femme, he's got no business being married to a woman who doesn't want a feminized sexual partner. Both partners in a relationship have a responsibility to participate in their shared sexual life, and if a CD is unable to do this, he should be single—and thus free to find outlets for his sexual desires. Ideally he could find a woman who would indulge him, but many don't. The crossdresser who can function sexually en homme within a heterosexual relationship is less likely to have problems in his relationship, unless his wife or girlfriend is threatened by his even harboring those desires.

Some women are offended by the idea of their men fantasizing and masturbating about anything or anyone other than them. For the record: that's absurd. It is perfectly normal for any person—male or female—to have fantasies or desires about acts or people outside their relationship.

Some women are offended by pornography on principle. Some think it's obscene. Others have political issues about how porn depicts women and are concerned about the porn "actresses" who often "work" without condoms or health insurance, and who face numerous other inequities and risks.

It's my gut feeling, however, that most women who are offended by their crossdressing partner's online activities are actually threatened not so much by the fantasies but by the behavior that accompanies them. That is, if a woman is so offended by her husband's desire to be feminized that she simply does not want him thinking or fantasizing about it, she probably shouldn't be married to a crossdresser, because he can control his fantasies about as successfully as she can control being disgusted by them. If she is going to check his Internet history and ensure that he never indulges his feminization fantasies by reading fictionmania erotica—even the "G" rated variety—his frustration will surely end up aimed at his wife. He may get to the point where he feels damned if he does and damned if he doesn't. Eventually, doing what he wants will become the more attractive option, as his wife will be angry with him whether he harbors the fantasies or actually indulges in them. The crossdresser is responsible for telling his partner how he feels, and together they have to find a way for him to indulge his fantasy life without threatening their relationship. The woman has to be flexible, too, and together they have to find ways for her to feel less threatened by his sexual thoughts—as long as they remain only thoughts. If she is more offended by him flirting in chat rooms, then he can avoid that practice and only look at pictures or read stories. I am not defending a man's poor decisions, and I do not think the long-suffering crossdresser who never told his girlfriend or fiancée or wife about his desires and then springs them on her deserves much slack. However, we are all of us a little repressed when it comes to sex, and many of us have a hard time articulating what we want, much less taking steps to get it.

When it comes to the crossdresser who has "fictionmania syndrome," as I call it, there are other factors at play, too. When a girlfriend writes to me about her husband's online porn hunts or IM/chat room flirting, I usually find that what bothers her is not the activity per se but the rest of the behaviors that surround the activity. She is more often upset by how much time he spends online, or that he lies about what he's doing, or that he is neglecting familial or romantic responsibilities. As is often the case in relationships involving crossdressing, the crossdressing is blamed for the surrounding behavior, even though the crossdressing is not problematic in and of itself. If a man has sexual fantasies that bother his partner, his response should not be to lie about them, but to tell her how he feels and let her voice her fears and jealousies. When there is a problem with online activity, it is usually because of the man's stubborn disregard for his wife's feelings and his failure to consider the repercussions of his behavior on their relationship. Women are most often upset when their relationship is threatened, and a man must remind his partner regularly that his sexual fantasies do not threaten their relationship. Otherwise, she will see the problem as his desires in and of themselves instead of focusing on his inability to reassure her of his love and commitment. A wife gets angry when her husband is failing her as a partner, not just because he is a crossdresser. Kelly summarized what I and many other girlfriends have felt:

I hate that there's something he craves that I can't provide for him. Not that I can provide everything he wants in his life anyway . . . but it's just how I feel.

I realized that that's a lot of what bothers me, other than the freak outs about the weird sex, and the worries about the bi-curiosity . . . because even though there are things you can't provide to each other in a relationship, this is such a big one for him, I feel like I'm always going to be climbing uphill.

In all relationships there are things one person can't provide for the other. That's normal. The question is how the couple decides to fulfill needs that can't be met inside the relationship, and whether or not the relationship can sustain the kind of honesty that's required to discuss them. Neither partner should ever feel less valuable because he or she can't discuss particle physics, for example. Whether the needs are sexual or conversational doesn't matter, because the same jealousy or feeling of "climbing uphill" can happen either way. I knew acting was the most important thing in my husband's life. I worried that my lack of experience in theater would prevent me from giving him the kind of insight or criticism that would help him improve as an actor. I told him how I felt, and together we figured it out: as I became immersed I learned more, and he found ways to include me in his theatrical life, like asking me to read lines with him. In the meantime he reassured me that my lack of theatrical experience didn't damper his love for me. He experienced similar feelings when it came to the difference in our libidos. Mine is high, and he worried I would have an affair. Over time he came to understand I would end a relationship before I cheated, and I would never end it due to sexual problems, but only if he didn't put in the effort to improve our shared sex life. My reassurances eventually helped assuage his worries. In this way, partners can verbally confirm their commitment to minimizing their differences.

Worries about a partner's bisexuality are often unfounded, not only because often the bisexualism is only a fantasy, but also because the fears are based on the incorrect belief that bisexual people are incapable of being monogamous. Bisexuals are perfectly capable of having monogamous relationships. A female and bisexual friend tells me she has no worries about getting married to a man, and explained, too, that her dating habits had always been cyclical: she'd go through a period when she dated only women, and then for a while would date only men. She was perfectly capable of being monogamous within those relationships, even though she might break up with a man and find herself dating a woman next.

III. LACK OF INTEREST/AVOIDANCE

I'm not sure if the third problem crossdressers experience sexually is a separate problem from the other two, or simply one that comes about as a result of the other two, and I'm not sure that it has anything whatsoever to do with crossdressing. It can certainly accompany either the autogynephilic type or the fictionmania type. Crossdressers' wives tell me that their husbands often have no interest in sex at all. They avoid it at all costs, providing "reasons" not to have sex no matter what the circumstances. "Honey I've got a headache" is only one of many excuses crossdressers have used to avoid sex. I don't know if their avoidance stems from the lack of acceptance they feel from their partners and the world in general, or if their shame about being crossdressers is the problem, or if they have a lack of sexual confidence that stems from issues entirely unrelated to crossdressing. For some men, it might be simply their own special manifestation of what a lot of men experience: that it is difficult to keep the spice in a long-term relationship or marriage. Whatever the reason for it, some crossdressers find a way to avoid sex. Angela explains that her husband was once a great lover, but over time has entirely retreated into his autoerotic habits:

> *Things were GREAT when we first started dating . . . he was the best sex I ever had and I have had many boyfriends before I married Jerry (I was thirty years old when we got married). I also think after so many years of marriage, they all resort back into themselves for self gratification and dressing. I never needed a vibrator all my life and here I'm married . . . talking about getting a vibrator! I do get mad sometimes thinking about this because why should I have to learn to use a vibrator when I have a husband who should be having sex with me? This does suck and I don't know if I will ever get to a happy place in my heart over this sex issue. It just seems like I'm fighting a brick wall over having sex. Jerry doesn't want me like a real man does when it comes to sex and I have to accept the fact. It's hard but I have been doing it for thirteen years and I realize it isn't going to go away.*

Angela even had to set aside hopes of having a baby because her husband so deeply avoided sex, so not only did it impact her sexual fulfillment, but it also greatly affected their future as a couple and family. It could be argued that he was avoiding sex because he didn't want a child, but his avoidance of sex started long before he and Angela realized they wanted to have children. Even his desire to make his wife pregnant didn't help him stop avoiding sex, which to me indicates exactly how deep that avoidance is.

Jerry is a kind of "textbook case" in that he exhibits symptoms of all three of the sexual problems crossdressers can experience: he prefers to be seduced, prefers autoeroticism to intercourse, and avoids sex in general. It is relatively easy to see how these three types of problems intersect: the autogynephilic man is turned on by the idea of being a woman, and since he can't bring that to the bedroom he finds an outlet for his fantasy in erotica, and because he is more satisfied by his fantasy sex life than in his actual one, he starts avoiding sex altogether. For a while Angela begged and pleaded with him to figure out what was wrong, especially when they were trying to get pregnant, but eventually she just gave up and bought a vibrator. She wasn't able to play the seducer in the bedroom or tell him stories of feminization, and she found even if she downloaded fictionmania stories to read to him, she would be so turned off by them that she didn't want to have sex. The result was a complete halt in their sexual relations.

Angela is cynical about my efforts, and has come to believe it's just in some crossdressers' natures to prefer autoeroticized fantasy sex over what she considers "the real thing." She is convinced her husband Jerry has a fetishist's sex drive, one dependent on his crossdressing and the fantasies of being a woman and that doesn't involve her at all. She thinks he used to be interested in sex because he had a high enough libido to accommodate both, but now that he has gotten older, and his libido has decreased, he limits his sexual activity to what really turns him on. She is young, looks great, takes good care of herself, and is practical and confident enough to know it's not about her looks.

One of the problems that can occur when a man is shy about sex—due to episodes of erectile dysfunction or myriad other issues—is that a woman who is not sexually satisfied can become quite aggressive and belittle her husband for not having sex with her. Or, if he is not very experienced and she finds their sex life unfulfilling, she may unconsciously send off signals—or say bluntly—that he's not satisfying her. For the man with little sexual confidence, this reflection of his inability compounds the problem. Often it sounds the death knell for their relationship altogether.

It is not, however, an unconquerable problem, but the first thing that's required is that the couple go to a sex therapist. They can't just read books, although books—like Bernie Zilbergeld's *The New Male Sexuality*—might help. They need a counselor because so much bad sex is caused by a lack of communication. A couple may not know which words to use to describe what they would like to do or have done to them, or they might be too ashamed of their desires to tell a partner about them. Furthermore, they might—if they haven't had good sex for a long time—have a lot of emotional baggage to examine.

When Angela is angry that her husband won't have sex with her, she's not angry because he won't have sex with her today. She's angry because he hasn't had sex with her "today" for the last five years. Likewise, he has shut down because his wife says his lovemaking technique doesn't satisfy her, and he sees no point in trying because he is obviously incapable (in his mind). With counseling, she might be able to express her anger over those years of sexual rejection she's suffered, and he might learn that most men—and most couples—have bouts of sex that is not satisfying for one or both of them. That is, the crossdresser may also be blaming his sexual problems on his crossdressing, when in fact they are much more common than he might imagine. He might also go to a medical doctor to rule out hormonal or other health issues that might impede his libido. Sex, as they say, is 10 percent physical and 90 percent mental, so it seems more likely that the reason a crossdresser avoids sex with his partner is that something in his mind is not turned on by the idea, and only with a therapist's help can he figure out what it is that keeps him from enjoying sex with his partner.

LET ME BE clear about the fact that not all crossdressers have sexual problems. Some crossdress and have perfectly good sex lives with their wives or girlfriends. Others are practically asexual, autoerotic, or oversexed. Some, like Jayne, don't understand fictionmania stories because they don't see that their being crossdressers means that "anything goes" with them sexually. Others are masochists, or fetishists, and others just like the sight of a beautiful naked woman. The variety is endless. Just as I have pointed out that some men are good partners and some are not so good, and that crossdressers can be either, so it is with crossdressers' sexualities. Their individual sexual lives may have more to do with upbringing than with crossdressing per se. Others may have developed sexual problems as a result of hiding their crossdressing from loved ones. It is very difficult to sort out one problem from another, but the very fact that there are crossdressers who have perfectly vanilla sex lives that have nothing whatsoever to do with their crossdressing indicates that it is possible for a crossdresser to have a satisfying sex life with a partner. How the ones who have sexual problems might become satisfied in their sexual relationships takes time, openness, and maybe a little creativity.

WHAT IS HETEROSEXUAL, ANYWAY?

When I venture into the TG community, poring through personal ads, websites, profiles and chats, and see the vast majority of MTFs I encounter intentionally attracting male attention in a sexual manner I do not believe the party line that most TVs/CDs are heterosexual. When they're en homme, perhaps that's the truth. But once the makeup comes out and the breast forms go on (even if only in their heads) all sexual orientation bets are off.

—Fem, an Alpha female who dates MTFs

Personally, I see a lot of "straight" CDs that engage in sexual activity of some sort with men. I have friends that outright have sex with them and tell me they are still straight, because when they are with men they are "a girl." I try to understand this point of view but really struggle with it. I personally think that 98 percent of them are gay men in denial, and I tell them so. Of course it bristles quite a few feathers when I do, but I tell it the way I see and don't expect people to agree.

—a crossdresser

I think 80 percent of all CDs have thought about men, or I should say a man's attention. It's not so much being bi as it is just another piece of clothing (in a sense) that the CD puts on to complete the look. Think about it. Which looks better? Or should I say more feminine, a CD walking down the street looking around, just a bit worried about a confrontation or a CD walking down the street holding hands with a man, looking happy because not only does she have his attention, but his protection and his power and all that goes with it. Which do you think stands out more? Not the one with a date for sure.

Just like 90 percent of all men who have ever donned a dress have thought about a sex-change, I'm sure they think about being gay, bi and a bunch of other things. I know I did, but in my day, being fifteen and "trying" to crossdress, I did not know there were others like me. So I had the right to question everything. Today I know better and that is no longer true.

Has a man ever bought me a drink? Yes. Did I like it? Yes. Am I gay? No, but it looked great sitting at a bar chatting with a man. Just like donning a gown looks great. So even today, if a man asked me for a drink or some chat or even a dance, would I say yes? You bet because it looks great and it's the greatest compliment a CD can get. Would I leave with him? Heck no, I'm not crazy you know.

—Victoria, a transvestite

There is an ongoing debate in the crossdressing community: are crossdressers straight or not? Often this is a wife's number one question, and she can find plenty of evidence either way. Crossdressers' sites proclaim hetero-sexuality, but there are plenty of online groups where so-called straight crossdressers post photos of themselves in next-to-nothing, and are available for chat with men. One of Bobbi Williams' fictionalized but autobiographical stories in the book *Me, Bobbi, & the Gyrls* describes two MTFs who meet at the bar during the Southern Comfort conference. One older and one younger, they sit at the bar within earshot of Bobbi and make plans to meet later in the older one's hotel room. It is obvious to Bobbi they will have sex.

What about the CD members of the "Enforced TV Cocksucking" group? And the many fictionmania stories that end with crossdressed men having sex with other men? One crossdresser told me he said yes to a ménage-a-trois with a heterosexual couple mostly because "she" wanted to experience giving a blow job, and got to, despite the fact that his wife was totally unaware her husband was a crossdresser, and who certainly didn't know he wanted to give a blow job en femme.

When we started going out to CD events like the Silver Swan (described further in the EpiScene chapter), I witnessed the pickups and flirtation, and noted the lack of genetic women. My first impulse was to assume that the participants—both the crossdressers and the "admirers"—were repressed homosexuals. Most gay men would probably agree with me. Others—including many wives and girlfriends of crossdressers—assume that if a man wants to wear a dress he is out to have sex with men. But as I've gotten to know the community a little better, I am convinced it's not—as nothing is in this community—that simple.

As we've already established, crossdressers don't just want to dress like women. They want to feel like women. They fantasize about being a woman sexually. They are certainly heterosexual in mind because they conceive that being a woman sexually means being with men. Some crossdressers, like Victoria, use men as a "prop" more than anything else. Having a man buy them a drink or offer his arm when they are en femme makes crossdressers feel validated as females. The man is the final "accessory," to be put on like a wig or stockings, and taken off just as easily. Many single crossdressers who are free to experiment may still be in the process of discovering their true sexual orientation. Some of these crossdressers may have sex with men and go back for more while others reaffirm that they are straight. In some cases, crossdressers may find that dressing is the perfect excuse to find the casual sex they desire—for example, the bathroom blow job. It is ironic that they need to dress as women to indulge in the kind of casual sex they desire as men, but the reality is that only by interesting male partners will they be likely to find that kind of sex.

I'm not interested in labels very much, especially when it comes to sex. Most of the time I think they're used to put people down. I don't think sexual behavior is dependent on gender identity, though gender roles are powerful enough to affect desire in significant ways. Yes, I've used terms like "male" to mean dominant in this book because that's the popular notion of male sexuality. It is just as fully male to be submissive, and no less womanly for a woman to want to be on top.

I don't care if a crossdresser who, en femme, has sex with a man is homosexual or heterosexual or bisexual or closeted or deluded or drunk. I don't care what he calls having sex with another crossdresser, either. What I do care about is whether his behavior is responsible. If he's fooling around with anyone (male or female) behind his wife's back, he's a jerk. If he's doing so without using protection and still having sex with his wife, he's an evil jerk. The HIV virus—and other STDs—don't differentiate between homosexual or heterosexual behavior: they simply infect healthy bodies. If he's flirting with men or women online and he knows his behavior hurts his wife's feelings and threatens their relationship and continues to do so anyway, he's a selfish bastard. If he wants to have sex with men and tells his wife he doesn't, he's a liar. Sometimes he's lying to himself, or in denial, or so deeply repressed that he doesn't even know he wants to have sex with men. Crossdressers themselves declare they get no arousal from dressing, but Blanchard found even the ones who deny that arousal have increased blood flow to their penises: biological proof of arousal. Still they deny it. I'm not a crossdresser, so I can't say for sure if Blanchard is right or wrong. I have met crossdressers who have never experienced orgasm as a result of crossdressing. Perhaps they don't recognize a more subtle arousal as a sexual feeling, or perhaps they really aren't turned on by crossdressing. My gut feeling is that Blanchard is right, but I'm not fond of "diagnoses" that second-guess anyone's sexuality. How we all define terms like "arousal" is personal.

I think everyone has the right to know themselves sexually and to experience sexual pleasure. I don't think there's any shame in having "deviant" sexual desires, either. I do think that not being able to own up to those desires and to address them causes a lot of harm: for single men it can result in alcoholic bouts and safety risks because some men see a drunk guy in a dress as a perfect victim. For married men it can lead to blackmail, self-hatred, and a miserable wife. The repressed, self-hating gay man calls homosexuals "faggots" in front of his friends and later in the night goes back to have sex with one. Fem, the alpha female who is actively looking for an MTF partner, summarizes the problems with the declared heterosexuality of crossdressers as concerns their identity, relationships, and public acceptance:

> *If someone wants to have sex with a Land Rover I don't really care. I'm sure there are a lot of people out there that would call me a sexual deviant for being turned by the sight of a guy in a garter belt and stockings underneath me with his legs in the air. The difference from my perspective is that I'm not out there promoting myself as a conservative, traditional, het female to anyone EVER.*
>
> *I'm wildly speculating here, but I'm beginning to think that the stringent denial-of-homosexuality-at-all-cost position MTFs frequently take is greatly responsible for their lack of credibility with GWs, and possibly society at large.*

Sex columnist Tristan Taormino wrote a column for *The Village Voice* recently about the emergence of the "queer heterosexual."

> *. . . the evolution of an out, proud, vocal, and visible transgender community has turned everything on its head, making the term "opposite sex" practically meaningless, or at best confusing. What's the opposite sex of a male-to-female transsexual? Is the lesbian lover of a male-to-female transgender person bisexual or something else entirely?*
>
> *. . . these advances have ushered in a new identity: the Queer Heterosexual. How does one spot a QH? In some cases, it's based on either one or both partners having nontraditional gender expressions, like she's tough-as-nails butch (yes, straight women can be butch—have you been to Montana?) and he's girlish and lets her take charge (which may or may not include bending over), or they actively work against their assigned gender roles. Some queer heterosexuals are strongly aligned with queer community, culture, politics, and activism but happen to love and lust after people of a different gender. I also consider folks who embrace alternative models of sexuality and relationships (polyamory, non-monogamy, BDSM, crossdressing) to be queer, since labeling them "straight," considering their lifestyle choices, seems inappropriate. Then there are those folks who may be straight-looking and straight-acting, but you can't in good conscience call them straight.*

Exactly. The whole idea of being straight implies vanilla sexual tastes, which are not something I see a lot of in crossdressing culture. If crossdressers realized what is going on in the rest of the world, they might realize that it's very possible for them to find relationships in which they can be committed to a partner and still find themselves sexually satisfied.

BDSM AND CROSSDRESSING

HEATHER AND MINNA are involved in the BDSM (Bondage, Discipline, Sadism/Masochism) community where they live, and I have found that·many other crossdressers, because of their desire to be submissive, find their way to the BDSM community as well. Minna, who is a dominatrix, found that many BDSM practitioners were ignorant about crossdressing and she prepared a Frequently Asked Questions list reprinted below for their enlightenment. She would have me add, no doubt, that if you are interested in experimenting with role-playing or other BDSM sex-play, that you educate yourself. The BDSM community insists that BDSM sex-play be safe, sane, and consensual. Any couples and/or individuals need to know how to keep their "scenes" within those boundaries. She recommends the book *Screw the Roses, Give Me the Thorns* by Philip Miller and Molly Devon as a good introduction to BDSM.

CROSSDRESSING WITHIN BDSM —FANTASY VS. REALITY

I was asked to do a FAQ about Crossdressing and what I deal with as Wife and Mistress of a crossdresser. This is by no means totally inclusive and is based on my experiences only. Your mileage may vary.

Real life: Why?
There are many reasons why someone crossdresses; here are some of them:

- **Sexually exciting**—*It is a hell of a turn on for some to wear taboo fabrics (satin, silk and lace) and taboo clothing. There are many men for example who say they are not a crossdresser, who wear panties under their business suits every day because it turns them on and it's a thrill.*

- **Permission to act weaker/slutty/sexy**—*Some men need to have a way to safely express "feminine" emotions that they feel they can* *not in their daily, real world lives. Crossdressing gives them an outlet for this.*

- **Chivalry/Courtesy**—*Men traditionally are expected to hold chairs out, open doors, and basically do nice things for women. Crossdressing allows them to feel the same things and to be treated as though they are special, pampered and loved.*

- **Disguise effect**—*"No one knows it's me." Crossdressing allows an escape from the real world and all its pressures. My husband says often that "Heather can't be caught, only I can," and if you think about it, it's very true. The disguise gives a freedom from responsibility and a kind of confidence that isn't normally present to some men.*

- **If I can't find a girl . . .**—*Yes, for some that are shy and lonely, when they first started dressing it was a way to role-play having a girlfriend, or to accessorize a masturbatory fantasy. If you don't have a girlfriend, make one.*

- **Gender dysphoria**—*Whether it's mistaken gender assignment at birth, a hardwire difference in the brain, genetically a different sex than the body portrays or nurture, the bottom line is that the inner being of the person does not match the outer body of that person. Crossdressing makes the person feel more like "themselves" and correct.*

- **Bisexuality/Homosexuality**—*For some, crossdressing gives them permission to experiment and explore their sexuality. Being a crossdresser is confusing and there are lots of questions. Going out dressed and meeting people of the same gender to experiment with can answer those questions.*

The most common CD fantasies:

Crossdressing in BDSM is common, especially among male submissives with female dominants. There are many reasons for this fantasy and here are the most common ones with what they entail:

- **Sissy Maid**—*the person is dressed in ultra feminine maid attire (French maid being the most common), high heels, slutty make up and nails, lots of frills and perfume. They are then to clean up Ma'am's*

(Madam's, Mistress' . . . *Goddess'* . . . *whatever) home from top to bottom meticulously, including doing menial tasks like hand washing of undergarments. After doing all said chores, the work is inspected, demerits tallied, punishment given for poor work (there is always something not right), and groveling to appease Ma'am. Reward for good work and/or groveling is usually allowance of orgasm.*

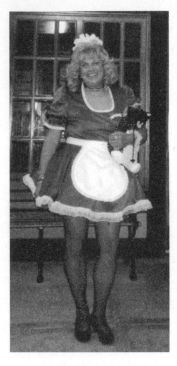

Stephanie, a Sissy Maid

- **"Forced" Feminization**—*This can be included in the Sissy Maid fantasy but not always. This is where the Dominant "forcefully" makes the male submissive over as a woman, meaning they have discussed this fantasy that he desires and she surprisingly restrains him in some manner later and makes him up. Usually this fantasy includes trashy lingerie, heavy makeup, slutty wigs and hair. Then they are "trained" to be a woman, which can include waist training, walking, talking, sissy maid, shaving, etc. All inadequacies are punished in training and usually include humiliation. Good performance usually ends in the allowance of orgasm.*

- **Roleplaying/Reversal**—*A specific scene where not only the crossdresser but also their partner switches roles and perhaps even gender. One of the more common is the CD going to a bar to be picked up by a "man" and when they get home find out its really a woman who is crossdressed like they are. Often kidnap fantasies; rape fantasies and other BDSM "forced" fantasies are included in this type of scene. This does entail a lot of planning by both parties on where and what is safe in public.*

- **Girlfriends**—*This is exactly as presented. The CD's partner treats the CD as a special girlfriend and they go shopping, do makeovers on each other and other things usually women do with special friends. It has very little sexual content but it is one of the more favored fan-*

tasies because it gives a lot of love and acceptance of who the cross-dresser is.

- **Dominatrix**—*Not all male-to-female crossdressers feel submissive when dressed. Dressing makes them feel more comfortable and gives them confidence. Also, in western culture women hold the power of permission for sex. (They are the ones that say no.)*

"TRANNY CHASERS" AND THE THIRD SEX

THERE ARE A lot of "straight" men out there who are interested in dating trannies, including crossdressers, MTF TGs, and pre-op transsexual women. When I first encountered these men at events we attended, I assumed they were—like the crossdressers who have sex with men or other crossdressers—closeted gay men. But it's never simple. Colleen was the first crossdresser who told me he had a sexual interest in she-males, and it was this interest that led to his own enlightenment that he was a crossdresser: years of drinking and repression had shoved his childhood dressing into the back of his mind, forgotten. But having sex with a pre-op MTF transsexual—a female-identified person who had retained her penis—was what "reminded" him of his crossdressing experiences as a child and teenager. Colleen is single and tells me his sexual preference is for females first, she-males second, and males last. He is also convinced that as transgenderedness becomes more accepted, more people will find themselves attracted to pre-op transsexuals, whom he refers to as having "the best of both worlds"—that is, breasts and a penis. He calls them "the third sex."

What I didn't realize until Colleen opened my eyes is that many of the men who court trannies—"tranny chasers" as they're derogatorily called, "admirers" when they're appreciated—are often transgendered themselves, and who either choose not to express their transgenderedness or are simply unaware of it.

One admirer I corresponded with, Ken, responded with such articulate answers, and with such depth and thought, that I know I could never look sideways at an admirer again.

*   *   *

INTERVIEW WITH AN ADMIRER

Helen: *You mention that your interest in t-girls stems somewhat from your own desire to crossdress. Would you say that is true for many other admirers as well? A few? Do you feel it's a "likely" cause for male interest in t-girls?*

Ken: *Of course, I can't speak for all other crossdressers, but I strongly imagine that the correlation is true for at least some of them. Once you've come to accept the existence of a "third sex" or of an "in between gender," then you can begin to have feelings about whether you find them attractive or not.*

Helen: *You also say that you have never "had the desire for a long term relationship with a male" which by default means that your interest in t-girls is more sexual. Am I misinterpreting here? Do you generally find your interest in t-girls is more about "dating" than "marriage"?*

Ken: *I think my interest in t-girls is perhaps a little more sexual. Were it to be more than sexual, I'd be driven to try to not label them. I am, though, a human, and have sexual desires. I find that t-girls are often, in some way, more feminine because they've become that way by CHOICE instead of by culturalization. That, and to be honest, there is some of the taboo factor, of a beautiful woman with a penis. Not to make it sound tawdry, but I would be lying if I did not admit that part of the attraction is because they are "different." I am attracted to the physical presence of a variety of genitalia in a variety of packaging, and titillated when they don't match stereotypes.*

Helen: *In order of preference, would you rather be intimate (i.e., have sex with) a) genetic women, 2) men, 3) t-girls? In what order? Likewise, for a relationship?*

Ken: *In a perfect world, I'd probably rather be intimate with a t-girl (given that her male genitalia were still functional) because we would both be equipped to physically give and receive in the same manner. That doesn't, of course, take into account if we'd want to switch roles, but it would at least leave the door open. In actuality though, I see no need to latch on to a preference, no more than we see the need to latch onto a preference of food or drink—tastes change, often frequently.*

Helen: *How do you feel about the CD/TG community in general? Do you feel welcomed, ignored, tolerated?*

Ken: *Contempt is the closest word I can come up with at the moment, sadly. There is a large portion of the CD/TG/TS community (e.g., Tri-Ess) which insists that cross-dressing is a primarily heterosexual activity. Then there's the drag community within the GLBT community, who will say "Honey, if you wear a dress it's because you're looking for a man." Then, in the serious transgender community (e.g., IFGE) who basically don't see it as having a sexual element, and in the medical community, there are "professionals" who dismiss those who don't pursue SRS as "not being serious." For myself, none of it is that simple. The "Tri-Ess types" can't accept my homosexual side, the "drag types" can't accept my straight side, the "IFGE types" can't accept that any of my sides want to have sex, and the medical community just sees me as sexually deviant since I don't want a sex-change.*

Helen: *Do you ever encounter crossdressers who are "hetero" & married? Do you find they are interested in you romantically/sexually? That is, do you "buy" the idea that there are straight CDs who do not want to have sex with men when they are en femme? How many CDs do you think are interested, or might be if they weren't married?*

Ken: *There is a LARGE community of hetero (and often married) crossdressers. The ones who grasp the labels of "hetero" and "married" aren't quick to admit if they are interested in men sexually or romantically. Occasionally they will admit to interest in other crossdressers. I do believe that many lie to themselves, however, and that many CD/TV/TG/TS types who say they have no interest in men do to some extent. Numbers? Personally, and this is a terribly uneducated guess, I'd say that 75 percent or more would at least be interested in experiencing the romantic or sexual intimacy associated with being in a female role **IF** there were no other pressures (societal, psychological, marital, social, religious, etc) influencing their behavior. On the other hand, I'd guess that less than half of the CD/TS/TG/TV community acts on that interest.*

Helen: *If you've ever had contact with women who are married to/date CDs, how do they treat you? How do you treat them? Is there a camaraderie or competition? Do you feel like a threat?*

Ken: *I have had contact with many girls who knew of my CD activities, and they love it. I'm not even going to begin to dissect the phenomenon, but watch "Will and Grace" or hang around gay men for any length of time, and you'll find no shortage of accepting straight women. This is true for crossdressers also—many even see it as an opportunity to have a "little sister" or "play dress up." Sadly, though, they almost always engage in this type of relationship behind a veil of limits—when it comes time* *for their own romantic and/or sexual intimacy, they retreat to "normal" men. And they seldom let the two worlds meet.*

Helen: *Do you prefer CDs, the transgendered, or transsexual women? Do you have any particular desires one way or the other?*

Ken: *Generally, I don't like those who dress infrequently, because their female persona is shallow—it doesn't get enough life to give it depth. In addition, those types often tend to try to do a bare minimum at their job of passing. Those who live life as a woman are often reluctant to pay much attention (or have much attention paid) to their penis, so thus there's a built in problem with how I approach the whole experience—I don't center on their penis, but I don't want it excluded, either. The type of t-girl I think I would most appreciate, (and sadly, a type I've never been with) is the one who still maintains some life as a male, but chooses to spend most of her time as a female.*

Helen: *Where do you meet t-girls most of the time? How?*

Ken: *It would be unfair for me to make this sound like I'm a real "player" in meeting t-girls. I can count those I've been intimate with on any level on my fingers. Let me think—bars, "support" type meetings, personal ads, and online (sometimes online ads, sometimes chat rooms) are the places that I've met people. As to how, I basically just say that "I like t-girls" and go from there.*

Helen: *Do you think your shyness as a male has anything to do with your desire to crossdress?*

Ken: *I think I'd be shy even if I didn't crossdress, but the crossdressing is among the things that make me shy. Shy—yes—but that does bring to mind a point to ponder— Why does every t-girl, even those of us who don't look that good, have this obsessive urge to have their pictures taken and show them off? That's one that I own up to, but can't begin to explain.*

Helen: *A lot of CDs do not "pass" or look very good en femme, but they go out anyway. You give this as a reason why you don't dress much and like dating t-girls (the "soft spot" you have for them). Why do you think others dress anyway, despite how they may or may not look? Why do you think it keeps you from dressing? How well does dating t-girls fulfill your own need to crossdress?*

Ken: *Let me clarify—I still dress, and still get my thrills out of it, and still have all those desires, but it does take a certain amount of the thrill away when you don't* *look the way you want to look. I'm not that hot, but the desire to be is still there. Others are perhaps less realistic or more outgoing than I, and can find thrills in it despite their shortcomings—I can't, but that's just me.*

Ken added a final comment:

> *I think perversion is nothing more than each of us living our perfect world in our head, and occasionally making forays to try and make our perfect world a reality. As everyone's reality and fantasy is different, I guess our world will never be perfect, except perhaps for each for a while.*

If there is any impression I get from talking to the wide variety of sexually diverse people for this book, it's that two things are important in sexuality: self-acceptance and responsibility. When a crossdresser can't share his fantasies with a female partner, it is very difficult to find his way to self-acceptance. A partner's help is not the only means, of course: plenty of people have found ways to accept their sexual selves through conversations with friends, books, or maybe just by going out and exposing themselves to new experiences and tastes. Once when buying a rubber skirt for a fetish event we were going to, I felt terrifically embarrassed, but the man in front of me was proudly purchasing a large anal plug, and in comparison I didn't feel like a pervert anymore. It wasn't that he was: it was that he wasn't ashamed of his sexual desires—and I was. And yet too there are plenty of people who couldn't have ever walked into that store in the first place, and others who wouldn't be caught looking in the window. Accepting that sexual desire is unfathomable and complicated may be the first step.

I'll end this chapter with a column by Dan Savage, a syndicated sex advice columnist, who takes on Dr. Phil, whose advice to the wife of a crossdresser upset most of the CD community.

WHAT YOU DON'T WANT
by Dan Savage

> *I was watching Dr. Phil on television the other day with my wife. He was talking to a woman who discovered, after marrying her husband, that he was a crossdresser, or at least had crossdressing tendencies. Dr. Phil counseled the woman to leave the man because of his "perversion," and told her that no one could ever be sexually satisfied with a*

crossdresser for a husband because he would always be masturbating while wearing her underwear, and so on, instead of sexually pleasing her. Mind you, the woman had three kids with this guy, and she actually didn't say that they didn't have sex. Then Dr. Phil got the husband on the phone and yelled at him for being dishonest.

From reading your column for a long time, I was under the impression that just because something turns someone on, it doesn't mean that nothing else turns them on. If I like blow jobs and my wife doesn't, does that mean we are sexually incompatible? How is this different? Or is Dr. Phil just projecting?

—Perverts and Nylon Tights

As the mental image of a crossdressed Dr. Phil is too horrible to contemplate, let's assume he isn't projecting. Besides, it's more likely Dr. Phil is simply doing what daytime TV talk-show hosts are paid the big bucks to do: Tell women in the audience exactly what they want to hear. In this case, he's telling the wife of a crossdresser, and, by extension, all the wives of all the crossdressers watching at home, that their husbands are dishonest perverts, that the wives are wronged innocents.

Yes, yes: In an ideal world people would make a full disclosure of their secret sexual fetishes before getting married and making babies. But most straight people with "shameful" sexual fetishes deny and suppress them for years in what almost always proves to be a futile attempt to control and deny their sexual desires and live "normal" lives. (Out gay people, as a rule, don't suppress their kinks. Compared to a desire for same-sex sex and love, a "perverse" desire for leather, dress socks, stuffed animals, spankings, piss, Ashton Kutcher, etc. just doesn't seem that scary.)

And why do straight guys with bizarre sexual fantasies and fetishes try to keep them secret? Why do they suppress them? Because of people like Dr. Phil.

It's the Dr. Phils of this world who run around telling people that anyone with a sexual fantasy wilder than whipped cream on the wife's nipples is a freak. It's the Dr. Phils who spread the lie that people with wild sexual fantasies are not interested in "normal" sexual activity, no matter how much "normal" sexual activity they've engaged in over the course of their lives. It's the Dr. Phils who tell women with small children that the discovery of a run-of-the-mill sexual fetish is grounds for divorce.

Gee, color me Bill Bennett, but it seems to me that the damage of divorce for all involved (especially kids!) is so great that the wife of a crossdresser might want to take a stab at accepting or accommodating her husband's fetish before filing for divorce. And perhaps the woman on Dr. Phil's show might have gone there if the not-so-good doctor took the trouble to do a little research before he stuck his big, bald head up his big, white ass. (Hey, that's perverse!) Then Dr. Phil could've told her that crossdressing is a common fetish among straight men, and that most crossdressers are only interested in indulging themselves from time to time. Dr. Phil could've told her that most crossdressers enjoy normal sexual relations with their wives. He also could've told her that there are support groups for the wives of crossdressers, books she could read, and Internet chat rooms she could visit.

And he could've told her that while it may not be pleasant to contemplate her husband in women's clothes, she doesn't have to contemplate it constantly. If she can't go there, as the kids say, the least she can do is give her husband permission to indulge on his own during solo masturbation sessions. If his occasional indulgence takes nothing away from their sex life, she should be encouraged not to dwell on the mental image of her husband in panties, just as we chose not to dwell on the mental image of Dr. Phil in panties.

It's Savage's last sentence, in my opinion, that is the most important: IF his crossdressing takes nothing away from their sex life, a woman can look the other way if she doesn't like it. But when his pleasure in crossdressing not only interferes with but entirely precludes a couple's mutual sexual satisfaction, there is a problem. When we admit there's a problem, we might find a solution, and too many wives have to find that solution on their own because their boyfriends or husbands are too ashamed to talk about what turns them on. It's a sad state of affairs when a woman—no matter her age—gives up on the intimacy in her committed relationship because her husband won't force himself to be honest—with himself, and with her. It's one thing for a man to be aroused by things that don't necessarily include his wife, but another entirely if he is unwilling to find creative ways for both of them to have a satisfying sex life.

CHAPTER 7

EpiScene*

FOR HALLOWEEN 2002 my husband and I dressed as two of the characters from Neil Gaiman's *Sandman* stories: I went as Delirium, since I'd just dyed my hair bright red, and he went as Desire. Desire is an androge, able to be male or female, or both. S/he is a temptress, a seducer—a home wrecker in either gender. My husband made up like a glamour girl but did not wear a wig. He wore a waist cinch, a tuxedo jacket, fishnet stockings, and high boots. His male chest was bare, nipples occasionally visible when his jacket slid to the side. I found him desirable, and I wasn't the only one. We were going to a Halloween event thrown by our favorite party promoters, Chi Chi Valenti and Johnny Dynell. We went with friends, and as I was getting seats for us all, Betty stopped to talk to a friend near the entrance. A young, attractive gay man approached him. I was busy talking but heard my husband shout my name. He was pointing me out to the man, who came over to talk to me a moment later.

"So you're his wife?"

I nodded.

"As in married?"

I nodded again.

"As in married married?" Again, I nodded. I showed him my wedding band and engagement ring. We talked for a little while about clubs in New York, and he introduced me to a friend of his. It was all very amiable. Then he asked for my husband's phone number. I must have looked surprised, because he asked if our phone numbers were the same.

"Well of course they are," I explained, "we're married!"

"Oh, like really married?" he asked.

---

*ep·i·cene ('e-pə-,sēn) adj., 1: having an ambiguous sexual identity [syn: bisexual] 2: having unsuitable feminine qualities [syn: effeminate, emasculate, cissy, sissified, sissyish, sissy] Source: WordNet ® 1.6, © 1997 Princeton University

"Like really married," I added. "With papers. Monogamous. All that. Married."

As if to clarify, he pointed at my husband, who was standing about ten feet away. "You're married to him."

I nodded again.

"But he's gay," the man said.

"No, he's not." I explained. "I'm married to him. We have sex like married people."

"But he said he does drag."

"He does. He's a crossdresser. He's a straight guy who does drag."

At that, the man laughed. "Oh, you're putting me on!" He decided I must have been pulling his leg the whole time. He glanced back at my husband again. "So what's his number?"

"The same as mine."

"You're not kidding."

"No," I explained again, "we're married. Husband and wife. Didn't he tell you I was his wife?" (I know my husband always does.)

"Well, yes, but I figured he meant 'wife,' you know, not really. I mean a lot of guys have 'wives.'" I understood what he meant; gay men have often met married men who are not as straight as their wives believe them to be.

"But do guys who 'have wives' usually introduce you to their wives?"

"No, but—look at him." And I did. My husband is beautiful as a man or a woman, but unbelievably beautiful when he's something in-between. Others have compared him to a young David Bowie, which is about the highest compliment an androge can get. I think I eventually got it through the guy's head that really, my husband was straight, we were married, and we were monogamous. He shook his head at me every time we ran into him that night as if to say "poor girl doesn't know her husband's gay." His reaction isn't atypical.

We have been asked by lesbians how we have sex. We were once asked by a Hassidic Jew at a bondage club if we were into S/M. Most often we're asked if we're looking for a third. When we clung together at clubs in the early days of our romance, we didn't get approached at all. We were wallflowers in the Versailles Room, as Rose Royalle, a downtown denizen, once described us, and we kept to ourselves: we dressed, we came, we watched, we left. But now that we've been together five years, we split up at clubs. We bring friends. We have started to recognize faces, and we mingle. As a result, it's much harder for people to understand that we're a couple. But we are; as devoted and loyal as we were when we didn't talk to anyone but each other.

* * *

IT'S ONLY IN the past few years that a significant number of crossdressers started going out in public at all. Many have wives and girlfriends who are unwilling to participate, so they often venture out alone or with "sisters." As a result, few people realize that crossdressers are mostly straight ("mostly" as in: 1) most of them are straight; but also as in 2) most of them are "primarily heterosexual." Because of their public presentation and behavior, they're usually read as homosexual. Many crossdressers en femme have fantasies of being with men, others let men buy them drinks, and some are bisexual, so when people see them in bars, they're often flirting with men. Crossdressers have been welcome in gay clubs, where boys in dresses are assumed to be gay. That they are usually unaccompanied by girlfriends "confirms" their sexuality.

But the majority of crossdressers prefer women. The only problem is, women don't often prefer crossdressers. And even those women who wind up married to crossdressers usually forego public outings, which means my husband and I are often the first heterosexual couple composed of a genetic female and her crossdressing boyfriend that other people have met. They've never heard of such a thing. If they can accept the idea that the guy in the dress is straight, then they still have to jump the hurdle of trying to understand why on earth I'd want to be with a guy who is "less than a man." And that's often too much to ask of a person who's had a few drinks. Snow, a woman in her early twenties who I interviewed for this book, says it's easier for people to accept the fact that she's polyamorous than it is for them to understand that both of her boyfriends are t-girls: the concept is too new, even for the younger generation.

Of course, other people just get it, like the lesbian woman who asked us how we have sex. She loved the idea. "They both get to play both parts," she explained to a friend who'd joined us. "I'd love that—I wouldn't have to lead every time."

A night out for us is often an "outreach" opportunity, and the other wives and crossdressers who have been out as couples know exactly what I mean. We are the first of our kind people have met, and we end up informing others of the existence of straight crossdressers. We end up answering more and more personal questions as the night goes on. Crossdressers aren't expected to be out. They're supposed to be at home, in the closet, whether their wives know or not. No one expects crossdressers to be out at bars having drinks with their wives—that would be obscene. Sometimes other people's assumptions make me feel like the Loch Ness monster: something between a myth and a joke.

TRI-ESS AND THE OLD ORDER OF THINGS

ONCE A CROSSDRESSER is determined to step out of the closet, he's still baffled as to where exactly he can go. Traditionally, his first step was a support group, like Tri-Ess, or the Society for the Second Self. Tri-Ess is a national organization for crossdressers which reports a membership of about 1,300. Tri-Ess was formed by Virginia (nee Charles) Prince—who was running a group called FPE (Femme Personality Expression) and who had formerly started the "Hose and Heels" club back in the 1950s—and Carol Beecroft, who was running a group called Mamselle Sorority. In 1976, after some negotiation, the groups merged to form Tri-Ess.

Tri-Ess is a national organization with local chapters, or "sororities," which like all sororities use Greek letters for their names. Before Tri-Ess started forming local "sorority" chapters all over the nation, most crossdressers didn't even know there were other crossdressers. Once they joined, they started getting magazines like *Transgender Tapestry* and *The Femme Mirror* mailed discreetly to their homes or offices or post office boxes. These magazines were their only contact with any others of their community. As an organization, Tri-Ess has always been a "safe" place for married crossdressers. A crossdresser could bring his wife and receive support in convincing her that she was not facing life with a crossdresser alone, and that if kept a secret, crossdressing could be tolerated. In this, Tri-Ess has accomplished wonders. Tri-Ess deserves credit for single-handedly alleviating the misery in crossdressers' lives.

Local Tri-Ess chapters are required to follow the national charter, but they elect their own officers, schedule meetings, and collect their own dues. Generally speaking, chapters meet monthly in a discreet space so that members arriving en femme don't have to feel too conspicuous. There is usually a changing room for those who can't dress elsewhere and a main room for socializing. Usually one of the veteran CDs makes a few announcements and asks for reports on "sisters" who are absent. Otherwise people eat, drink, and mingle.

The Chi Delta Mu (CDM) chapter meeting my husband and I attended was held in two rooms of a motel in New Jersey. My membership in Tri-Ess prevents me from giving more detail than that. We were told where to find the hotel and given these mysterious instructions: *There is an outside staircase behind a wall, opposite the swimming pool.*

Entering a nearly vacant motel via a back entrance is depressing. The secrecy quickly translated into a sense of shame. Why couldn't we walk through the main entrance? Why wouldn't the guy at the desk greet us and direct us to where we were going? Was this discretion part of the group's agreement with the motel?

We crept around back, and walked up the stairs surrounded by the scent of cold chlorine from the nearby pool. The door was open a crack.

A roomful of crossdressers is a real sight. There were "sisters" gathered in the usual social groupings: three or four chatting around the coffee, one or two engaged in private conversation in the corner, a few talking amiably around a table while others sat and listened. Most of them didn't even look up when we walked in. There was no "new members" corner for us, so we took seats near the door while I had a look around. One of the members, Tammie, had been a member of CDOD, but I'd only met her once in person and wasn't sure if I'd recognize her.

A lot of crossdressers come to CDM for a safe place to dress. They cannot dress in their own homes because their wives forbid it, or because they have not told their wives they are crossdressers. Meetings like these are often referred to as "a bigger closet" in that many of the attendees are still not known as crossdressers to anyone other than their "sisters." They have found a place to crossdress and to be treated as women for one night a month, and that is incredibly satisfying to many of them. Their participation has a tremendous impact on decreasing their shame.

At the meeting we attended, there were a few bad wigs but otherwise most of the "ladies" were dressed appropriately for their age and body type. A younger blonde "woman" wore tight jeans and a tight shirt; an older "lady" with a blunt brown wig wore lime green pants and blouse. (I always notice when crossdressers wear pants: If a genetic woman wearing pants is cross-dressing, a crossdresser wearing pants is a man who's crossdressing as a woman who's crossdressing?) There were also a few crossdressers who looked like they were transitioning transsexuals, and I found out later they were.

Eventually someone asked us if we were new, and we started mingling and being introduced. Just when we'd gotten into a conversation, one of the elected officers announced a trip to Dress Barn. The store had closed an hour early to accommodate exclusively the "girls" of CDM.

Shopping with crossdressers is very different from shopping with genetic women. There are no complaints about fat butts or big hips, and when a blouse pulls on its front buttons, a large back is usually causing the trouble, not breasts. I am not an avid shopper and can usually evaluate the mer-chandise in a medium-sized store in about five minutes. I spent another five minutes perusing the racks for my husband, and then, with nothing else to do, waited outside the dressing rooms where the other ladies were trying things on. I gave advice where I could, and for the fun of it, tried a few things on myself. I started to feel like someone's chubby kid sister because the other "women" around me were all on the tall side with men's long thin legs, and that pretty much ruined my fun. I bought a tuxedo-front white blouse, which was probably the only man-tailored item purchased that night.

When we returned to the meeting, "girls" who hadn't come to Dress Barn were already eating pizza, showing each other pictures of recent outings, calling each other names and generally behaving like a group of people who have known each other a while. I was congratulated on being an accepting wife. One of the younger CDs told me his wife came to meetings but wasn't at this one for want of a babysitter. As it was, I was the only genetic woman in the room besides a Mary Kay lady, who had gift baskets for Valentine's Day set up on one of the tables. We were both wearing comfortable shoes.

As the meeting wound to a close, we found out some of the "sisters" were downstairs at the motel's bar. We went down to say hello and have a drink, and the mood in the bar was considerably different. These "girls" were the ones who regularly went to bars. As René explained to me, she didn't need to come to a "support" meeting like CDM: she went out all the time. But she had made friends at CDM, and liked to support the new arrivals. I was quickly informed that some of the Tri-Ess rules are bent by local chapters:

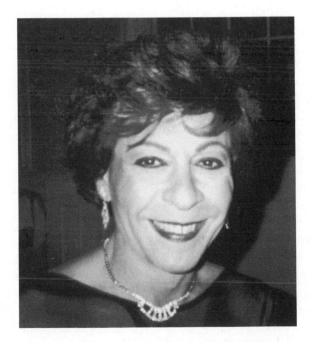

René

one CD told me he considers himself bisexual, and another verified my suspicion that one of the meeting's attendees was in fact a transitioning transsexual woman. When I asked why these rules were bent, one of the other
crossdressers pointed out that it's impossible to police sexuality (*tell that to
the Religious Right,* I thought), and that most members were not interested
in prying. As long as everyone understood that propositioning other members was unacceptable, variance in sexuality was covertly accepted. "Do
we expel those who would like to do it in order to prove they are women?"
one member asked. By "do it" she meant "have sex with men." Ditto for
those who might be experimenting, or trying to find out—once and for all—
if wearing a dress means they are gay, as they've been told their whole lives.
As for the transitioning woman: she was an active and long-standing member, and no one was going to ask her to leave. She was, after all, a friend, and
she would need the support of her "sisters" during her difficult transition
period. No one had the heart to deny her that support, knowing what she
would be up against with the rest of the world.

René convinced the bartender to let us order drinks even though it was
almost closing time, and we finished them quickly. I spoke to a lovely CD
who told me "she" had only told his own (genetic) sister about "her"
crossdressing in the event "she" died suddenly, so as to spare their parents' finding his boxes of women's clothes. The sister didn't want to see
him en femme face to face, but she had seen pictures. She didn't ask questions, but she did pass sample perfumes and discarded clothes onto her
crossdressing brother.

I don't think I've ever heard anything more depressing, and yet the way
"she" told the story was so matter-of-fact I didn't pity him at all. I was
struck, instead, by how practical he was about it. These were the facts of his
life as a crossdresser and he had decided that his parents would never know.
I respected him for that. He told me about a few of the resort weekends for
crossdressers he'd been to. He didn't expect to meet a woman who could
accept him as he was, and couldn't be with someone who didn't know the
whole truth about him. He was hardly old enough to toss in the romantic
towel at forty-something. He wanted kids, and knew he'd never have any.
Aren't there thousands of women out there dying for a partner?

I continued to think about his story once we were in our car heading
home. And all I could think was that no eligible woman I knew would ever
consider dating him, despite the fact that he made a decent living and seemed
like he'd make a reasonably handsome man. His romantic prospects weren't
dim just because he wears a dress, but because he believes himself—and is—
unloved for wearing a dress. He is a Tri-Ess member, and is still not getting

the support he needs. I wondered if that had something to do with the fact that he cannot openly admit his bisexuality.

Something is wrong with this picture.

CDM ALSO THREW a spring dinner/dance at a hotel near to the one where the meetings are held. It was something like what I imagined all those Kiwanis dinners were that my mom and dad used to attend. Or maybe a bad wedding. Either way, it wasn't full of couples but instead mostly single crossdressers, trannies, and transsexuals. In a room of more than a hundred people, six of us were genetic women. One CD was there with his girlfriend and it was "her" first time out; Meredith was there to see her husband Victoria en femme for the first time; the third woman was Michelle, Tammie's wife; a fourth was the wife of a crossdresser I knew, the fifth was Karen of Femme Fever, and then there was me. The first two I assumed would never return. Michelle would come as long as Tammie, a real veteran who has given many years of her service to Tri-Ess, would come. The fourth wife I met only briefly. I didn't get to meet Karen, who wasn't an SO but the owner of an organization that caters to CDs. Where were the rest of the wives and girlfriends?

Something is wrong with this picture.

THERE ARE OTHER problems experienced by members of Tri-Ess. Valerie is a closet crossdresser and does not go to her local Tri-Ess meetings, because he didn't feel he was getting any help. He explains:

> The other support groups in this locale are diluted with hetero, homo, and bisexuals. That doesn't bother me as much as their dress code, i.e., they require crossdressing to attend meetings, which I cannot do. Tri-Ess has no such requirement. Since my wife is nonaccepting of my proclivity, I cannot take advantage of what Tri-Ess has to offer in the area of spousal cooperation and social activities . . . and my chapter "sisters" have been of no support for me. Their attitude has been one of "Crossdress and come join us!" without regard of my circumstances of a) having no experience in the fine art of feminine presentation to the point of going out in public, and b) having no female wardrobe which precludes dressing at the meeting's location. I don't even have a decent wig. So I still remain in the "closet" at home, rather than attending meetings in only a larger "closet," i.e., a sequestered and secluded hotel suite.

He does dress at home but doesn't think his feminine presentation is acceptable for a more public gathering. His, of course, is only one crossdresser's story. I do not know which Tri-Ess chapter he is referring to, but clearly the idea behind the organization is to give exactly this type of crossdresser somewhere to go. He explained to me that he hasn't pushed himself to ask anyone for help, that it's no one's fault but his own. He has no community, when he is supposed to be exactly the kind of crossdresser Tri-Ess is out to make feel welcomed.

Something is wrong with this picture.

I'M SURE MANY other inconsistences with Tri-Ess fall onto the shoulders of the local chapter leadership, but there are other problems that seem to be caused inadvertently by Tri-Ess's membership restrictions. Tri-Ess's intention to cater exclusively to heterosexual crossdressers was explained to me by Gerri, a crossdresser who runs the Chapter Outreach division of the organization:

> *The reason Tri-Ess is primarily a Hetero-CD organization is to try and get timid spouses to attend meetings and learn to be a little more open minded. As Victoria Prince put it, When a spouse attends a Tri Ess meeting for the first time to try and learn why her CD husband wants to*

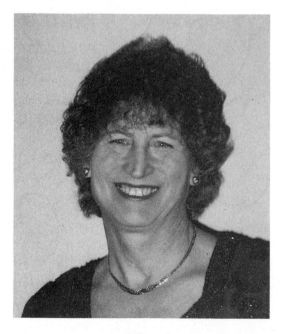

Tammie

*dress up like a girl, she doesn't want to sit next to a TS person that wants
to talk about SRS. I know that I attended a Tiffany Club meeting in the
Boston Area and the TS folks there scared the hell out of me. So I went
looking for a group like Tri-Ess.*

Crossdressers and their genetic female partners are often an exception within
the larger TG community, and I appreciate Tri-Ess' attempt to address our
particular issues. To me, however, barring transsexual women—many of
whom spend their lives thinking they are "just crossdressers"—isn't a productive response.

Apparently barring transsexual women from full membership doesn't
necessarily encourage wives to come. Valerie, whose wife is not willing to
participate, doesn't feel comfortable socializing without his spouse. "She"
explains:

*As for going out to chapter social activities, as I said, I prefer to go
places with my spouse. We are also newlyweds, forty-one years worth!!
Seems most of my "sisters" are divorced or separated and dating. The
ones who are married seldom bring their spouses . . . that's their choice.
So it turns out to be more of a "guy's night out" for the group anyway,
with a few GGs attending.*

I want to be clear that I fully appreciate Tri-Ess's purpose and the role it
plays in the crossdressing community. Tri-Ess intends to keep its membership restricted to heterosexual crossdressers precisely so it can offer support to a very specific set of people and directs its magazines, website, and
conferences to them. This targeted approach—and the motives behind it—
can't be faulted: I know wives who can't even look at pictures of crossdressed men. Crossdressers who spend their time and energy making sure
other "girls" have somewhere to go for support—and maybe just a place
to dress—have my full appreciation. Tammie has put in twelve years of
service at CDM, despite the fact that she probably hears more criticism
than praise, and despite the fact that she identifies as a transsexual who
has withheld from transitioning out of love for her wife. Other members
of local chapters are equally generous of their time and effort. There are no
doubt hundreds of such unsung heroes as Tammie in the crossdressing
community: those who have found some peace with their crossdressing
and wish to share it with others. Barbara Van Horn's local chapter, Chi
Epsilon Sigma, recently did a presentation about crossdressing for a
Human Sexuality class at a local college. It proved an educational and

liberating experience both for the crossdressers—who found themselves accepted by the students—and for the students, who appreciated getting to meet a few crossdressers in real life and not just in textbooks.

Older crossdressers who have just come out to their wives find Tri-Ess a kind of found paradise, a place where they can, once and for all, truly be themselves, but many also—upon seeing opportunities to transition that didn't exist when they were younger—can cause a late realization of transsexualism, or a crisis of transsexual feelings. Are members who have spent years nurturing a chapter to be told they can't vote anymore? Younger CDs could benefit from their experience and knowledge.

The relief of walking into a room where everyone not only knows your secret but shares it can be liberating for both the crossdresser and his wife. I'm sure Tri-Ess will continue to serve people who, for one reason or another, need to be more secretive about their crossdressing. For them, conversations about how to stay successfully in the closet will be useful. However, nearly every younger couple I've interviewed tells me their experience at Tri-Ess meetings felt "creepy" or "scary" or "uncomfortable." I know I don't want to meet people in motel rooms, no matter how friendly they are. It just seems seedy and full of shame. I also want to be able to tell someone where I'm going in case of car trouble or some other emergency.

Perhaps instead of having one big group, Tri-Ess could welcome more types and tailor meetings to suit the varied membership. A spouse like me, for instance, who wanted to know transsexuals in order to understand if my husband was different from them, and what made him different, might want to be able to meet transsexuals within the supportive community Tri-Ess can be, so I would have other wives and crossdressers to confide in to talk about my experience. Crossdressers have told me they sought out transsexual meetings for the same reason—to finally answer the difficult question of their own transgenderism for themselves—and that they only found the answers once they heard what transsexual women had to say about their own experiences. If the group's discussion for one month was transsexualism, those who were not ready or able or interested in such could stay home. When CDM went to Dress Barn, some of the crossdressers chose not to come: meetings could be scheduled similarly, with some in one room opting for a discussion of these topics, while the others did their usual socializing in another.

Likewise, there is a new generation coming up that could be served by more open communication about sex and coming out, which might start on the basis that new couples are more likely than the old generation to be more at peace with their crossdressing. One CD told me recently it has never occurred to him that he should feel ashamed or guilty for being turned on by crossdressing, and that when he went to a meeting whose topic was about shame and guilt he started to wonder if he should. Younger women now often know about their partners' crossdressing long before marriage, and start in a more accepting place. They feel uncomfortable talking about their acceptance with women who are still angry about being betrayed. The younger women I've spoken to absolutely understand why the others are so angry, but they're not. They don't want to make the women who weren't told upfront to feel any worse, and stay silent about feeling accepting. As a result, they may feel they don't belong in Tri-Ess in the first place. Again, tailoring a local group's discussion might help. Announcing that the group's conversation will be about sexuality will allow those who aren't ready to stay home, or have a separate meeting. It will let those who are ready for the conversation talk about it openly.

It is clear that the problem with Tri-Ess is not its members, but its outdated approach and its stubbornly narrow focus. As one of the members of CDM recently told me, "If Tri-Ess keeps insisting on only their definition of heterosexual crossdressers, there's going to be ten people left in the organization." I've heard the same kinds of thoughts from others in the community, some of whom put the number closer to three. In a nutshell, what Tri-Ess needs, in my opinion, is a community within the community, something like Tri-Ess's "next generation." Younger crossdressers do need an organization that's specific to them, and so do their wives. Likewise, I've heard wisdom from older crossdressers—a lecture on hormones by Jane Ellen Fairfax comes to mind—that would be incredibly useful for crossdressers who, tempted by illegal hormones and easy access to them, have a more difficult minefield to step through than even a previous generation. They need to hear this stuff, but they're not coming to the conferences. Perhaps by encouraging younger people to join and to be honest about what they want, Tri-Ess will find ways to change in order not to become vestigial. As it stands right now, Tri-Ess's membership has steadily decreased since the 1980s.

ALTERNATIVE MODELS

WE ALSO WENT to another meeting sponsored by Renaissance, another transgender association. Renaissance was founded by JoAnn Roberts, Angela Gardner, Alison Laing, Trudy Henry, and Melanie Bryan in the spring of 1987. Renaissance is the definition of inclusive:

*Everyone who identifies as transgendered, is close to a transgendered
person, or has a professional interest in transgendered people is welcome
at Renaissance: transvestites, transsexuals, counselors, therapists, and
clergy—male or female—are all invited to learn more about this behavior. Spouses, partners, and friends are especially welcome to participate
at chapter meetings. Renaissance is not concerned about your political
affiliation, ethnic background, religion, education, economic status or
sexual preference. It is concerned, however, about respecting the rights
and privacy of its members and expects everyone to act accordingly.*

The members of the Mid-Hudson Valley Transgender Association—or
MHVTA—chose Renaissance's affiliation because Renaissance would allow
them to include the entire transgender spectrum, and Jan, the group's founder,
says the membership is 60 percent crossdressers, 15 percent transsexual, and
25 percent who are unsure where they fall on the TG spectrum. Her logic for
creating a more inclusive group is based on her belief that "we are all in it
together." When MHVTA was just starting out, inclusiveness helped boost
membership, and Jan was aware that the group would fill a void for those
otherwise bereft of TG support. Also, they had several active members who
were TS early on, and Jan hated the idea of expelling "sisters" who had
become friends. MHVTA invited someone to speak about electrolysis, a topic
that might not be as welcome in a group exclusively for CDs since many
wives of CDs draw the line at permanent physical changes. The "girls" who
attend MHVTA are not all transgendered, however: Jan is a crossdresser, and
he founded the group before he even told his own wife he crossdresses.

We had to go to the back of the motel again, of course. I'm convinced at this
point that crossdressers just like to be near water, as the motel rooms in which
they hold their meetings are always near the pool. It was the same setup: a
small changing room connected to a larger meeting room, with soda and chips
and donuts. Melissa's girlfriend Denise was the only other genetic woman
present, and again, she and I were the only ones wearing comfortable shoes.

Unfortunately, Renaissance—whose policy is more inclusive and whose
focus is outreach and education—serves a more limited region than Tri-Ess.
Renaissance has 500 to 700 members in Pennsylvania, New England, and
the New York tri-state area. They have chapters in only seven states, while
Tri-Ess has thirty-five chapters nationwide but only double Renaissance's
membership. Surely that indicates that Renaissance's more inclusive policy
is more attractive. Renaissance doesn't run any online support groups for
couples or partners as far as I'm aware, and in 2004, that's where most people are getting their support and community.

THE INTERNET REVOLUTION

IRONICALLY, IT MAY be that crossdressing organizations have suffered more from the birth of the Internet than from anything else. The closet at home is still being replaced by a "larger closet," but now that larger closet is cyber. The traditional network of secret support groups may, as a result, fall by the wayside.

The Internet may be the biggest single factor in changing the cross-dresser's world. Young men who don't like sports end up on computers, and the incidence of "geeks" who crossdress is astounding. As a result, there are many, many sites for crossdressers on the Internet, from those sponsored by groups like Tri-Ess to private sites maintained by individual crossdressers. There is TG Forum, an online transgender magazine started by Joann Roberts (a crossdresser, and one of the co-founders of Renaissance), Cindy Martin, and Jamie Faye Fenton (who is now transitioning), where cross-dressers can get information, education, and community resources. There are online stores that sell to crossdressers with discreet billing, chat rooms, mailing lists, and any number of other forms of "online community." Anyone who has a computer can use a search engine and with words like "crossdressing" or "transvestite" will find resources too numerous to mention. Typing in the search word "crossdressers" in Yahoo yields 161 groups. There are Mormon crossdressers and Florida crossdressers and groups from Indonesia and India. There are groups that serve as "bulletin boards" for the local sororities of Tri-Ess. Lacey Leigh moderates a list called "Closeted Crossdresser," and the list I've run for the past few years, CDOD, shows up, too. These communities represent the entire spectrum of crossdressers' interests. There are support groups for couples, support groups just for partners, and groups where the exchange is all about how to look your best en femme. In others, crossdressers share erotic stories featuring crossdressing. When I first went online, there were only a handful of groups, but while I've been running CDOD, several more have emerged and flourish.

There's a New Yorker cartoon by Peter Steiner in which a dog at a computer says to another dog, "On the Internet, nobody knows you're a dog." no one knows you're a crossdresser, either, or a woman or a man. Plenty of crossdressers go online en femme to meet others. Others go online with femme names and never tell a soul they're men. They get the satisfaction of "passing" even if they're six feet two inches and 240 pounds, which they probably never would in real life.

But passing online is not the same as passing in the Real World. The Internet may be a useful substitute for many in small towns, but most crossdressers desperately want to go out. They want to be out in the world and hear the sound their heels make in the gravel of the parking lot, feel their skirts blown against legs in pantyhose. They want to drop their car keys casually into their purses as they wait for the maitre d' to open the door for them. They want to go out in the world as women. They'll probably do so by getting their "support" online and in books, and skip the "larger closet" of support groups altogether.

PASSING

SO WHY DOESN'T the crossdresser just stay home? Getting all dressed up with no place to go is just no fun. Crossdressers all want to be out. I can't tell you why. Maybe it's the thrill of it, the masquerade, or maybe it's just the experience of being able to be their true selves and be accepted in public. No matter the reason, almost all crossdressers I've met want to be out en femme. The veterans carry pictures of themselves in public places in their purses, and if you ask, they'll show you: "Here's me at the Washington Monument, here's me in Times Square, and here's me in front of the Houses of Parliament." It's a veteran's badge. Crossdressers are very proud when they've been out en femme, much to the dismay of CDs who are still in the closet. The closeted CD is often convinced the out crossdressers "pass" no matter what the out CD might say about going out. The closeted CD tells "herself" that "she" can't pass, and that's why—"she" explains to herself— "she" can't go out. It's not that simple. Some of the CDs who go out fail to pass but go out anyway. Conversely, crossdressers who could pass still might be too terrified to go out. Others are just perfectionists who, if they can't achieve their personal feminine goal, won't let another soul see them.

A crossdresser is passing when "she" goes out en femme and comes home thinking everyone who saw "her" actually thought she was a genetic woman. Some crossdressers pass some of the time, others pass none of the time, and almost none of them pass all of the time. When my husband and I walk into a dinner party for crossdressers and the attendees wonder who the two lesbians are and if we're in the wrong room, my husband has just "passed." When a crossdresser goes up to a Macy's register en femme to purchase a scarf and the clerk only looks up when "she" gives the clerk a credit card with a male name on it, "she" was passing until he handed over the card. Most of the time people register gender from the most obvious clues: breasts, lipstick, and nail polish. My husband was called "ma'am" on a flight once even though the only femme thing about him was his painted nails. We realized afterward that the flight attendant probably only ever looks at hands when he's serving food. (Either that, or the steward had transgendered friends.) It can be harder to pass when the expectation in a certain situation is that you are a man in a dress, and all the other "girls" are men in dresses, too, like at crossdressing events or clubs.

My husband doesn't aim to pass, though for years the fear that he wouldn't or couldn't was his chief reason for not going out. He is sometimes still disappointed when he doesn't. He is still a perfectionist about how he looks, however. He aims to go out as his femme self, and it's more important for him to feel feminine than to "pass." He wants to go out and be treated as his femme self and that might be exactly why he passes at all. He smiles a lot. He also happens to be an actor and that doesn't hurt: I've seen him play "bad guy" roles and even I hate him for the two hours he's onstage. He brings that talent to his femme side. He's also not very tall or broad-shouldered, and he doesn't have very large hands or feet. He's relatively hairless, and he's got well-shaped lips. Tweezing his eyebrows helps a lot. He wears good wigs and natural makeup, and, like a genetic woman, he dresses appropriately for the occasion more than for his own pleasure, which means he wears flats and no stockings when he's out shopping on a warm afternoon. All of these aspects help him pass, but there is no one single thing that "does the trick."

My husband has also been "read" or "clocked." One of the first times I got him to leave the house, he made it about half a block before a woman looked at him a little too closely and he wanted to go back home. Children and teenaged girls are especially good at clocking crossdressers. Kids are still learning about gender and haven't learned yet that it's impolite to point and ask questions. Teenaged girls are constantly sizing up other women for fashion tips and for help in acquiring their own (fashion) identities.

My husband's voice is usually what gives him away. Sometimes he remembers to soften his tone, which is enough to do the trick, but he often forgets and out comes his big, gorgeous, booming actor's baritone. Though his aim isn't to pass, he is always amused when someone takes him for a woman before he opens his mouth. Recently we were waiting for an elevator and a couple stepped aside to let us get on first. He looked us both over head to toe in the discreet way a married man does when his wife is right behind him. The elevator went up, and as we came to our floor, my husband—without even thinking about it—said "This is us." As the elevator doors shut behind us, we heard the man yell: "Holy shit!"

That's passing. It may occasionally be amusing, but it can be dangerous, too: a crossdresser doesn't want to attract the attention of a man whose homosexual panic is going to kick in the minute he hears a male voice. People usually don't appreciate being fooled, and it's the foolhardy crossdresser who thinks he's fooling anyone. Most crossdressers, like Lacey Leigh, advise CDs to refrain from expecting—or trying—to pass. "You'll never be mistaken for a genetic female 100 percent of the time," she writes in *Out and About,* "so get over it." Leigh especially deplores the way crossdressers who "pass" in public express embarrassment about their "sisters" who don't, suggesting that any crossdresser who feels that way might have some of her own shame left. She advocates a big smile and professional clothes and advises a crossdresser to work her way through the world with confidence. Most crossdressers—especially novices—might not be ready to smile and sure as hell don't feel confident, so what are they supposed to do?

They fake it. Only the rare person feels genuinely confident walking into a job interview, and no crossdresser ever went outside for the first time feeling confident. The idea is to go out and have fun en femme, not to pass.

Gina Lance of *Girl Talk* gets a little ruffled when readers assume that "she" and her staff all pass. "Because of the magazine, people think we pass all the time. We don't." She points out that the difference for her is that she's out. Her local post office knows who "she" is, and knows her as a guy, too. She also has a sense of humor about being out: once she brought a group of crossdressers to a busy L.A. lunch spot, and told the Maitre d' the entertainment had arrived. When a crossdresser boasts to Gina "I was at the mall in six-inch heels and a miniskirt and I passed!," Gina points out that it's more likely that no one cared, not that no one knew. If my conservative grandmother wasn't shocked at watching a quarterback-sized man try on size 12 pumps while helping my sister shop for her wedding shoes nearly twenty years ago, no one will be. (She only advised he get a lower heel so he could walk more comfortably. She was always practical about shoes.)

"Passing" sidesteps the whole issue of acceptance, anyway. It may be a thrill to feel like everyone thinks you're a woman, but the more experienced crossdressers simply want to be accepted as crossdressers. Lacey Leigh offers:

> Crossdressers who wish to pass physically *are aiming too low. They would be much better served developing the confidence, character, grace, and manners which will allow them to pass* socially. *The former is living in the shadows; the latter is blossoming in the light.*

In other words, the crossdresser who passes socially is being accepted as a crossdresser, and is doing herself, and her sisters—a world of good. She is showing by example that being a crossdresser is nothing to be ashamed of. Despite the fact that crossdressers adore being treated respectfully as women—and are amused at their occasional successes at passing—plenty realize that everyone around them is in on the "secret." Besides, taking people by surprise can get old, and it can be dangerous. It's always best for a crossdresser to go out in the world with the mind-set that "she" isn't passing, otherwise he may delude himself when it comes to safety. Just as women are assaulted and attacked merely for being women, transgendered people face similar threats. The reality is, if you're perceived as a woman or a crossdresser, either label could make you a "victim." Crossdressers would be wise to check Leigh's book for excellent safety advice before going out, and reread it periodically to remind themselves of the risks.

THE FIRST TIME OUT

THE FIRST TIME a crossdresser goes out—whether to a Tri-Ess meeting or to a restaurant with a more experienced friend—is an event the crossdresser remembers for the rest of his life. Dixie, a closeted crossdresser, offers this account of her first and only experience out en femme:

> On March 14th, as I drove the short distance back to my hotel, I let my mind wander back to the chain of events which had led to this day. I had e-mailed Karin a couple of weeks before to let her know that I would be in her area soon and asked if she would like to meet and have dinner together. She said she would be delighted. She had already told me quite a while back that she often goes out en femme for dinner after work. She went on to tell me that many of the local restaurants were fully aware that she was a crossdresser, had made good friends with her, and really looked forward to having her come in. Karin suggested I go out as Dixie: at first just the thought of it scared the daylights out of me. But Karin's enthusiasm and confidence planted a little "seed" in the back of my mind that maybe, just maybe, I could do it.
>
> I reached my hotel and took a good long shower. Then I shaved as close as I could with a new blade. Next, I "underdressed" as much as possible and finally put on a shirt and pair of jeans. After loading all my "goodies" into the car—including the outfits I was going to get Karin to help me select from—I closed the door and hit the road.

More than once as I drove down the interstate I questioned my sanity. Karin had asked me, "So what if someone does recognize that you're a crossdresser? You've never seen any of these people before, and will never see them again, and they don't know you from Adam's house cat." She was right. Excitement mixed with fear gripped me as I entered the hotel. I stood at her door for a few seconds contemplating what I was about to do. It was now or never. I tapped on the door. The door opened and there stood a neat and smartly dressed lady. In a low and uncertain voice I asked, "Karin?"

"Dixie?" she replied. We talked for nearly an hour about our marriages and our conversation had put me somewhat at ease. She had so encouraged me that I knew that the time had finally arrived. I went to the car and got my things. I hung up the outfits I'd brought; she chose a simple long-line, long-sleeved red dress I had bought only the day before. I was pleased as I could walk comfortably in the red pumps with the two-inch heel that went with the dress. The next step was hair and makeup. I took great pains in getting everything just right. Karin zipped up the back of my dress and told me I'd do just fine. I picked up my little purse (money, ID, compact and lipstick, cigarettes and lighter). Karin opened the door and out we stepped: that mixed feeling of fear and excitement again. We walked the short distance to her car. The air was circulating around my legs and my shoes were making that distinctive clicking sound as we walked. I was exhilarated!

I pulled my dress back down from where it had "ridden up" from sitting, and we walked toward the restaurant's door. "What am I doing?" again entered my mind for a brief moment and my knees actually got weak. The hostess seated us at a corner table. The nearest customers were three tables away and if they had noticed anything odd they certainly weren't acknowledging it. I am certain the waitress knew we were not the women we were presenting ourselves as, but she was very professional about it and never even looked at us strangely. We did have to ask for straws, as women would, so as not to leave lipstick on the glass. Beads of perspiration formed and I knew what would happen to my makeup if I started to sweat. Once or twice I ventured a quick look around at the other customers, but not once did I find anyone staring at us or hear any derogatory remarks. Since it appeared that we weren't going to be stoned to death I was actually beginning to enjoy myself. I ate, even though I wasn't that hungry. My stomach was still too nervous from the excitement of it all.

At the end of the meal I took my compact out of my purse and proceeded to touch up my powder and freshen my lipstick. Right out there in public! How awesome and feminine that was!

I had about an hour's drive to get back to my own hotel so I decided to remain dressed and drive back that way. I have been out driving many times while en femme, but this time it would be the icing on the cake. During the drive back I smiled as I went over the night's events in my mind. It occurred to me that I had experienced a lot of "firsts" that night. Obviously going out en femme for the first time was the most monumental. But there were other firsts. This was the first time I'd met Karin, the first time I'd met another CD who was dressed, the first time another CD had ever seen me dressed, the first time anyone had ever helped me get dressed, and the first time I had passed anyone's "inspection."

All good things must come to an end: so it was for my debut. As I lay there in bed trying to settle back down from the thrill of the evening I found myself already planning to do this again sometime. I've been told that going out en femme is very addictive and I am quickly discovering that is the truth.

Dixie's "first" is not unlike those of many crossdressers.' Many report surprise at how others didn't seem to notice or to care and how professionally they were treated by store clerks, wait staff, and doormen. My husband's first time out was similarly successful, but a lot of people think that's because we live in New York City. It's not. When someone does notice a crossdresser, it's often to express curiosity, pay a compliment, or ask a question. Some are blunt, but others are very polite, especially if the CD has chosen age-appropriate clothing. Anyone—male or female—wearing a skirt slit up to the hip is going to get a lot of attention, especially if he or she doesn't remember to keep his or her legs together. On the other hand, two demurely dressed "women" at a restaurant won't command attention; they're assumed to be married ladies out to lunch. (There is a rule, known as the Rule of Threes in the CD community: that two "girls" out in public will pass, but three together will be read. My husband and I have found that to be true. If a crossdresser is so intent on "passing," he'll miss out on a lot of fun parties with other "girls"!)

There are alternative ways of going "out" as well. There are businesses that "serve" crossdressers who have never been out by supplying makeovers, wigs, clothes, and even undergarments (with padding). Usually for an exorbitant price, they will transform a man into the best woman he can be. Many of them will also escort the "woman" to a restaurant or club, or to a salon for a manicure, or on some other "fantasy" outing the crossdresser has always dreamed about. Some crossdressers feel ripped off by these services once they realize how little the items they provide otherwise cost, but Colleen says despite having outgrown such services, she was glad she used one for her first few times out. The extra cost, I suppose, buys you peace of mind.

Miss (Veronica) Vera's Finishing School for Boys Who Want to Be Girls is one of these establishments. Miss Vera offers makeovers, and teaches classes in deportment, flirting, and even ballet. She's comfortable with fetishes and will even train a man to be the perfect maid. Her location in downtown Manhattan allows students to shop by day and club by night. She also welcomes significant others.

Karen's Femme Fever, located on Long Island, New York, is a combination makeover service and support group. Karen has a background in both Social Work and Cosmetology, which means she can help a crossdresser with his makeup and counsel him and his girlfriend on issues that arise in their relationship. She holds monthly meetings, and also offers shopping services and photo shoots. The "girls" adore her. Her attitude is indicative of the New Paradigm in the crossdressing community. She explains:

> My philosophy of all this? Simply put is acceptance and loving life—and I guess that's why the Femme Fever gals (all 1,027 of them) are "known" to be the belles of any "ball" they attend. I have no rules like many other organizations—my only rule is that one is respectful and accepting of whatever differences anyone else in the group may have . . . and that they have a good time and support one another. The ages vary greatly, the mind-set of where each gal is "at" with dressing varies greatly as does sexual preference and style etc—and again, none of that matters. . . . All that really matters is to enjoy and accept. And hopefully, it's what I do 24/7 that sets the example.

THE NEW PARADIGM

I'M OFTEN TICKLED to see websites by crossdressers who proudly defend their transvestism but haven't taken a step outside the door. Are these crossdressers "out" because they have managed some degree of self-acceptance, even if it's never been challenged in public by being "clocked"? I wonder if all of the guys who have sites and proclaim themselves out are even out to their own wives. There is great variation as to what "out" means to different crossdressers. Some define it as their victory in the struggle for self-acceptance, others with having overcome shame. By calling themselves "out," others mean they go to Tri-Ess meetings and know other crossdressers. Others' wives are in-the-know. These different definitions reflect personal choices, compromises between desire and practicality. I don't disrespect anyone for being in the closet if that is the only way he can come to terms with his crossdressing. I just wish they wouldn't post advice to other crossdressers on their websites and via mailing lists. They tell others how relieved they are to not feel ashamed but they've never had to ask a bartender for a beer, en femme.

Others are *out*. Their post office, bank, parents, children, coworkers and friends all know they crossdress. Some are politically active—there are two crossdressers on the board of the NTAC (National Transgender Advocacy Coalition)—and others are making inroads with the rest of the transgender community.

The New Paradigm is best expressed as being out and proud, of leaving secret societies behind and being known to the rest of the world. It's about reaching out to other communities, which have been through similar struggles for self-identity. It's about leaving shame behind and embracing a positive attitude. It's not about apology or explanation, but a simple statement of fact: I'm a crossdresser, and I want to be respected for who I am.

The best and most widely known example I've found of the New Paradigm, on the national stage, is Gina Lance's *Girl Talk*. It's a full-color, bi-monthly, glossy magazine aimed at the entire transgender community: from crossdresser to transsexual woman, from straight closet case to out gay man. Gina Lance is the editor-in-chief and a crossdresser. The magazine may be produced in Los Angeles, but it serves a community spread all over the country, from small towns to big cities and everything in-between. The magazine delivers support in a way that vastly differs from the historic model: there are no groups or secret meetings. Readers write to Gina to tell her the magazine has helped them feel good about themselves. Because it's not pornographic or depressing, the magazine can be shown to girlfriends and wives. It shows—by example—that crossdressing is "not something you have to be embarrassed about." *Girl Talk's* photo spreads of TG women in public places are proof that a crossdresser "can go out and do things."

The glamorous quality of the magazine is part of Lance's plan. She modeled it on the old Hollywood magazine *Photoplay* (and admits to other influences, including *People, Allure,* and *Harper's Bazaar*). *Photoplay* in particular celebrated the glamour of movie stars. As Gina puts it, Joan

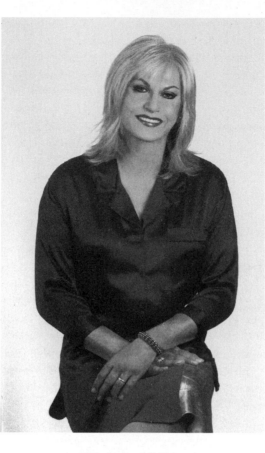

Gina Lance of *Girl Talk*

Crawford was photographed dressed to the nines even to buy groceries. They were staged photos, of course, but *Girl Talk* continues the tradition: to show that TG women can be as beautiful and fashionable—and attractive—as the genetic women they admire. *Girl Talk* has interviewed Genetic Glamour Girls like Eartha Kitt and Julie Newmar and Beverly Garland (who, Gina laughs, wanted a few extra copies to send to her crossdressing friends). They've also featured important figures in the TG community like Eddie Izzard, the comedian, and Patricia Field, who has been designing clothes for club kids and trannies for decades. (Patricia Field's store in Manhattan was the first place I ever saw a transgendered person, and "she" was a salesperson. I have no idea if she was transsexual or a drag queen or a crossdresser, but I very clearly remember my friend saying after we left, "She was a man." It was my first experience of the lovely sentences transgenderism can produce. I was about fourteen years old, and immediately intrigued.)

When Gina and I spoke, what most impressed me was her interest in encouraging the diversity of both her staff and the crossdressing community at large. Her staff is made up of men, women, transsexual women, gays, lesbians, straights, crossdressers—you name it, she's got someone who fits the label working for her. She thinks that this range in perspective only benefits the magazine's large and diverse community of readers. On a more local level, Gina was faced with devising a solution last year to the closing of The Queen Mary, the famous L.A. drag club. Crossdressers didn't know where to go, as the club had been open every night of the week. She scouted three different clubs, and one of them happened to be a forty-year-old gay bar, whose patrons suddenly found their space newly injected with 200 crossdressers. It took a while, but the gay men and the crossdressers got used to each other, and Gina believes that the experience served to help many of the crossdressers overcome their homophobia.

That kind of proactive guidance is exactly what the crossdressing community needs.

Integration with other communities happens in smaller ways all over the country. CDI, or Crossdressers International, is a group local to New York City. It is open to the whole TG community. They held their Valentine's Day dinner last year at the Stonewall Inn, where the Gay and Lesbian Civil Rights Movement was born—started, some like to forget, by drag queens. It seemed only too appropriate to me that a new generation of men who wear dresses should celebrate Valentine's Day there. Watching otherwise-closeted and some heterosexual crossdressers flirt harmlessly with gay bartenders represented a full circle of acceptance. It was the kind of event that indicated—in its own understated way—which way the future lays.

MY HUSBAND AND I have never felt uncomfortable at gay bars or in lesbian spaces, but we also call ahead and ask if the transgendered are welcome. As any drag queen can tell you, some gay bars do not welcome drag queens or crossdressers. In smaller towns, there tends to be more solidarity within the GLBT scene: crossdressers and drag queens are usually welcome in bars with a gay and lesbian clientele. In big cities like New York or Los Angeles or Chicago, there is room for "splintering": different types of bars and clubs for each specific type of clientele. Gay men have their bars, lesbians have theirs, and the transgendered are sometimes forced to choose. Many of these bars do have "tranny friendly" nights, but New York is large enough that these events even seem to serve different types of MTFs. At some, crossdressers feel comfortable.

New York's tranny scene was heavily impacted in recent years by two events: the closing of a bar called Edelweiss, and the gentrification of the meat-packing district. Edelweiss had been a tranny bar for years, and if a crossdresser happened in, "she" might have discovered that a lot of her she-male sisters were there to "work." But Edelweiss closed, and the "girls" had to find a new scene. Likewise, TS working girls (known in street parlance as "tranny whores") were booted out of their neighborhood when the meat-packing district—which had long been an area clubs catering to fetishists, trannies, and the BDSM community—gentrified. Now that the "normal" people are going to restaurants in that area, the alternative sex community has had to find somewhere else to go. (Many of these clubs are still looking for permanent homes, in fact.)

En masse, the "girls" of Edelweiss and the meat-packing district's street-walkers eventually found club events that were conducive to their trade: Glorya Wholesome's nights at NOW bar are rife with what my husband and I call "pros." To be fair, Glorya herself has tried to attract a broader range of the TG community, but the presence of the working girls will likely keep crossdressers and their partners away. Why? I have found that TS "working girls" resent the presence of a genetic woman and her crossdressing husband. My husband has gotten a lot of what gay men call "shade" from TS working girls as well, maybe for looking good, maybe for having a female companion. Even when a crossdresser and his girlfriend make it clear that they're not there to infringe on anyone's business, it can be a hugely uncomfortable environment. I don't have an issue with women—genetic or otherwise—working as prostitutes, and have long thought prostitution should be made legal for the safety and health of the "girls" and their johns. I also understand that a lot of TS women work in the sex industry because transitioning is expensive and rarely covered by health insurance. I'm not there to judge anyone—I'm the one married to the guy in the dress, after all—but I've found a lot of the pros are so ready for me to be judgmental that they start throwing attitude before I've even taken off my coat. There is also a weird ambience created when some women are advertising themselves as objects to the "chasers" who are there; I find myself ogled in very discomforting ways as a result, which is no fun. Whenever we've been to evenings at NOW bar, I've insisted on accompanying my husband to the bathroom, where we use the ladies' room together. (Why? Because I know the kind of pressure oversexed and dis-respectful men can lay on a girl, and my husband isn't as experienced in dealing with it. By going with him I don't have to worry, and we get a moment's private conversation, to boot.)

There are clubs where crossdressers might feel more at home, and where male admirers treat the "girls" like ladies. The Silver Swan—German restaurant by day, t-girl hangout by night—hosts one of these nights. Crossdressers can gather to dress up, dance, and chat. "Admirers" are welcome, as are genetic women, friends, or dates, or anyone else. The atmosphere is a little closeted, but has opened up in the time we've been going. Early on, there was no sign on the door, and I felt like I was entering a speakeasy during Prohibition. Now there's a big Silver Swan and a sign out front. Ina's friendly face collects cover charges at the door, and it feels much more welcoming and less seedy as a result. When admirers chat up my husband, some of them will even chat with me once they learn I'm his wife. (Others, who are looking for sex, realize they're barking up the wrong tree and find a graceful, or occasionally graceless, way to exit the conversation.) Some of them are unaware that t-girls are often heterosexual, and the idea that a genetic woman would enjoy being with a t-girl usually tickles them pink. A recent visitor from Hong Kong couldn't understand our relationship. I finally told him that when my husband is dressed as a guy, we're straight, and when he's en femme, we're lesbians. Finally the metaphorical light bulb lit over his tourist's head. (His interest only redoubled.) Another man engaged me in a long conversation about why genetic women can't accept their husbands' crossdressing.

There are always genetic women at Silver Swan—some obviously as supportive friends, others as dates. I'm certain I've even seen a few sisters and moms. I have not met many genetic women at these outings, but it's usually because I'm at a loss for an introduction, and it seems odd to just approach someone and say hi. (Sometimes, too, you're not sure if a "girl" is genetic or not.) These nights have had more of a European pub atmosphere. Everyone is drinking, dancing, and dating, but nothing feels "dirty." I worry that may change, because so far I enjoy this scene. The only thing it's still missing is your basic "heterosexual" element.

There are, of course, the admirers, but I'm not sure they count as your ordinary heterosexuals, because they usually don't hit on genetic women. In fact, crossdressers hit on women more frequently, in my experience, than male admirers do. Watching Colleen, a crossdresser, in her tight little black dress flirt with a cute blonde woman—and watching the cute blonde woman flirt back—made me happy to see that it is possible for a hetero CD to get a date en femme.

We didn't want to hang out with only crossdressers, so our only alternatives were gay and lesbian bars, or the bars frequented by folks who enjoy other alternate sexualities: the BDSM, goth, and fetish scenes. For us, all of them came together in a place called Mother.

Mother spoiled us. We started dating when Mother was still in operation as a place, and the weekly themed night Click + Drag was more than any crossdresser and his girlfriend could hope for. Unfortunately, it was one of the many places ousted by the meat-packing district's gentrification, and its loss is still deeply felt. The community of Mother-lovers is online these days, and Mother's organizers—Chi Chi Valenti and Johnny Dynell—still throw parties on special nights (Halloween, New Year's, or Betty Page retrospectives) at various clubs around town. These nights were by far the best club experiences we have ever had. An older friend to whom we showed pictures

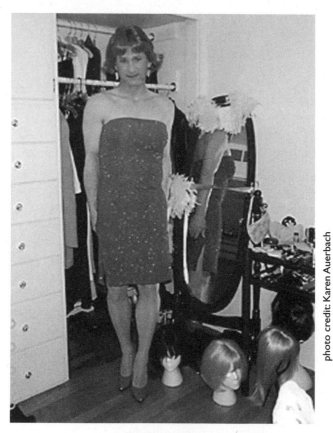

photo credit: Karen Auerbach

Kimmi in red dress.

said that Mother was the only place that seemed reminiscent to her of the wild days of the 1970s New York club scene. That is no small compliment: before AIDS devastated NYC's population in the 1980s, the club scene here was purportedly only rivaled by Weimar Berlin's.

Unfortunately, we don't know of any club that has filled the void: where crossdressers mix with drag queens, where latex and crinoline fetishists can exchange notes at the bar, and where masters can command their slaves without anyone batting an eyelid. Colleen said she would only ever feel comfortable hitting on a genetic woman while en femme at Mother. Straight men may come to watch the burlesque, but they know they might get hit on by men when they're there, too. Anything can happen—and everything does. I think my favorite moment of all time at Mother was a night themed Dog and Pony Show, during which (mostly) women showed what good ponies they can be. The members of the incredibly diverse crowd, "weird" by most standards, seemed to be looking at the stage thinking "Well I don't get it but if it turns them on . . ." That kind of tolerance—even without understanding—is priceless. It was at Mother that I realized that with the right attitude—and a little effort—it's possible for a scene to engender diversity in real ways that affect real people. My feminine husband felt affirmed, and so did I: there were women at Mother twice my size who were obviously making the men around them hot. I'm thankful that when we first started going out, we had Mother. Unfortunately it set a very high standard, one that I've not seen met anywhere else by anyone else.

The sad reality is that being the wife of a crossdresser can be remarkably lonely, and some days I feel too much in common with Ken, the admirer I interviewed for the sexuality chapter: the drag queens don't necessarily understand that my husband and I really are straight, Tri-Ess doesn't understand that I really do enjoy my husband's crossdressing, and most straight people—especially ones who don't know me—can't possibly understand how I can love my husband at all. But if Ken feels lonely, and so do I, and so do many crossdressers—surely we can work together to figure out how not to be. The answer may be creating a community the old-fashioned way: by setting common goals and working to achieve them, together.

CHAPTER 8

Gendered Politics

IF ONE MORE crossdresser complains to me about how unfair it is that crossdressers can't wear what they want and tells me I don't understand because I *can* wear whatever I want, my head might explode. First off, women cannot wear whatever they want. If a woman dresses too provocatively she's assumed to be a whore; if she's not sexy or feminine enough she's a man-hating lesbian. Ditto if she won't wear high heels. She may get picked on if she wears revealing clothes without being "model skinny," or she may get gently chastised for not dressing "more attractively" if she prefers practical, comfortable clothes. It is true that I don't get ridiculed for wearing jeans in public the way a man would for wearing a skirt. But what the crossdresser doesn't recognize is that he's not yearning for the right to wear certain items of clothing: what he wants is the right to be his transgendered self in public.

After five years of talking to crossdressers online and in person, I've developed a standard response to a CD who bemoans his lack of sartorial freedom. When he wonders aloud why he can't wear what he'd like to, I just say, "because you haven't earned it yet." I've made more than one crossdresser angry with that statement, and some just do not want to face the truth of the situation. The problem is, the crossdressing community has virtually cut itself off from all the groups who could otherwise educate and liberate them: the feminist community, the gay and lesbian communities, the alternative sex community, and the transsexual community. There are many people whose experiences and histories could inform the crossdresser's, but a variety of circumstances have prevented that exchange. Crossdressers have isolated themselves from these groups in different ways, but the result is a minority of straight men who don't understand that the only way any group gets their rights is by fighting for them.

* * *

WOMEN AND FEMINISM

I'M A FEMINIST, but not a particularly doctrinaire one: my feminism derives more from my experiences than my education. I am what my husband likes to call a "pragmatic feminist," which I think is his way of saying I like sex and have a sense of humor (so do most feminists, but we've been misrepresented for so long that these traits are often overlooked). Just as "crossdresser" means a lot of different things, so does "feminist": There are feminists who actively engage healthy attitudes about sex, political science feminists, feminists who work in child care, and feminists who are gender activists. We're a pretty diverse group, but the basic tenet of feminism is that women should be accorded full human rights, get equal pay for equal work, and have the right to define themselves in whatever way they choose: executive, slut, goddess, witch, jock, mom. Fat, thin, muscle-bound, or differently abled. All of the above and none of the above.

A woman's right to dress in pants did not come out of nowhere. It was our insistence that we could do men's jobs that women opened the doors to our so-called sartorial freedom. When women went to work in munitions factories during World War II, they had to wear clothes that were appropriate to the job at hand. Thus, images like Rosie the Riveter were born: a strong woman, muscular arm raised, fist clenched, hair tucked under a bandana. Her image was accompanied by the slogan *We Can Do It*. At first there were feminine versions of all the uniforms required in different industries, but step by step women insisted that they needed pants—not skirts—to do their jobs, and that they needed those jobs in the first place. It was the change in our gender roles—politically, socially, and economically—that granted us the relative sartorial freedom we currently enjoy. This freedom—so envied by crossdressers—wasn't handed to us. It was earned over 150 years of activism: before Rosie, the Suffragettes fought for the vote, and before that, women organized for the abolition of slavery. Currently, women are confronting the corporate "glass ceiling." The women who are aware of this struggle—how it happened, why it worked, when it didn't—are the women of the feminist community. (In fact I'd argue that the difference between a liberated woman and a feminist is that the feminist is knowledgeable about Women's History, whereas the average liberated woman is less aware of the historical context behind the rights she enjoys.)

The problem with the crossdressing community is how little understanding it demonstrates of genetic women. Crossdressers are like most guys in that they don't really know what makes women tick, but they claim to. The single most difficult thing about being a woman who is married to a crossdresser is dealing with a crossdresser's fetishized ideas of femininity. When they dress, many choose to reflect the Victoria's Secret version of womanhood, and many wives and girlfriends are duly offended. There has been a shift toward crossdressers dressing in an age-appropriate, dignified, and ordinary way, but there are still plenty who want to wear spike heels and pounds of eye makeup and skirts that barely cover their butts. (Of course, there are women who choose to dress like that as well, but they're not usually the ones crossdressers marry.) I pointed out in an earlier chapter that the more independent, modern woman is best suited to life with a crossdresser: a woman who is stable in her own identity doesn't rely as much upon her husband's identity to feel good about her life or herself. She has often struggled to accept her body image and self-presentation as a compromise between how she feels comfortable and what she is told daily she is supposed to look like. Such acceptance is hard-won, but many women make peace with the fact that the images of women portrayed in the media are downright ridiculous.

The problem is, men buy into pop-culture images of women whether they're crossdressers or not. In an insightful book called *The Centerfold Syndrome,* Gary R. Brooks argues that men's ideas about women's beauty prevent the potentially genuine and loving relationships men and women *could* enjoy by positing an image of a woman that does not exist, that is, the Centerfold. He claims that men have been taught by the culture at large to distance themselves from women in ways that prevent intimacy, and that a man's desire for "the Centerfold" is comprised of five principal elements: 1) *voyeurism,* where men get to look at women in sexual ways without being looked at in return; 2) *objectification,* where the man's voyeurism effectively removes the woman's personality from her physical form; 3) *validation,* which is when a woman's sexual power—based on her ability to meet cultural standards of beauty and sex appeal—validates the man's sex appeal; 4) *trophyism,* where men compete with other men in terms of "how beautiful" a woman they can date or marry; and 5) *fear of true intimacy,* which arises when men's love for the feminine in the form of the mother's body is "trained out of them" in order that they not be perceived as vulnerable or weak. For the average man, this syndrome is problematic, but for the crossdresser—who expresses his notions about women's beauty by dressing himself as a woman—it's a nightmare. Joanne, the genetic female partner of a transitioning transsexual woman (who once thought she was "just a crossdresser"), sums it up in a nutshell:

> *CDers model themselves not on real women, but on the* Vogue/Elle/Playboy *sort of anorexic, overdone, dream-girl in dream clothes. These are also the very intimidating images with which we*

genetic women struggle, even though we know that they are ⅒ of 1 per-
cent of women, and that even that small percentage is airbrushed in the
magazine photos. When CDers take on the attributes of these unreal
women, it breeds insecurity in that manner, as well. So many women ask
themselves whether the CDer is acting out in response to their own lack
of or insufficient femininity.

In his actual life, where he's a man who loves women, my husband has always preferred *actual* women. Based on our relationship and the other women who have turned his head, I know that my husband is more interested in women with curves than in skinny models. He thinks Kate Winslet is the hottest woman in the movies, and she herself complained that someone on the staff of the British *GQ* airbrushed her thighs in a recent photo spread to make her legs appear thinner. My husband is also sensitive to women's body image issues: his mother has been overweight for most of her life because she's asthmatic, and his sister had breast reduction surgery when she was seventeen.

Despite this sensitivity, and his love of and desire for actual women, my husband still often opts to emulate the media-driven images of women—the Victoria's Secret models, the Christy Turlingtons—when he chooses to dress himself as a woman. I have wondered if my husband even realizes the political ramifications of the images he wishes to emulate. I don't think he does. I understand his choice as an unconscious manifestation of Centerfold Syndrome. However, when that kind of self-presentation emerges in combination with the common sexual issues some crossdressers experience, wives end up convinced that they are not good enough for their husbands: not feminine enough, not sexy enough, not thin enough. Many have guessed that the reason their husbands need to crossdress is to create their own girlfriend, and so they create the most sexualized woman they can imagine, a fantasy woman. This may be fine when the crossdresser is single, but when wives and girlfriends of crossdressers are faced with "her," many gain weight, convinced that their own appearance is irrelevant to their husbands' sexual desires. (There are women, also, who return to previously conquered anorexic or bulimic behaviors in order to meet what they assume their husbands' expectations are. Whether she gains weight or loses, the woman is experiencing a profound loss of control in her life as a result, and her body will often reflect that.)

What crossdressers need to face is that the oppressive image of the anorexic woman sends the message to all women that they are not good enough. When crossdressers emulate those images, they are validating them.

Their love affair with this kind of female image is resented by their wives, whether the wives are anorexic or obese or anywhere in between. My husband can tell me he would love me if I weighed 300 pounds, but his enjoyment of Victoria's Secret catalogs—whether he looks at the models or emulates them—makes his reassurances seem untrue. I don't want to be loved *despite* the fact that I don't fulfill his image of a dream woman: I want to be the most beautiful and sexy woman in the world to him. In that sense I am no different from any other woman in any other relationship.

Despite the fact that liberated, independent, self-confident women are the best partners for crossdressers, the crossdressing community doesn't celebrate women who embody these traits. There are no images of three-dimensional, successful women in the crossdressing community. Drag queens and female impersonators tend to model themselves after women like Liza Minnelli, Madonna, and Marilyn Monroe, and they celebrate the women's beauty and their talent (and often their struggles). Crossdressers, on the other hand, dress like archetypes, instead: sexy secretaries, French maids, slutty schoolgirls, teenaged tarts. The choice of these oversexed stereotypes of women is not accidental, but is, rather, another manifestation of the Centerfold Syndrome. The irony perhaps is that even Victoria's Secret models are probably more proud of the salaries than in how well they pout and get men off. Getting men off is just what brings home the bacon, and being able to earn top dollar is empowering.

Where are the wives and girlfriends of the crossdressers themselves? I didn't find any featured in the pages of *Girl Talk,* and that might be exactly because it's a glamour magazine—and genetic women are more interested in escaping those ridiculous standards than indulging in them. I felt as oppressed turning its pages as I would looking at *Cosmo.* Are glamour girls the only women that crossdressers and transsexual women admire? Are they all that shallow?

I am half convinced the reason that there aren't more women involved in the crossdressing community is because the images of women crossdressers love are all the same old crap. Why would we want to be part of a community that advances and celebrates images of women that make us feel bad about ourselves? How can we feel welcome when all crossdressers want to talk about is shoes and makeup?

Dixie, a crossdresser, relays what he hears when he hears women talking, and the envy he feels from being excluded:

> Has anyone in the group ever paid any attention to the usual topic of conversation is when a group of women get together and start talking?

Just be quiet sometimes and listen. Not every time but quite a bit it has
to do with fashions, what's that perfume you're wearing, where did you
get those cute shoes, there's a sale on at Penney's, who is your hair
dresser, blah, blah, blah. . . . But for a CD, admission into these feminine
topics is a godsend and is almost like being invited to join a very private
and very exclusive club.

What he doesn't realize is women switch to these more "neutral" topics
when the guys are within earshot; as soon as the men leave, we have entirely
different conversations. We do talk about shoes, but what women really
want to talk about—especially with their husbands and boyfriends—are
their lives, their feelings, their hassles at work, or conversations they've had
with family and friends. We don't want to feel like advice columnists for
Glamour or *Cosmo* or *YM*. Women have actual issues and problems we
need to be able to discuss with our life partners. We've got psychotic ex-
boyfriends and PMS bloating and dads with Alzheimer's. We want to know
how the tax cuts will affect us and our community. We want a world and a
community where we are our husbands' equals, and they ours: where we
foster mutual respect. The very idea that men crossdress in order to get away
from the Real World offends the heck out of most of us. Wearing women's
clothes *is* our real world. We don't escape to anywhere when we put on
heels, we just go to work. We don't escape when we take them off, either—
we do the housework, care for children, and make phone calls to relatives.

There are crossdressers who are more considerate men than the average.
There are those who take women's studies classes. There are those who will
get their wives ice cream when it's that time of the month. My guess, though,
is that the percentage of these "sensitive guys" isn't higher in the crossdressing community than it is among married men in general. That is, there
are good guys and bad guys, and there are crossdressers in both groups.

I once read an essay by a crossdresser explaining that crossdressers make
good partners because they understand what it's like to be a woman. One of
the examples given was that a crossdresser knows what it feels like for your
bra strap to slip off your shoulder. It's become a joke between my husband
and me: whenever either of us feels a bra strap slip, we say, "Well, now I feel
like a woman." What a joke. Tell me how it feels to get paid less for doing
the same work, and then maybe we can have a conversation.

I would feel a lot better if crossdressers, who use breast forms that were
originally invented in order to replace breasts removed by mastectomies,
would donate money to charities that promote breast cancer awareness and
research. Many men know women who have been diagnosed with breast can-

cer, and I assume some crossdressers are included in that count. I would love to hear a CD even mention the subject, and I'd be doubly pleased to hear a crossdresser use his status—as a man and often as a professional—to put pressure on the government to fund research. They don't have to admit they're crossdressers to do that. Likewise, any crossdresser with a website could provide a link to a breast cancer website or other websites dealing with women's issues. I don't feel willing to go to the mat for their right to self-expression when they fail to demonstrate a concern for women's real lives.

It even took Tri-Ess a while to come around to the idea that genetic women are a vital part of the crossdressing community. Early on, wives were accorded only "guest member" status and they couldn't vote or hold office until the early 1990s. Even at that time, making women full members was a controversial idea. Shirley Kay, a crossdresser's wife, argued in *Transgender Tapestry* #56 (a publication of the IFGE) that wives and SOs should be granted full membership on the grounds that they could not only help other wives accept crossdressing but also provide a more legitimate image so that "Tri-Ess won't just be dismissed as an organization for crazy men wearing dresses." Fantastic: we were being invited in so that the guys wouldn't be so reviled. I'm reminded of something Virginia Woolf once wrote, in her brilliant essay *A Room of One's Own*:

> Women have served all these centuries as looking-glasses possessing the magic and delicious power of reflecting the figure of man at twice its natural size.

And that's what we get to do at Tri-Ess, too, huh? No thanks. With a crossdresser, it's like having to reflect him back at himself as *her* and as *him*. Interesting that Woolf should use a mirror metaphor, because crossdressers spend so much time in front of theirs.

The biggest problem caused by the crossdresser's disconnect from the real world of women is the missed opportunity of being able to be educated and liberated by feminists' knowledge about what it takes to gain respect in a world that doesn't respect you. We know what it's like to be disrespected for wearing a skirt; we get how it feels to be reviled simply for being feminine. When a judge hands down a ruling that a rape victim in a short skirt was "asking for it," how many MTFs understand that they, too, could be victims of such discriminatory rulings? There is a wealth of experience to be tapped in the feminist community, and a lot of feminists—despite the now-infamous examples to the contrary, like the author of *The Transsexual Menace*—understand something about how narrow the gender boxes are and how unfair it is not to be appreciated as a whole person. A natural empathy exists between crossdressers and genetic women, just as it does between genetic women and gay men, but until the crossdressing community gets hip to real women's lives, that empathy will go untapped.

Crossdressers often envy my husband because he's got an accepting wife. What they don't realize is that while I may be half Gwen Stefani, I'm also half Gloria Steinem. He has had to learn about real women's suffering: about pay disparity, sexual assault, domestic abuse, and Female Genital Mutilation. He has been asked to read (though has not always read) books by women I admire: Virginia Woolf, Naomi Wolf, Natalie Angier, Eve Ensler, bell hooks, and Ursula K. LeGuin. He knows who the Suffragettes were and when women got the vote. He can tell you why I admire Emma Goldman, Edna St. Vincent Millay, and Simone deBeauvoir. He understands that I believe the world keeps women tied up in knots over how fat they are so they don't get on with their lives. He now knows more about women's history and politics than a lot of women do. When he sees crossdressers look at him with those "you're so lucky" puppy-dog eyes, he knows that he's earned an accepting wife, not just miraculously "found" one.

None of this, of course, is to say that men shouldn't want to feel pretty. They should. So should women. But any man who loves or lives with a woman should know a few things about her and her history, and crossdressers should know a little more. They're inundating their wives with catalogs and websites, and the wives need to be reminded that their husbands know that we're more than what we look like. Women are unbelievably beautiful, but in more ways than most crossdressers imagine. All of us in the crossdressing community, including genetic women, might want to offset the celebration of vacuous beauty that surrounds us. Read these:

- Natalie Angier's *Woman: An Intimate Geography*
- Virginia Woolf's "A Room of One's Own"
- Naomi Wolf's *The Beauty Myth*
- Eve Ensler's *The Vagina Monologues* (you can cheat and see a performance of this one)
- A biography or an autobiography by a woman of your choice

This is a reasonably good introduction to women's lives: our bodies, our minds, our beauty, our souls. When crossdressing evolves into something more than "wanting to feel pretty," maybe more genetic women will join the community. Genetic women are tired of accepting crossdressers for who they are without feeling like they are accepted for who *they* are. Once crossdressers start to understand that women didn't magically become "modern women," women can start informing crossdressers as to how one goes about earning respect in a society that doesn't take you seriously.

TRI-ESS'S HISTORICAL IMPACT

THE CHASM BETWEEN genetic women and crossdressers is more incidental than historical, but the crossdressing community is also missing out on finding ways to accept and liberate itself because of its own history. When Virginia Prince formed Tri-Ess, the founding ideas of the organization were based on her own. Those underlying beliefs go a long way toward explaining the current state of the crossdressing community. The Bulloughs explain:

> Prince argued that most transvestites were normal heterosexual men who sought only to express the beautiful "woman within." When pressed, however, she would admit that some homosexual transvestites existed, but she excluded them from her definitions of transvestism, and, whenever possible, from her groups. She did not approve of masochism, bondage, sadism, fetishism, or even references to sex. She also disapproved of Sex Reassignment Surgery.

This passage makes clear that Tri-Ess's founder and her personal beliefs greatly impacted Tri-Ess's value as an organization. It also illuminates how Tri-Ess, and the average crossdresser, ended up estranged from three more communities—the gay and lesbian community, the alternative sex community, and the transsexual community—whose input and experience could have helped the crossdresser accept himself for who he is and fight for his right to be himself in society. Whatever Tri-Ess's current value as an organization, its history has shaped the way crossdressers define themselves. They have been the only game in town for many, many years, and as a result, Tri-Ess's "definition" of its own membership has evolved into a general definition of the term "crossdresser." Many CDs internalize Tri-Ess's membership policies to the degree that Tri-Ess culture is crossdressing culture. That Tri-Ess does not represent the entire spectrum of the crossdressing community is a fact seldom noted. Since most crossdressers are ignorant of their own history, they don't realize that their ideas about being a crossdresser stem from three huge "myths" that arose out of historical necessity. The first myth is that crossdressers are never homosexual, the second is that sexuality has nothing to do with crossdressing, and the third is that crossdressers never transition. Why and how those myths helped create the abyss that keeps crossdressers from connecting with other communities is vital in understanding how crossdressers can change course and start reaching out to the people who might respond with empathy and aid.

THE GAY AND LESBIAN COMMUNITY

IN 1976, WHEN Tri-Ess officially came into existence, there was a standing history of confusion about homosexuality. A gay friend, in his fifties, told me a story that gives crossdressing some historical context. As a preteen, in the early 1960s, he saw a show he thinks might have been hosted by Mike Wallace. Around a table with the interviewer sat four other men with paper bags over their heads. At the bottom of the screen was the word "homosexual." My friend listened for a while, and, recognizing himself in some of the descriptions, went to his mother—who he describes as having been a 1950s kind of mom—and asked what the word "homosexual" meant. "Don't ever say that again," she said. "Who taught you that word?" He pointed to the living room, abashed, and admitted he heard it on television. Since television is some kind of authority in American culture, she decided to explain to her son what the word meant: "Homosexuals," she clarified, "are very sad men who wear dresses."

Imagine, then, starting an organization for crossdressers within that cultural context. People thought that gay men wore dresses, and that any man who wore a dress was gay. Therefore, Tri-Ess's first attempt at educating the public was to clarify that crossdressers weren't homosexual and that homosexuality had nothing to do with crossdressing. It was an unfortunate choice. In its attempt to defend crossdressing by putting down homosexuality, Tri-Ess spread homophobic ideas. In *The Transvestite and His Wife*, Virginia Prince explains five ways in which crossdressers differ from homosexuals. Number two is: "Practically no femmiphile would advise, induce, or influence another to become a transvestite. . . . Most homosexuals, however, have no hesitation about indoctrinating and initiating others into the practice." Yikes! This was published two years before the Stonewall Riots but it's not hard to guess what kind of damage it did. Any latent homophobia in crossdressers and their wives found confirmation in the "facts" provided by Virginia Prince. ("Femmiphile," by the way, was yet another substitute for "transvestite," but thankfully it was never widely used.)

Tri-Ess's current "don't ask, don't tell" policy doesn't do enough toward rectifying its unfortunate, historic mistake. Jane Ellen Fairfax, Tri-Ess's Chair, explains the current policy:

> Tri-Ess focuses its work on crossdressers and their families, and we use a heterosexual family model in everything we do. We believe in truth in advertising. We inform people clearly about our focus, and expect that they will be honest with themselves and with us. We do not ask people how they identify, or what their sexual orientation is. Anyone who enters under false pretenses soon finds that Tri-Ess does not offer any programs to those outside the focus.

This policy may not explicitly exclude gay members, but it sure isn't welcoming of their sexuality, either. The reality is that some of the only places crossdressers feel welcome are in gay bars and lesbian restaurants, and for Tri-Ess to insult the gay crossdresser by excluding him—discreetly or not—from its organization seems incredibly ungrateful.

We recently went to a TG/CD weekend at Rainbow Mountain, a gay and lesbian resort in Pennsylvania owned by two gay men. The whole weekend was designed to put the CD at ease; the wait staff had been instructed to refer to the CDs as "ladies," and a voluntary group outing was planned for CDs who may not be able to go "out" at home. I was struck by how incredibly welcoming the employees and owners of a gay and lesbian resort were toward us straight crossdressers and wives. The gay and lesbian community may not always understand us, but they do welcome us, and not just when there's money to be made.

At the GLBT Center in Manhattan, crossdressers and their partners are also welcome. This is a space where gays and lesbians and bisexuals can feel "safe" and find support. How incredibly generous of them to open up their doors to straight, albeit transgendered, people who do not necessarily know or understand the issues of the gay and lesbian community! That is not to say that they understand us either, because they often don't, but the reality is that we have a shared experience: gays and lesbians have been struggling as perceived "deviants" in our culture for decades. They've actually gained some measure of acceptance and have figured out how to live without shame or guilt and sometimes even without fear. We in the CD community could be learning how to accept crossdressing and gender variance by listening to their experiences and by educating ourselves in gay history. Gay people, like CDs, have faced rejection from family and friends, been prevented from obtaining jobs and homes, and faced real fears about harassment.

When I started researching Magnus Hirschfield online, where did I find information on him? Not on a single crossdresser's website, but rather on several gay history sites. Because gays and lesbians started seeking their own history several decades ago, they have found leaders like Hirschfield who, it turns out, is one of our leaders, too, but very few crossdressers know who he was. Hirschfield was, after all, trying to decriminalize both crossdressing and homosexuality, and should rightly be honored for both. Gays and lesbians have already unearthed much of this history, and crossdressers can not only take advantage of that, but can learn how, as a community, they might unearth their specific history as well. Transgendered academics, for example, can read Eve Kosofsky Sedgwick's *Epistemology of the Closet* to learn how transvestites have appeared in literature and film, and how those portrayals have informed the public consensus about crossdressers in general. Exploring the results of how living in secrecy and shame—of living in the closet—can affect a person, is the kind of work that gays and lesbians have already done.

There are innumerable ways in which gay and lesbian people can share personal examples and experiences that could help the average crossdresser and his wife. I have an old friend (we'll call him Kevin) who is gay who was once dating a man (we'll call Richard) who did drag occasionally. Kevin had the same visceral—"but I want a man"—reaction that straight wives of crossdressers experience. Richard didn't even want to make love in drag; for him, drag was more political than personal. But Kevin still wanted a guy, even in public. Kevin had only recently come out. I wondered if Kevin was more worried about what others thought of him when they saw him with Richard than anything else. My guess was he didn't want others to think he couldn't accept his homosexuality and dated a man in a dress to assuage his guilt about it. He could not articulate what bothered him about Richard doing drag, so he couldn't explain it to Richard, either. Richard was left feeling rejected for his feminine side. Every crossdresser can relate to his experience. But Richard is neither allowed to join Tri-Ess in order to talk about his experiences nor permitted to bring his partner to meetings, so his perspective is seldom heard by the people it might help the most.

During the Rainbow Mountain weekend, my husband and I talked with one of the drag queens who performed on Friday night. His stage name is Anita Mann. He was once married with children, but five years ago he came out as gay, got divorced, raised his younger daughter, and started doing drag. He was at first apprehensive about entertaining crossdressers and wondered if his glamour would jive with the crossdresser's sensibility. It turned out that most of the CDs and their wives who saw Anita's show enjoyed it, and afterwards he was full of questions for us: Was crossdressing about sex? Or glamour? He didn't know that crossdressers have deep feelings of transgenderedness and wish to pass as women. He didn't know that most crossdressers start dressing at an early age. There was a lot he didn't know about CDs, but what he did understand—implicitly—was what it was like to live in the closet, repressing one's true self. He immediately wanted to help in any way he could: by offering makeup and fashion tips (my husband learned how to make shoes bigger without taking them to a cobbler), and by hosting group outings. A drag queen's attitude—that confident, catty, sarcastic quality—is something that crossdressers might armor themselves with when facing the real world. An exchange like the one we experienced—between a gay drag queen and his partner, and a crossdresser and his wife—is not so difficult to achieve. It may only take circumstances that allow such a conversation to take place.

Likewise for the lesbian woman who wants a partner who is feminine, not butch, because she likes women, not men. Her experiences of her partner's transgenderedness is similar to the way the wife of a crossdresser feels, the objection that "this is not what I signed up for." Kate Bornstein found herself facing her partner's FTM transition, and keenly felt the loss of her identity as a lesbian as a result. There are lesbian communities where the butch/femme dynamic is the standard, just as it is in heterosexual relationships, and for butch lesbians to date each other is not always considered okay by the rest of the community. The commonality is that transgenderedness is upsetting to all of us—not just heterosexual couples. A lifelong lesbian identity is as much a part of a woman's life as is a wife's heterosexual identity, and its loss is as acutely felt.

Lesbian couples also provide role models for crossdressed relationships. They have figured out how both partners can feel feminine without either always playing the "wife" or "husband." They can negotiate their relationship based on the strengths of each partner—not based on expectations of who is *supposed* to do what. A lesbian woman is not shocked or offended that her partner is feminine or wants to feel submissive in bed. But what the crossdresser's wife might not realize or guess is that a lesbian doesn't come by this acceptance naturally. Every lesbian is raised a woman in this society just like genetic women, and has to find ways to accommodate the other woman in her relationship and accept that she is not the only one who expects to be seduced.

There are, of course, significant differences between the crossdressing and gay and lesbian communities. Crossdressers and their wives can legally marry, often have children together, and do not face job or housing discrimination based on sexual orientation. Same sex couples do not have power of attorney, can have children taken away—and sodomy laws are often unfairly applied to gay and lesbian couples when plenty of heterosexuals break sodomy laws. (Sodomy is not, as many people think, specifically anal sex. Sodomy is any sex which is not intercourse, including oral sex, anal sex, and any use of sex toys, or, in general, nonreproductive sex.) Same sex couples face legal and institutional challenges that most straight couples never think about. Crossdressers and their partners do, however, face similar cultural and social challenges as same sex couples, and certainly will face more as they come out.

Crossdressers pass as ordinary straight men. What we don't always realize is that most gay or lesbian individuals can "pass" in similar ways. Individuals going for job interviews do not wear labels identifying themselves as gay or lesbian. A friend of mine, Zoe, recently had a job interview. When the prospective employer called Zoe's apartment in response to her request for directions, she spoke to Zoe's girlfriend, Abigail, and later mentioned talking to Zoe's "roommate" during the interview. Zoe was tongue-tied: Should she correct the woman and clarify that Abigail was not her roommate but her girlfriend? Would outing herself prevent her from getting the job? Did the employer really need to know she was a lesbian? If she didn't tell the woman the whole truth, did that mean she was ashamed of being lesbian? Or just that it wasn't anybody's business?

For the straight crossdresser and his wife, there are probably no instances that are completely analogous with my friend Zoe's predicament. Imagine, however, that I get a job and at some point or another am expected to bring my spouse to an office party, or we are invited to have dinner with the boss and his wife. I have never told anyone my husband is transgendered because "it is none of their business." If my husband's transgenderedness is part of his regular presentation—say he keeps his nails long or polished and his eyebrows shaped—what do I do? Do I ask him to "look more straight" for the work function? Do I make him promise he won't do anything feminine while we're there? If I do so, doesn't that mean I'm ashamed of his being transgendered? Are we really out if we "cover up" any signs of the reality of our lives every time something important comes up? When I was offered the contract to write this book, for instance, I wanted to tell friends and family, but doing so required me telling them what I was writing the book *about*. There was no way around it, and now most of our friends and family know Betty is transgendered.

There are less serious examples of similar situations, like when I'm shopping for a present for Betty. Do I tell the clerk that I need larger size shoes because the pumps I've picked aren't for me but for my husband? That a blouse with no stretch won't do because he needs the extra give for his shoulders? Zoe's story gave me a whole new insight into being part of a sexual minority. If you don't tell, you suspect yourself of being ashamed of who you are, but if you do tell you're "putting it in someone's face." It's not fair, but it is reality. A crossdresser doesn't need to be a crossdresser at work, but it could be argued that my friend Zoe doesn't need to be a lesbian there, either: it's not like she's going to be having sex during working hours. Right now, crossdressers are nearly all "passing" as ordinary heterosexual men at work. Zoe could have decided to "pass" as a heterosexual woman if she so chose. Why didn't she? Because she doesn't want to lie by omission and hide who she is, or find out later—if she likes the job—that her employers are uncomfortable with her having a picture of Abigail on her desk. She wants to be accepted for who she is.

ALTERNATIVE SEXUALITIES

EVEN IF THE crossdresser decides he doesn't need to be out at work, he must still accept himself in his private life so he can escape the web of shame and guilt. But as surely as they have alienated themselves from the gay and lesbian community, crossdressers have also failed to benefit from another community that could help them on the road to acceptance. There is a huge and diverse group of people who live alternative sexual lives but are not necessarily gay and lesbian, including the BDSM community, fetishists, and polyamorists.

Minna, for example, discovered that she came to understand her husband Heather's crossdressing by first understanding his desire to be submissive. She understands that he doesn't want to feel "traditionally male" in the bedroom: in charge, doing the seducing, making the decisions. She doesn't always like that submissive = female in some men's heads, because she knows that being a woman certainly doesn't make her submissive. She does understand that male submissives want to be lead to the bedroom, and some want to be feminized as well; they want to have sex with a woman who calls the shots. Most women in the BDSM community could probably "get" a crossdresser's sexual needs because they understand that being a "top" or "bottom" is not based on gender. They also understand that fantasy and role play are important elements in a satisfying sex life. How many wives of crossdressers could benefit from hearing what a dominant woman knows? Plenty.

Likewise, there are those in the fetish community who could share how they have adjusted to living with a spouse who requires more than another partner for arousal.

When the wife of a fetishist feels displaced by her partner's sexual needs, she might think to herself, "I am just an extra in this kind of sex." She might ask her partner, "Do you want sex with me or do you just want to have sex by yourself?" Many wives of crossdressers can relate to how this woman feels. Because crossdressers have been so tight-lipped about their sexualities, there is little acknowledgement within the community of the wife's feelings. The crossdresser's wife often feels rejected, hurt, insufficiently feminine, and insecure. Likewise with the fetishist's wife, who can never replace the object that excites him. At some point in the fetishist's history, his sexuality got connected to a practice or object that is not another person. This does not, however, mean that fetishists are incapable of loving their wives. Many wives of fetishists find that they can sustain romantic and sexual relationships despite their husbands' unusual desires. They may be able to share how they accomplish this.

Both the BDSM and fetish communities are friendly toward crossdressers. We are welcome at their club events as long as we learn and respect their own rules of behavior. Both of these communities are known, too, for accepting people—especially women—as they are. They've made peace with their own kinks, and found a way to live a private life that isn't "vanilla." They find a way to do so without feeling ashamed of their desires, and without trying to "normalize" them. They have accepted that their sexuality is an integral part of their identity, and that it's too deeply rooted to change. Heather explains why he never kept secrets from his wife.

> *In large part I credit this to O/our involvement in the BDSM lifestyle. One of the advantages of being into BDSM is that it requires a great deal more candor and trust than a typical "vanilla" relationship does. Since I have to literally trust Mistress with my life when W/we scene (when you're tied up, gagged and about to be flogged or whipped, this is not the time to have a serious difference of expectations of what is about to occur) it means that W/we talk in great depth about what W/we are looking for and how W/we are going to go about getting there. This means everything from day to day events all the way through the spectrum of sexuality and gender. You can't safely take part in BDSM activities if you don't know who and what you are dealing with.*

Since this kind of honesty is also required in a relationship involving crossdressing, the honest exchanges practiced by BDSM couples could serve as another useful lesson for CDs and their wives. However, since there is often skittishness and reluctance within the CD community to discuss these alternate sexualities, the possibilities are once again foreclosed upon.

THE TRANSGENDERED/TRANSSEXUAL COMMUNITY

TRANSGENDERED PEOPLE—ESPECIALLY those transitioning or opting to live dual existences—face discrimination in housing, and employment, and, of course, face threats of physical violence. The political strides being made by transgender activists are making the world safer for crossdressers as well, but crossdressers are rarely engaged in the struggle. Even when it came to protesting Winn-Dixie's firing of Peter Oiler for his off-site crossdressing, it was mostly trans activists—not crossdressers—who protested. Vanessa Edwards Foster, of the NTAC, explains:

> *Traditionally, there is not a lot of proportionate participation from cross-dressers. One of the primary reasons I theorize is that most people don't get involved in activism until they are personally impacted in some fashion. Most of those who are impacted are transsexuals who due to living full time end up with more opportunity for discrimination in its many forms—especially in the workplace. Most crossdressers are fairly well closeted, and do not wish to upset this delicate balance—and activism can be potentially noted publicly. We do have a brave few who do get involved, regardless of those concerns . . . but if I were to have to place an estimated percentage of our membership, it would likely be in the 10 percent range or less. We do have two crossdressers on our Board.*

The closet may be an explanation, but it's not an excuse. The gay and lesbian community have added the "T"—for transgender—into the GLB banner, but crossdressers are not answering the call. I see this as the worst side effect of the crossdresser's Fear of Freaking that I mentioned in the Introduction. If a crossdresser cleaves to his status as a straight man, he won't do himself any good, and should expect resentment for his lack of political activity. Gay, lesbian, and transgender activists should not have to fight crossdressers' battles for them. They don't want to feel like crossdressers and their partners will go back to their "straight" lives and leave them holding the ball.

Their need for secrecy and their political inactivity mean that CDs have more in common with transsexual men and women. Because of the bias against transsexual people, many transition only to become what's called "stealth." They live lives as people of the sex they've transitioned to, and keep their history a secret. Willow, for example, did not tell her fiancé she had been born with a male body even after he proposed. (When she did tell him, he said he loved her despite her past, and also admitted that he'd suspected the truth before she told him.) Katie describes it as running from one closet, where transgendered individuals are ashamed and repressed, to another, where they pretend they were never transgendered at all. Because many transitioned women date men, and many transitioned men continue dating women, they are publicly identified as heterosexual, just like crossdressers are. Transitioned FTM men are usually in relationships with women, as are some transitioned MTF women, as are crossdressers, and surely their relationships with genetic women—especially in the context of their transgenderedness—might be a great starting place for sharing common experiences. In that sense, crossdressers and transsexual people could engage in useful conversations, but again, there is no real openness toward transsexual people by the crossdressing community. Of course, chance exchanges do occur, but there is no national effort under way to facilitate such cooperation. Jane Ellen Fairfax of Tri-Ess quotes Benjamin Franklin when he says that "We must all hang together, or surely we will hang separately," yet Tri-Ess encourages transsexual people to go elsewhere.

Unfortunately, transgendered people often "hang" separately—or are shot, beaten, or strangled. At least two transgendered people are killed per month internationally for being transgendered, Monica Helms asserts. She based her statistics on the information compiled and posted by Gwendolyn Ann Smith on her website www.gender.org. The murders are often brutal. The Fourth Annual Day of Remembrance took place in November 2002. These are some of the people who were killed in the United States in 2002.

Amy Soos
Location: Phoenix, Arizona
Cause of Death: Murdered
Date of Death: February 16, 2002
Source: Phoenix, Arizona police report

Amy Soos lived all her life on the Salt River Pima Indian Reservation in Arizona, but often went into Phoenix in the evenings. After not returning home one such night, her body was discovered in a roadway. She died of multiple blunt force trauma. She had been beaten many other times before her death.

Arlene (Hector) Diaz
Location: El Paso, Texas
Cause of Death: Shot in the back
Date of Death: April 10, 2002
Source: *El Paso Times,* April 27, 2002

Arlene (Hector) Diaz was planning her upcoming transition, and attended a local transgender support group the night of her murder. She was fatally shot in the back, allegedly by Justen Grant Hall. The local police have classified this murder as a hate crime.

Paola Matos
Location: Brooklyn, New York
Cause of Death: Strangled
Date of Death: July 22, 2002
Source: *The New York Post,* July 23, 2002

Paola Matos had recently moved to New York after a series of transsexual-related surgeries done abroad. She was discovered in her home by her live-in boyfriend with a white cord wrapped around her throat. Police have ruled her death a homicide, and are seeking a suspect, Fernando Batista.

Deasha (Gerald) Andrews and Terianne Summers
Location: Jacksonville, Florida
Cause of Death: Shot multiple times
Dates of Death: August 8, 2002 and December 12, 2001
Source: WLTV 12, Jacksonville, Florida, and *Florida Times-Union*

Deasha Andrews was discovered in her car, after having been shot several times. Police are not pursuing this as a hate crime, and do not feel that there is any tie-in between it and another Jacksonville murder that took place in December of 2001, when Terianne Summers, a transgender activist in the Jacksonville area who had been very involved in efforts against discrimination at the Winn-Dixie food chain, was shot to death in her own front yard days after participating in the 2001 Transgender Day of Remembrance.

Ukea Davis and **Stephanie Thomas**
Location: Washington, DC
Cause of Death: Shot multiple times
Date of Death: August 12, 2002
Source: WJLA ABC 7, Washington, DC

Stephanie and Ukea were friends living in Washington, D.C., and had begun living in their preferred gender roles. Both were shot multiple times in a car they often shared. They were half a block away from home.

Gwen Araujo
Location: Newark, California
Cause of Death: Beaten to death, allegedly by four ex-classmates.
Date of Death: October 3, 2002
Source: *San Francisco Chronicle,* October 17, 2002

Gwen Araujo had been dressing as a woman since she was fourteen years old, and was murdered at the age of seventeen. During a house party, she was revealed to have been a male. After this revelation, at least three individuals allegedly beat her, dragged her into a garage, and strangled her, before disposing of her body in a remote location 150 miles away.

THESE DEATHS—AND the hundreds more like them—indicate exactly how much is at risk when it comes to being transgendered. Some of the people killed are drag queens, others are transitioning or transitioned transsexuals, still others are transvestites or crossdressers. A crossdresser is no longer a straight man when he's dressed as a woman, and the type of person who would kill a transgendered individual because of his or her gender identity is not going to ask questions about whether the man has a wife or family at home. For this reason, more "stealth" transsexual women and men and more crossdressers need to become more vocal and politically active. When some people are losing their lives, it is unconscionable that others in the community refuse even to write a letter to their local representative when a bill protecting transgendered people is up for a vote.

Even if a CD doesn't want to be out in public, he can write to his local politicians in favor of pending bills that protect transgendered people. In doing so, he is under no obligation to reveal that he's a crossdresser.

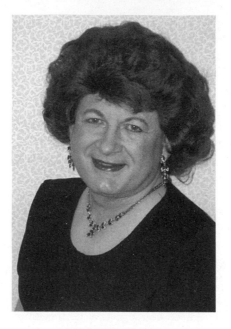

Barbara Van Horn

Alternately, he can bypass the political and take a more educational approach, by visiting a local college with some of his "sisters" in order to put a human face on crossdressing. Barbara Van Horn did so with other members of his local Tri-Ess chapter, Tri Epsilon Sigma. They spoke to graduate students earning degrees in Sexuality, and felt they communicated a lot more than what the students might learn from a textbook. The crossdressers left feeling affirmed and understood, and the students had been able to ask questions to which they might not otherwise find answers, since the literature on crossdressing is so sparse. At the very least, a crossdresser can join GenderPAC or the NTAC (National Transgender Advocacy Coalition) and keep informed on current legislation and court rulings.

During the six months of January to June 2003, many pieces of relevant legislation came to a vote, and quite a few court rulings came down. Here is a sample:

- *In New York:* Activists and elected officials have finalized language for the Gender Expression Non-Discrimination Act, a state bill that would ban discrimination based on gender identity or expression. The bill is expected to be introduced in the Assembly and State Senate in April.

- *In Illinois:* A Cook County, Ill., judge told a transgender father that he lacks the right to seek custody of his son.

- *In California:* Introduced by Assemblyman Mark Leno, D-San Francisco, AB 196 would expand the state's Fair Employment and Housing Act to include the transgender community. The bill's definition of "gender" includes "identity, appearance, or behavior, whether or not that identity, appearance, or behavior is different from that traditionally associated with the victim's sex at birth." On April 21, the bill passed the California Assembly 42-34 with all Republican members in opposition. The senate has yet to take up the bill, and Governor Gray Davis has not yet given any indication of his position.

- *In Texas:* The El Paso City Council voted unanimously on Tuesday, April 9, to expand its anti-discrimination ordinance. The amended ordinance will ban discrimination based on sexual orientation or gender identity, which Rep. Sumrall described as "one's gender being misidentified at birth."

- *In New Mexico:* The New Mexico legislature passed anti-discrimination and hate crimes bills that cover both gender identity and sexual orientation.

- *In Florida:* A Florida circuit court judge ruled that Michael Kantaras, a FTM transgender man, is legally male, and was legally married to his wife, Linda Kantaras. The ruling cleared the way for the judge to grant Kantaras primary custody of the couple's two children, one of whom he adopted after marriage.

Lisa, the wife of a crossdresser, points out that crossdressers can only benefit from forming coalitions with other groups whose issues are similar. She also warns of the disadvantages of being single-issue activists:

> TGs are a small crowd when viewing the population as a whole. I think it would be in the TG's best political interest to align with other, bigger groups, to address concerns about civil liberties. Otherwise their voice is so small no one hears it, or if they do, and if they are politicians, they don't care because they would rather curry the votes of the more numerous TG detractors than risk a political career over a few TGs.

> *There is a danger, in my opinion, in being single issue activists, i.e.,*
> *only being politically active when the cause is one which concerns your*
> *rights alone. If one only looks out for discrimination or restriction of*
> *civil liberties in small isolated areas a lot can slip by and not only do*
> *other causes suffer but one's own cause can suffer as well.*

Many people get involved in politics over a single issue and find they
become engaged with broader movements. Engagement on any level is a
great way to educate oneself about politics and local politicians. A crossdresser can certainly work on voter registration drives without telling anyone he is a crossdresser.

Incidentally, one doesn't have to be part of any political party to understand that there are issues with crossdressing in this society. Democrat or
Republican, liberal or conservative on other issues, the way people feel about
gender identity makes them an outsider in certain ways. Heather explains:

> *I see most people that are into fringe movements and lifestyles as a*
> *bunch of whiners who would rather try to legislate society's acceptance*
> *of their actions than try to make themselves valuable people who hap-*
> *pen to be crossdressers (or whatever other fringe they inhabit). To me,*
> *no one owes me acceptance, much less encouragement. If they are capa-*
> *ble of giving me that, bonus! But, it's not and shouldn't be a given.*
>
> *That being said, our government is based on the principles of life, lib-*
> *erty and the* pursuit *of happiness. That means do what you will so long*
> *as it's legal and makes you happy. If it's illegal and you don't think it*
> *should be then convince enough people you are right and make it legal.*
> *If it's not illegal but simply odd from the point of view of the majority,*
> *seek to make it seem less odd by expressing your view of what you do*
> *and pointing out the harmlessness or the similarities to other accepted*
> *practices.*

Heather's last comments are certainly relevant to the crossdressing community. Crossdressing itself is not illegal (unless one is crossdressed in order to
perpetrate a crime) but it certainly is considered odd. As Heather points out,
though, there is no guarantee of acceptance. Crossdressers are not going to
magically win the right to be who they are with impunity. They have to earn
society's respect, and that respect takes work. There are few feminists alive
today who experienced the early struggles for the vote, but there are plenty
who were rejected from restaurants or workplaces for wearing pants. Gay

and lesbian activists have been involved in more recent struggles and can share their ideas about what it takes to promote national acceptance of a minority. The crossdressing community must reach out to these other groups to learn what it takes both personally and politically, and until then I'm afraid I don't want to hear about the unfairness of the crossdresser's plight. As the wife of a crossdresser I met at Rainbow Mountain put it, "We had to burn our bras. You're going to have to wear yours in public."

A HEAD START

THE GOOD NEWS is that crossdressers don't have to reinvent the wheel. Numerous organizations and people are already tackling the legal and civic issues of being a transgendered person. GenderPAC, a lobby group, has a compelling list of *Myths and Facts* on their website, www.gpac.org.

GPAC: MYTH VS. FACT
ABOUT GENDER STEREOTYPES

MYTH
Gender stereotyping in the workplace is a woman's problem.

FACT
According to *The New York Times,* almost one in seven new claims filed with the EEOC are male-on-male gender harassment, double only a decade ago. For example, Joseph Oncale, plaintiff in the Supreme Court case *Oncale* v. *Sundowner,* was repeatedly menaced by oil-rig coworkers for being slender, blond, longhaired, and wearing an earring.

MYTH
Gender stereotypes are only a problem among adults.

FACT
Children of all ages from toddlers to teens complain of harassment or bullying to force them to conform to gender norms. And it can create long-term problems: a recent university study showed that adherence to strict codes of masculinity, hardness, aggressiveness, and emotional distance is a leading cause in academic underachievement among teenage boys.

MYTH
Only gay and transgender people are targeted for transcending gender stereotypes.

FACT
Anyone who doesn't meet expectations for a "real man" or a "real woman" can become a target, from a successful professional like Anne Hopkins in the Supreme Court's *Hopkins* v. *Price Waterhouse* case, who was fired for being "too aggressive," to African-American bus driver Willie Houston, who was killed while celebrating his engagement when a man became enraged at seeing him holding a blind friend on one arm and his fiancé's purse on the other.

MYTH
Federal legislation to stop gender violence already exists.

FACT
Gender is excluded from federal hate crimes legislation: the FBI is not authorized to collect statistics on it, and, as in the murder of Brandon Teena (memorialized in the movie *Boys Don't Cry*) showed, federal authorities are not authorized to act when local officials fail to ensure that justice is done.

MYTH
Gay, lesbian, and bisexual Americans are only discriminated against because of their sexual orientation.

FACT
In a recent GenderPAC survey, one third of gay, lesbian, and bisexual respondents who suffered workplace discrimination reported that it was due at least in part to their gender. For example, in New York's *Dawson* v. *Esteé Lauder* case, thirty-two year-old Dawn Dawson was fired for allegedly looking "too butch."

MYTH
Gender stereotyping affects few Americans, and mainly those who want to change their sex.

FACT
In fact, at some time in their life, almost every American is shamed, harassed, isolated, or even attacked because they don't meet someone's idea of a "real man" or a "real woman."

MYTH
Boys will be boys: bullying is wrong, but natural.

FACT
It's not only not natural, but it's increasingly violent. Five of eight assailants in recent school shooting incidents were reportedly students who had been repeatedly genderbashed and genderbaited in school. And last year, gay and transgender two-spirit Navajo teen Fred Martinez, Jr. was beaten to death by another student in Cortez, Colorado. School bullying doesn't stop with other boys: a recent Harvard University report revealed that 20 percent of teenage girls are assaulted by a boyfriend, increasing their risk of bulimia/anorexia, early pregnancy, drug abuse, and suicide.

This last fact brings me right back around to the transgender community's connection to the feminist community. Bulimia, anorexia, and early pregnancy have all been feminist issues for years now, and GenderPAC acknowledges that when a teenaged girl experiences this kind of harassment from boys, it is a gender issue—not just a feminist one. When transgender teens are kicked out of their homes, and find themselves without shelter, health care, or food, they are in the same position as teenaged girls who get thrown out of their homes for getting pregnant. (Not many boys get the same treatment for getting a girl pregnant.) Trans teenagers without support networks or financial resources are more likely to end up working in the sex industry.

Likewise, there are some transitioning TS women who, because they are without financial resources, may be forced to work as prostitutes. Health insurance doesn't usually cover the cost of hormones or surgery or perhaps they have no health insurance at all. Transitioning transsexuals who work in the sex industry stand primed to become the new victims of our repressed and undiscussed sexual impulses: as "men" they will be neglected by feminists who are otherwise engaged in trying to help protect women who work in the sex industry, and as "women" they will face sexual violence committed by johns. They're in a double-bind because of their trans-ness, and while that trans-ness may be their appeal to "customers," it's also what leaves them open to violence. Since prostitution is traditionally a women's issue, it's important that women with experience in these matters are courted by the transgender community. It has taken the feminist community a long time to realize that middle-class women are not the only group who need liberation, but that the problems experienced by women are more keenly felt by working-class women and women of color. The gay and lesbian community is criticized from within its ranks for overlooking the same issues of class and race. The transgendered community, as a result, doesn't have to make the same mistakes and can put measures in place from the start which are more inclusive.

The intersections of these various communities—gay and lesbian, transgender, feminist—could lead to a coalition that would help redefine how we think of gender in this society. There is a lot of internal education to be done: crossdressers need to learn gay history, women need to learn about transsexual women. Transsexual women have to find a way not to judge us all by the often vitriolic attacks feminists have made on transsexual women's existence. There are places where we can meet. Galen Sherwin, the former president of NOW-NYC, describes her experience organizing a conference to promote solidarity between the transgender and feminist communities:

> *The conference we organized was great and had as one of its goals stimulating dialogue between feminists and the trans community, and building momentum for positive collaboration/activism on gender issues. I think it really worked. There were quite a few trans folks there. I've worked with quite a few activists in NYC and around NY State and about local issues of concern to the transgender community, particularly hate crimes.*

Sherwin points out that the goal is dialogue—the ability for us to talk about our specific but also shared concerns. I see a great deal of potential, but the one requirement is that crossdressers abandon their "straight" identification. There is a difference between "straight" and "heterosexual": the former implies a kind of political identification, and the latter only sexual preference. Too often, crossdressers see their only "saving grace" as being that they're not gay, not transsexual, and not perverts. Whenever a straight crossdresser says "At least I'm not . . ." he has distanced himself from people who are likely to understand his suffering and open doors toward personal and political liberation. Crossdressers are struggling with deep, complicated feelings about gender. Furthermore, some are bisexual, and others have fantasies and fetishes that the BDSM community would understand. I find that the denial within the crossdressing community responsible for most of the side effects that accompany a life of secrecy and shame: sadness, depression, alcoholism. Is holding on to the "prize" of straightness worth all that? I don't think so. If crossdressers are really committed to being "out and about," they will have to confront their own prejudices: their sexism and homophobia, and their transphobia, in order to connect with a larger community that is already actively welcoming them. Crossdressers and their partners should feel lucky: not only do they not have to reinvent the wheel, but they're already standing on the shoulders of giants. Liberation may only require the ability to let go of the status that comes with being "straight." Since cross-dressers have shown a willingness to let go of the status of being "men," rising to this new challenge shouldn't be the hardest thing they've ever done, but even if it is, the freedom and self-acceptance to be had at the end of the day will be well worth the effort.

A Few Words from Betty

WHEN I WAS twelve years old, I remember sitting in a library somewhere in L.A. and surreptitiously looking up "transvestite" in the card catalog. I don't remember where I ran across the word, but I do remember opening the two books they had and finding some variation of myself reflected back. It was thrilling and it was depressing. Thrilling because I wasn't alone and depressing because I knew deep down inside that I *was* alone.

I remember looking both ways when pulling those books down, because I surely didn't want anyone to know that I was interested in books on "abnormal" sexuality. It was a secret and it was mine. I didn't know what was going on, I just remember looking at those books because I had to *know*.

If some person in that library had come up to me and said, "Young man, in twenty some years you'll be writing an afterword to a book that your wife has written on transgendered people" I would never have believed him.

I'd probably have told him that I wouldn't have a wife. No girl in the world could possibly be interested in my "secret."

Yet here I am in a small apartment in New York City, surrounded by dozens of books on the transgendered, writing an afterword to my wife's book.

What can I say?

I can't tell you why I'm transgendered. I know that. The only answer I can honestly give is "because I am." I wish I could do better than that. I could describe at length how it feels when I'm dressed, but others have already done that. My wife has presented all the theories so there's no point in reiterating, and they don't answer the question, anyway.

Hence: because.

All I know is that I'm an extremely lucky person to have found someone like Helen to live my life with. She's smart, she's always asking questions, and I think she's the most beautiful woman to ever walk the planet.

She's worked long and hard on this book. It's been a labor of love, because, truly, without love, this book would never have been written. We've had many conversations, many laughs, and many fights about my tranny-ness. It just isn't an easy thing.

At the end of the day it all boils down to human beings struggling to be themselves. That's all we are: human beings. I'm pretty sure Martin Luther King, Jr., didn't have the transgendered in mind when he said he had a dream, but he sure did illuminate the hopes of this boy.

I'd like to think that maybe some twelve-year-old out there might find this book and won't feel so alone when he goes searching for the answers to the questions within.

We can dream, right?

Glossary

OKAY, LET'S GET the definitions I use all in one place. Fold down the corner of the page if you're new to this stuff, so you can refer back here whenever you need to. These definitions are neither all-inclusive nor excruciatingly thorough: they are merely an introduction to common terms, and a Rosetta Stone for my personal usage.

I have tried to be as sensitive as I can to any and all of the issues involved in defining terms, which are so deeply personal, and where possible have chosen definitions provided by or approved by members of that particular community. Where there is disagreement within a community, or when the use of a term has changed historically, I have tried to indicate as much. This is a new and developing community, and any definition listed here is sure to be clarified or changed even in the time it takes to write this book and publish it.

I must emphasize as well that the terms CD, TV, TS, TG, etc. are not exclusive categories. Some crossdressers feel they are more transgendered, and a lot of TS women spend some time thinking they are crossdressers. This is a spectrum, a continuum. Think of it this way: if a crossdresser is in category 1, and a transsexual is in category 9, there are endless amounts of numbers between 1 and 9, like 1.65, 4.224593, 6, 7.9999. Each transgendered person is his or her own number between 1 and 9.

Each of those individuals deserves to be called what he or she prefers to be called. Some TS women prefer to be known as "women who transitioned" while some younger TS women proudly define themselves as "transsexual women" and never leave off the adjective that they feel makes them the special people they are. Other TS women prefer only to be known as women, especially when a great deal of time has passed since their transition. I offer only this piece of advice: when a person introduces him or herself to you as a crossdresser, don't call him or her anything else. Likewise with someone who introduces him or herself as transsexual, or genderqueer, etc. There is far too much denial of transgendered realities in the world as it is, and the only person who can inform you of his or her reality is, and what he or she prefers to be called, is the transgendered individual in question.

Likewise, make sure the pronouns you use when referring to that person match their gender presentation. When a crossdresser is en femme, that crossdresser is a she, and her slip is showing, not his. It's a sign of respect that doesn't go unnoticed. (In this book I do refer to crossdressers as "he," for the sake of clarity. In person I would never do such a thing.)

Crossdresser, or **CD,** has two main definitions. 1) The first is the more general term used to describe anyone who dresses as the opposite sex for any reason. Joan of Arc was crossdressed, as were Marlene Dietrich in *Morocco* and Jack Lemmon and Tony Curtis in *Some Like It Hot*. The members of Monty Python, Flip Wilson, and a score of other comedians crossdressed for the sake of comedy. (The only exception, of course, is our own beloved "executive transvestite," Eddie Izzard, who is a comedian and actor who just happens to be a transvestite.) Crossdressing is a very general term, to be used to describe anyone who for any reason wears the clothes of the opposite sex: theatrically; for practical reasons (like the way women did in order to live lives of greater freedom); for comedy; or for sex or even just for masquerade (like on Halloween). That is, a man who dresses as a woman for Halloween crossdresses, but he is not necessarily a transvestite.

2) I will use the more specific—and recent—definition of the term *crossdresser* in this book. A crossdresser is the new term for what most people think of as a transvestite, a man who wears women's clothes in order to feel like a woman. Because the term *transvestite* came fully loaded with sexual connotations and mental illness, America's crossdressers—sometime in the 1970s—started using the more neutral term *crossdresser* to define themselves. They emphasized that transvestism wasn't about sex, that crossdressers were not homosexual but were in fact largely heterosexual, and that crossdressing is, for the MTF crossdresser, more about expressing "an inner feminine." Eventually they stopped using the word "transvestite" altogether, and substituted "crossdresser." That said, the term transvestite is still used by the rest of the world. As this book is being written for an American audience, I'll use the term crossdresser so as not to offend accepted sensibilities. In general the term has stuck within the crossdressing community, so I use crossdresser and its shorthand, CD, to mean a man who dresses in women's clothes, often with the intention of being mistaken for a woman. Most of the time he is heterosexual, and he may or may not experience sexual arousal as a result of his crossdressing.

Drag queens are generally gay men who are all about glitz, performance, beauty, humor, sex, and sometimes politics. RuPaul is a drag queen. Drag queens are performers, either traditionally as lip-synchers (like NYC drag legend Sweetie) or—more and more so—with their own voices, such as Justin Bond or Joey Arias. Drag queens started the Gay Pride movement, by finally getting fed up with the regular and frequent police raids at the gay and lesbian club The Stonewall in June 1969. The lesson? Never underestimate a drag queen: she's more man than you'll ever be, and more woman than you'll ever get. (Note: All gay men who dress in women's clothes are not drag queens. Some gay men who dress as women are transgendered, and dressing as a woman is not about performance, but about identity.)

En Femme is the term used to refer to a man who is dressed as a woman, used in the TG and CD communities. **En Homme** is used more rarely, and used to describe a CD when he's not in women's clothes and not presenting as a woman.

FTM (female to male) is a person who was born female, and dresses as, or has become, or is becoming, or lives as, a man. **MTF** (male-to-female) indicates a person was born a man, and dresses as, or has become, or is becoming, or lives as, a female. Both of these terms are directional, to indicate the gender someone is starting from and arriving at.

Fetish is something, such as a material object or a nonsexual part of the body, that arouses sexual desire and may become necessary for sexual gratification. The popular usage, "to have a fetish for" something, is not accurate.

Gender dysphoria is a term used to describe a person whose gender role, or presentation, or cultural expectations related to gender cause them feelings of anxiety, depression, or unease. This is the older version of the term that appeared in the *DSM-III*. Dysphoria is the (Greek) term for the anxiety, depression or unease: "*dys*" like in dysfunction meaning not, and *phoria* (like in euphoria) meaning "joy." The term was changed entirely, for *DSM-IV,* to *Gender Identity Disorder.*

Gender Identity Disorder, or **GID**, is psychologists' current term for transgendered feelings, what they had previously called "gender dsyphoria." The APA (American Psychological Association) defines it like so:

The patient strongly and persistently identifies with the other sex. This is not simply a desire for a perceived cultural advantage of being the other sex. In adolescents and adults, this desire may be manifested by any of:

- *Stated wish to be the other sex*
- *Often passing as the other sex*
- *Wish to live or be treated as the other sex*
- *Belief that the patient's feelings and reactions are typical of the other sex*

There is strong discomfort with the patient's own sex or a feeling that the gender role of that sex is inappropriate for the patient. This is shown by any symptoms such as:

- *Preoccupation with hormones, surgery or other physical means to change one's sex characteristics*
- *Patient's belief in having been born the wrong sex*
- *The patient does not have a physical intersex condition.*

These symptoms cause clinically important distress or impair work, social or personal functioning.

People who have transgendered feelings often resent being classified as having a disorder at all, exactly because it implies mental illness. Some argue for the removal of *GID* from the next *DSM*, on the grounds that their minds are perfectly fine: it's their bodies, or the culture, that isn't what it should be.

Oh, right, then there's my group: **Genetic Girls (GG),** or—much improved—**Genetic Women (GW).** I've also seen the term **FAB,** which means "Female At Birth." That's for women like me, who were born female and identify as women. Because etiquette within the TG community often dictates that a MTF crossdresser be called "she" in public and often has a femme name, the term *genetic girl* was termed in order to distinguish the husband from his wife. I am not sure who coined the usage, but it is useful because crossdressers change their gender, and transsexuals change their sex, and at a previous time it was thought the only sure thing was chromosomal sex, but of course it turns out that chromosomal sex is not a guarantor either (see *Intersex*). I will use GW because—as I often remind my father—no female over the age of eighteen is a girl (a point which is often forgotten in the TG community, as well). To put it bluntly, GGs or GWs are what most people would refer to as "regular women": those of us who were born and raised female.

T-girl and **transgirl** are short forms of Transgendered Girl/Woman. Transgirl is used by MTF transgendered/transsexual girls, especially younger ones. It is used widely within the Trans community. T-girl is also used by men who are both MTF transgendered and gay. Not all men who are gay are drag queens, and I find this is the term many of them use to describe their own gender identity. She may live as a woman 24/7 or she may not. She may be on hormones or she may not.

Tranny is a short form for transvestite, transgender, or transsexual. It is considered derogatory in America (the most common usage stateside is in the term *Tranny Chaser* which I'll get to in a moment) but around the world this is another umbrella term, and can indicate crossdressers, transsexuals, and the transgendered. (Vickie Lee's *Tranny Guide* is a good example of the global use of the term; it's a guide that reviews safe places for t-girls of all varieties to party, dine, and shop.) When used within the community, "tranny" can be acceptable and playful, but when used by an outsider is considered an insult, like queer in the gay community.

Tranny chasers, or **Admirers** are the men or women who seek the company of MTF TGs and go looking for them. They can be male or female but the female variety is rare. Often spoken about contemptuously by crossdressers and their wives, Tranny chasers are infamous for being oversexed and quite blunt about it. They're to be found in Internet chat rooms, at nightclubs and bars, and sometimes are welcome in T-friendly spaces. Tranny chasers are the big bugaboo in the crossdressing community, because their very existence suggests that crossdressers are not all as straight as they claim to be. Chasers are willing to give crossdressed men the kind of attention they desire, and that attention (a drink, a compliment) validates the crossdresser's experience, and completes the fantasy of feeling like a woman.

Transgender, or **Transgendered**, is probably the trickiest word of the lot. Generally speaking, it describes people who experience a gender identity of the sex opposite the one they were born into. How they choose to identify as a transgendered person depends on what kinds of feelings they have about their gender, how acute those feelings are, and how frequently they have them. The term can be used in a few ways: 1) as an umbrella term which encompasses the whole of the community, transsexuals, and cross-dressers, t-girls and drag kings, e.g. "The Transgender Community"; 2) as a way of indicating someone who does not fit into the classic "types," i.e., someone who is transgendered is not "just" a crossdresser but not a "classic" transsexual woman either, sometimes because they are not opting for the "traditional" path toward changing sex. In fact, they may not be interested in changing sex in any kind of permanent way. To me, a transgendered person doesn't fit neatly into pre-ordained categories, but still presents a gender that is different from their birth sex. For example, a crossdresser who has deep gender dysphoric feelings, and is pretty sure he is not transsexual, may try hormones for a while and refer to hirself* as transgendered—Katie tells me it's the term Elle used before she began transition; or 3) to refer to a person who might have previously been called a pre-op transsexual, who is on hormones, lives 24/7 as a woman, but who has otherwise held back from genital or other surgery for a variety of personal or medical reasons. Transgendered people can be genetic men who use hormones and have feminine bodies but who live as men, or alternately, the term might be used to describe a MTF crossdresser who lives as a woman 24/7. I use transgender in all three ways, and context should reveal which one it is: when I refer to the transgender community I'm using it as an umbrella term, but when I refer to someone being transgendered that is in the specific, singular sense.

Transitioning, in front of Transsexual or Transgender, is a way of indicating that a person is in mid-journey from birth sex to desired or internal sex. I will use it to describe anyone who is "on their way" to living full-time as the other gender and doesn't quite yet—however that might manifest.

Transsexuals are—as the term suggests—those who cross the boundaries of gender and the boundaries of sex. MTF Transsexuals, for example, are born male and eventually transition—via hormones and/or surgery but sometimes neither—so that they live and work as female.

---

*hir, hirself, s/he are pronouns used when the gender of the person is in question or otherwise not indicated. Some Genderqueer activists use these terms exclusively, basically just to tell anyone who comes along that their gender will not be made clear and never will be made clear, and if you need to know that badly you shouldn't know hir, anyway. I'm glad I have them to use in a book like this one, but otherwise I do often wonder if they will go the way of the feminist-inspired, politicized spellings of woman/women: there are precious few wimmin's groups around these days.

- **Pre-op Transsexuals** want and plan on having SRS. They are usually on hormones but haven't had surgery yet.

- **Post-op Transsexuals** are usually on maintenance hormones and have had surgery.

- **Non-op Transsexuals** live 24/7 as the sex which they were not born. They have no intention of ever getting SRS. It is not part of their transition plan.

The short form—for this book—is **TS**. My use of the term "usually" is no accident. These are meant to be general categories only. I, like many others, reject the idea of the "true transsexual" as essentialist and mean-spirited. It is too frequently used to belittle the identities and struggles of people who for one reason or another rejected some part of the traditional transition path. In order to qualify my very-limited definition above, I offer this personal account, by a friend who asked not to be identified.

> My sustaining mantra is that I am who I am supposed to be. I borrowed it from a close friend with "obsessive-compulsive disorder." I find that it molts shame, it extends my space, it curtails the need for intellectual defenses of my identity, and it smoothes the craters of my heavily bombarded sense of self.
>
> I am transsexual—I suppose. I know that I am a woman because I feel it. But, transsexuality bears a very heavy burden of definition. It is a line in the sand that people demand in order to rank and file me—a counterpoint and dexotifier to create distance. It is viewed as a disorder of the mind. Like a woman's body, it is somehow everyone's business. And it is the supposed secret that "dupes" or beguiles the onlooker.
>
> I, like Dr. Harry Benjamin, view transsexuality as a congenital disorder of the body, not the mind. That is not to say there are only two sexes or two genders. It is to say that I have a body that does not convey either my own gender and sex as a female woman. Physicians consider me a woman with a physical disorder, while psychologists consider me a man with a mental disorder. And despite a few decades of lobbying, I am clearly designated a second-class woman by my society. Only a scant group of attorneys, medical professionals, and politicians defend my right to self-determination. I am exotified in popular media. Yet I remain the same woman regardless of this all.

Transsexual women do not feel their transsexuality. They feel their womanhood and act to express themselves. When they sometimes transition and "disappear" into society, they are not letting go of their transgender identity. This is because the majority of transsexuals hardly identify as one during the implementation of their womanhood.

I am a recent fan of the idea that once a transsexual woman transitions, she is then an ex-transsexual. As in healed—cured.

This is, of course, only one TS woman's opinion and experience. There are as many definitions, and self-definitions, of TS identity as there are TS women.

Transvestite (**TV** for short) is the traditional term for a man who wears women's clothes. *Trans-* meaning across, and *–vestite* from the Latin verb *vestire,* to dress. The term usually applies to men. The term was coined by Magnus Hirschfield in 1910, who coined the term with interest and empathy, not to label crossdressing men "deviant." Unfortunately, over time the "deviant" label cleaved to the term, despite the fact that the "deviant" variety of transvestism is more accurately referred to as *Transvestic Fetishism.* Transvestism, in and of itself, does not appear in the *DSM-IV.* Transvestites, as a result, started using the term *crossdresser* instead, which has come to specify a man who wears women's clothes, but not one who does so for sexual pleasure. If this seems extraordinarily and unnecessarily confusing, it is, but it was a political effort on the part of American Crossdressers to self-identify, and political endgames always make language a kind of double-speak.

My husband prefers the term *transvestite* over *crossdresser* and is distinctly in the minority of American crossdressers as a result. He prefers the term for four main reasons: 1) for starters he did and sometimes still does get a sexual thrill out of wearing women's clothes and he doesn't mind admitting it; 2) he feels it connects him to history, to the work of Magnus Hirschfield who was the first to identify and respectfully present transvestites, in his seminal 1910 work *Transvestites;* 3) my husband appreciates that the *Trans* in transvestite connects him to the rest of the rest of the Transgender community; and 4) in the rest of the world, most men who wear women's clothes—for sexual or other reasons—call themselves transvestites. His using the term *transvestite* is something like the way some gay men and women chose to identify as queer, which they did to take back the word from the people who would use to slur them with it. Out of respect for the majority of the community I will use the term *crossdresser* throughout this book, except when I refer to my husband or others who self-identify as transvestites.

Transvestic Fetishism is in the *DSM-IV*, and it is defined like so:

> Repeatedly for at least six months, a heterosexual male has intense sexual desires, fantasies or behavior concerning crossdressing. This causes clinically important distress or impairs work, social or personal functioning.

Because of the psychological community's use of the word, the term Transvestite became associated with men secretly using articles of women's clothing to masturbate (that's a classic case of Transvestic Fetishism, but I've yet to meet anyone who does this), or, in other words, it came to mean men who dress in women's clothing for sexual pleasure.

SUPPLEMENTAL TERMS:

Autogynephilia is still a new word in the Transgender dictionary, and one that is little understood but hotly debated. The concept was first described by Ray Blanchard, a sex researcher. An autogynephile is a male who is sexually aroused by either the idea of having a woman's body or by the idea of being a woman. (*Auto* = self, *gyne* = woman, *philia* = love, or erotic love of oneself as a woman.)

The term has been described as the "unified field theory" of transgenderism, but Blanchard's application of it to transsexuals is the epicenter of the debate. From what I understand, MTF transsexuals often gain pleasure from imagining their female bodies, but that pleasure is more about the fantasy of finally having a body that will match their internal gender identification. Transvetites and crossdressers also often admit to autogynephilic feelings, but because of the newness of the term and the general lack of research on crossdressers, there are no statistics. As one crossdresser put it: "Some guys are only ever in love with the woman they see in the mirror." Further discussion of this term appears in two chapters: *Slippery Slope?* (Chapter 5) and *Sex and Sensibility,* (Chapter 6).

BDSM is short for Bondage, Discipline, Sadism, and Masochism.

Diagnostic and Statistical Manual, or **DSM** is the cornerstone reference manual used for psychiatric diagnosis and classification. Such diagnosis and classification is meant to be done only by trained professionals. The numbers afterward (usually III or IV) refer to the edition, and if an "R" appears, it stands for Revised. Therefore, *DSM-III* came out first, followed by *DSM-IIIR,* followed by *DSM-IV,* and so on.

Drag king is the female equivalent of the drag queen. She is usually a lesbian, and dresses as a boy or man for a variety of reasons: to feel more genuinely macho, as a result of gender dysphoria, because it turns her or her girlfriend on, or to deconstruct gender via performance. There are drag kings who perform, like New York's own brilliant Murray Hill and Mo B. Dick. They are not necessarily FTM transsexuals, although some modify their bodies with testosterone.

GLBT stands for Gay, Lesbian, Bisexual, and Transgender, and encapsulates the community created from the Gay Pride movement, which also included lesbians and later bisexual people. The "T" has only been added in the last year or so. In New York State, gay activists worked to get SONDA passed—the Sexual Orientation Non-Discrimination Act—and it did, but without including protection for transgendered people. As a result, GENDA—Gender Expression Non-Discrimination Act—has been drafted and will be pushed in the upcoming legislative season. Sometimes, too, a "Q" is added, as in **GLBTQ**, for Questioning, which was described by journalist Deborah Young as "a neologism coined for anybody who falls outside the traditional boundaries of heterosexuality."

Genderqueer, Genderfuck, Genderhack, Gender-bender, and **Gender-blender** are all the terms for the more subversive of the TG community. These are the folks who have read Kate Bornstein or Leslie Feinberg and who refuse to allow gender to be an either/or situation. If someone tells you they are a genderhack, you might not be able to tell what their genetic or biological sex is or was, or they have just chosen to identify as someone who insists that appearance, behavior, and roles should not and are not determined by gender. To be perfectly honest, this is my favorite category by far: it's loaded with political intent and puts the middle finger up at the traditional gender roles and a society that promotes that system. What can I say? I'm a punk rocker at heart. God bless the subversives.

Intersex is a term used to describe those who, at birth, have genitalia or chromosomes or an internal reproductive system that are not "standard." Sometimes they have ambiguous genitalia, and other times their external sex organs are quite decidedly male or female—but their internal organs are the opposite of the visible ones. There are many different categories of

Intersexuality. A genetic male (XY) may be born with female genitalia, and so raised as a girl. Sometimes the chromosomal coding is more complicated than a simple XX or XY. Traditionally doctors have decided, and often without even the parents' knowledge or consent, or in response to parents' distress, to surgically "fix" the child one way or another. ISNA, the Intersex Society of North America, provides information on Intersex conditions and actively educates the medical community on the error of this "tradition." They insist:

- *Intersexuality is basically a problem of stigma and trauma, not gender.*
- *Parents' distress must not be treated by surgery on the child.*
- *Professional mental health care is essential.*
- *Honest, complete disclosure is good medicine.*
- *All children should be assigned as boy or girl, without early surgery.*

SRS (Sexual Reassignment Surgery) is the surgery transsexuals get in order to align their bodies with their internal sense of gender. That is, an MTF transsexual woman will have surgery to replace her penis with a vagina. There are other associated surgeries. A TS woman describes them thus (though the comments in parentheses are mine, to explain the purpose of each):

> *Then I hack out my throat* (to remove a visible Adam's Apple), *shorten my vocal chords* (which makes the voice pitch higher, and so more traditionally feminine), *sand my brow bone* (men have more visible brow bones than women), *staple my hairline forward* (to revert the hairline to its place before Male Pattern Balding took effect), *invert my penis, and reshape my scrotum into labia* (the last two are genital surgery. The penis and scrotal sack are used to create a labia and vagina, inverted so as to make use of the nerve endings and hopefully enable the TS women to experience orgasm as a woman). Most *of what I'm suffering now would not be necessary if laws allowed the interruption of adolescence with simple pills. We "transsexuals" always knew we wanted those pills as teens. There's no controversy—as adults, we save $40,000 cash for procedures that intermittently disfigure us over three years in order to reverse adolescence. Then, we spend $20,000 more to deal with our groins once and for all. Pishaw. How can I not be angry at the government (and society) for a multitude of reasons? I could use the $40,000 for other things, like a house, and my employer could use me at work.*

All TS women do not get all of these surgeries, and in fact many do not get any of them. These are the ones that are currently available.

Some TS and TG women opt for another surgical option: the orchiectomy, which is the removal of the testicles. Without an orchiectomy or genital surgery, TS women have to take estrogen (usually in the form of Estradiol) *and* anti-androgens. By removing the testicles, the TS woman effectively removes the source of the male hormones, or androgens. She can then take only maintenance levels of hormones and cease taking anti-androgens altogether, which decreases associated health risks.

Surgery that converts male genitalia to female, or female to male, is referred to as GRS, *Genital Reconstruction Surgery*. Surgery for FTM transsexual men usually can often involve chest reconstruction surgery, hysterectomy, and GRS.

She-male is neither male nor female and (usually) likes it that way. Usually a she-male is a person who was born male but who has since developed breasts, either through the use of female hormones or via silicone implants or both. She often presents as female. The striking characteristic, you might say, is that a she-male retains hir penis. The best of both worlds, as some fans of she-male porn would say. This does not always sit well with pre-op Transsexual women, whose bodies are pretty much the same as the She-Males'. The She-Male is a sexualized body and sometimes hirself is in fact a pre-op transsexual. They're otherwise known as "chicks with dicks." She-males work primarily in the sex industry, often in order to afford the hormones and surgeries they are seeking. The target audience for she-male porn and sexual services consists of men, and usually men who publicly identify as heterosexual.

Third Sex is a term used to describe someone who is neither male nor female, man nor woman.

The Cast of Characters

THIS IS AN alphabetical list of all the people mentioned or quoted in this book. They are alphabetized by first name if no last name is given. Names have been changed by request.

Adrian/Ali is a crossdresser from the Southwest of England.

Amanda is a crossdresser, married to Kathy.

Charles Anders is the author of *The Lazy Crossdresser*.

Angela is the genetic female wife of Jerry, a crossdresser.

Natalie Angier is the author of *Woman: An Intimate Geography*.

Kevyn Aucoin was the pre-eminent makeup artist of our times, but passed away in May 2002. He frequently featured male to female transformation in his books. His book *Making Faces* is a standard of makeup application.

Michael Bailey is the author of *The Man Who Would Be Queen*. He is also a Professor of Psychology at Northwestern University.

Becca is a crossdresser who runs the Eureka En Femme Getaway with his genetic female wife Dixie (not to be mistaken with the crossdresser Dixie).

Carol Beecroft founded Tri-Ess jointly with Virginia Prince.

Harry Benjamin was born in Berlin, Germany in 1885 and emigrated to the United States. just before WWI. Upon arriving in the United States, he joined the Neurological Institute of Columbia University to study endocrinology. He did much to develop medical treatment of transsexuality and related TG issues in the United States and Canada, bringing his German knowledge to North America and emerged as the American leader in the field. In 1966, Benjamin published *The Transsexual Phenomena*. The medical standards and ethics body that governs treatment of transsexuals today is named after Dr. Benjamin: the "Standards of Care" or HBIGDA.

Ray Blanchard is the Head of the Clinical Sexology Program of the Clarke Institute of Psychiatry in Toronto. He is published in numerous academic journals dealing in human sexuality.

Kate Bornstein is an author and performance artist whose published works include the books *Gender Outlaw: On Men, Women and the Rest of Us* and *My Gender Workbook*. Kate Bornstein's books are taught in over 120 colleges and universities around the world.

Gary R. Brooks is the author of *The Centerfold Syndrome*.

Gerri Buchanan is the Director of Chapter Development for Tri-Ess.

Colleen is a crossdresser who was born on Long Island and raised in a middle class suburb. He has lived in Manhattan on and off for the last thirteen years, and currently lives on the West Side and loves it. He went to a Catholic grammar school and then to college down south. After school, he worked for a while in the corporate world, but now works as a freelance marketer. "She" tries to get out in the city as often as possible.

Lynn Conway is a woman who transitioned over three decades ago.

Corinne is the dominant genetic female partner of Kimmi.

Alyssa Davis is an older, married, closeted crossdresser and fictionmania story writer.

Simone deBeauvoir (1908–1986). French author, existentialist, and feminist. She was a friend, lover, and peer of Jean-Paul Sartre's, and there is much debate as to how much her ideas influenced his work. DeBeauvoir had a philosophy degree from the Sorbonne, and is most famous for her groundbreaking work, *The Second Sex,* in which she examines sexism in Western Culture.

Denise is the genetic female girlfriend of Melissa, a crossdresser.

Diane1962 is a former crossdresser who is now a woman. She was married in June 2002.

Dixie is a crossdresser from the Southern United States.

Richard Docter is Chair of Cal State Northridge's Psychology Department, and the author of *Transvestites and Transsexuals: Toward a Theory of Cross-Gender Behavior.*

Donna is a transgendered woman who lives publicly as a man. She hopes to continue transitioning so that she will eventually live full-time as a woman.

Johnny Dynell and **Chi Chi Valenti** are downtown New York luminaries.

Elle is a transitioning transsexual, the former husband of Katie.

Havelock Ellis (1859–1939), was an English sexual psychologist and a supporter of sexual liberation. His interests in human biology and his own personal experiences led Havelock Ellis to write his six-volume *Studies in the Psychology of Sex*. The books, published between 1897 and 1910, caused tremendous controversy.

Elizabeth is the genetic female wife of a crossdresser.

Emily is the transitioning transsexual woman to whom Kathryn is married.

Emma is the genetic female wife of a crossdresser.

Eve Ensler is the author of *The Vagina Monologues,* a play dealing with the issues of the female sexual body. The monologues themselves examine women's sexuality, violence, and procreation. Ensler has encouraged the discussion of women's bodies by making the rights to her play free to anyone who participates in V-Day, a yearly event in which groups perform the play and so raise consciousness about violence against women.

Estelle is the genetic female partner of Judy, a recently transitioned transsexual woman.

Jane Ellen Fairfax is the Chair of Tri-Ess, and a crossdresser.

Margaret Feinbloom is a sociologist and author, whose work *Transvestites & Transsexuals* was a significant contribution to the popular understanding of crossdressers and transsexuals in the 1960s when it was published.

Fem is a self-described "Alpha Female" who is seeking to date MTF TGs.

Neil Gaiman is the author of best-seller *American Gods* and *Sandman,* the graphic novel. His works often feature sympathetic portraits of transgendered people.

Gidget is the wife of Jayne, a crossdresser.

Emma Goldman (1869–1940), was a radical activist, writer and anarchist who was jailed for advocating the right of women to practice birth control.

Guy is a gay man, and friend, fellow writer, and wit.

Harry Hay was an activist, author, teacher, and visionary. He is famous for having launched the Lesbian / Gay liberation movement. As early as 1948 Harry Hay began pursuing his vision of forming an organization, the Mattachine Society, devoted to the welfare of Gay people. Hay was the first to propose the idea of Gay men and Lesbians as a cultural minority, the very basis of the Gay movement today. His essays have been published in the book *Radically Gay: Gay Liberation in the Words of Its Founder.*

Heather is Minna's crossdressing husband.

Magnus Hirschfield is the "Father of Tranvestism," in that he coined the word "transvestite" and did the first full-length work on transvestites. He also created the first institute for research on sexuality, the Institute of Sexual Science, which was razed by the Nazis. He actively campaigned for the legalization of both homosexuality and crossdressing, and often wrote letters of recommendation for transsexual people so that they could receive identity cards reflecting their correct gender identity. He is one of the heroes of the early transgendered movement.

bell hooks is a contemporary feminist writer, who regularly takes on issues of class, race, and gender in her works. Her books include *Ain't I a Woman*, and *Feminism is for Everybody*.

Eddie Izzard is a British comedian and actor who also happens to be a transvestite. His comedy shows *Dress to Kill* and *Glorious* are international hits. As an actor, he has appeared in such films as *Velvet Goldmine*. He made his Broadway debut in the spring of 2003 in Peter Nichols' *A Day in the Death of Joe Egg*.

Jayne is Gidget's husband, and a crossdresser.

Jan is a crossdresser who is only recently out to his wife, and who helped start MHVTA.

Judy recently transitioned. She is in her early fifties, and father of two, and is currently dating (genetic woman) Estelle.

Joanne is the genetic female partner of Donna. She has been encouraging and nurturing Donna's transgenderedness so that Donna can emerge as the woman she is.

Karen is a genetic woman who owns and operates Femme Fever, an organization that provides support and transformation services to MTF TGs.

Kathryn is the genetic female girlfriend of a transitioning transsexual woman.

Kathy is the genetic female wife of crossdresser Amanda.

Katie is the genetic female ex-wife of Elle.

Kelly is the genetic female girlfriend of a closeted crossdresser.

Ken is a male admirer of transgendered women.

Kevin is a gay man who once dated Richard, who did drag.

Kimmi is a tranny from the midwest, who is currently dating Corinne.

Richard von Krafft-Ebing (1840–1902) published the first edition of *Psychopathia Sexualis* in 1886.

Kyrie is a crossdresser who lives in Canada.

Gina Lance is the owner and publisher of the national tranny magazine *Girl Talk*, and a crossdresser.

Ursula K. LeGuin (1929–) is an author primarily of science fiction and fantasy. Her novels examine social and cultural constructs by putting them in imagined worlds. Her recurring themes, of anarchism and androgyny, suggest alternate but unconsidered realities for our own world. Her novel, *The Left Hand of Darkness,* is considered a classic of science fiction literature, and her short stories are often featured in literary anthologies, and feature a race of people who are genderless and whose sexual organs morph depending on their sexual partner, for procreation.

Lacey Leigh is a crossdresser and the author of *Out & About,* the crossdresser's field guide to getting out there.

Lisa is the genetic female wife of a crossdresser.

Liz is the genetic female wife of a crossdresser, Ann.

Luke/Elle—Luke was Katie's husband's male name. Luke is now Elle, and is transitioning.

Anita Mann is a drag queen who has won titles in the upstate New York region. She was recently invited to join the Imperial Court.

Melissa/John is a crossdresser from northern New York.

Meredith is the genetic female wife of Victoria, a crossdresser.

Michelle is Tammie's genetic female wife.

Edna St. Vincent Millay (1892–1950), was an openly bisexual American Romantic poet famous for her poetry and her "Bohemian" lifestyle. She supported her mother and two sisters on her literary earnings.

Minna is Heather's genetic female wife.

Viggo Mortensen is the man who plays Aragorn in the current *Lord of the Rings* movies.

Peter Oiler is the former employee of Winn-Dixie who was fired for cross-dressing in his free time.

Dr. Roger E. Peo was a gender counselor from Poughkeepsie, New York. He received his Ph.D. from the Institute for Advanced Study of Human Sexuality and was certified by the American College of Sexologists. Dr. Peo was a diplomate in sex counseling of the American Board of Sexology and a fellow of the American College of Clinical Sexologists, a member of the Society for the Scientific Study of Sex and of the Harry Benjamin International Gender Dysphoria Association. Sadly, Dr. Peo passed away in April 1994 after a brief illness.

Virginia Prince is a full-time transgenderist and cofounder of Tri-Ess.

René is an out crossdresser.

Richard is a feminine gay man.

JoAnn Roberts is a crossdresser, founding member of both Renaissance and TG Forum, and author of *Coping With Crossdressing*.

Rose Royalle is a TG woman, active in New York City gender politics, and denizen of Mother.

Peggy Rudd is the genetic female wife of a crossdresser. She has written books on the subject, such as *My Husband Wears My Clothes* and *Crossdressing with Dignity*.

Dan Savage is the author of "Savage Love," a widely syndicated sex advice column, and for two years he wrote the popular "Dear Dan" advice column for ABCNews.com. Dan also wrote *The Kid: What Happened After My Boyfriend and I Decided To Go Get Pregnant,* a memoir about becoming a father. Like most advice columnists—think Ann Landers and Abigail Van Buren—Dan has no professional qualifications, just lots of common sense, a sense of humor, and a pronounced inability to suffer fools gladly.

Galen Sherwin is a former president of NOW-NYC.

Snow is an androgynous genetic female who is in a polyamorous relationship with two t-girls. She is in her early twenties.

Gwen Stefani is the lead singer of the punk/ska/rock band No Doubt. Her platinum blonde hair and super-feminine looks are offset by her six-pack abs and the combat boots she wears. She combines an aggressive femininity with more glamorous looks, and her song "I'm Just a Girl" has become a new anthem for an upcoming generation of women.

Gloria Steinem is a writer and activist who has been a leader in the late-twentieth-century women's rights movement. Among her many achievements is the founding of *Ms.* Magazine, the first national women's magazine run by women. Her books, like *Revolution from Within* and *Outrageous Acts and Everyday Rebellions,* provide essays that encourage women to achieve equality in their personal lives.

Sue is crossdresser Ali's genetic female partner and the mother of their child.

Tammie is a crossdresser who identifies more as TG/TS and longtime treasurer of CDM, a sorority of Tri-Ess. She chooses not to live full-time or transition because she is happily married to her wife, Michelle.

Tristan Taormino is a writer, editor, sex educator, and sometimes fetish model, performer, and porn producer.

Valerie is a closeted crossdresser.

Barbara Van Horn is an out crossdresser who is active in her local Tri-Ess chapter.

Veronica Vera is the genetic female creator and founder of Miss Vera's Finishing School for Boys Who Want to Be Girls. She has authored hundreds of articles on human sexuality, performed internationally, lectured at Yale and Dartmouth, and testified for freedom of expression in Washington, D.C. She is a sex rights activist.

Victoria is a transvestite from the NY tri-state area.

Glorya Wholesome is a NYC transgender party hostess.

Bobbi Williams is the femme name of writer George Wilkerson, author of *Me and Bobbi and the Gyrls.*

Willow is a woman who transitioned a decade ago. She is in her early thirties, married, and is currently living where mountains are easily accessible.

Naomi Wolf is the author of *The Beauty Myth, Misconceptions* (about childbirth), and *Promiscuities.*

Virginia Woolf was the pre-eminent feminist and literary writer of her day. Her novels and nonfiction were profoundly concerned with issues of gender and the experience of women in a patriarchal world. Her essay, "A Room of One's Own," has continued to be a source of inspiration for women artists, and her *Three Guineas* is still the best explanation for why a genuine feminist revolution would do the world a lot of good. *Orlando,* a later novel, examines what would now be considered transsexual issues, though it's hard to believe she would have seen the book in that light.

Zoe and **Abigail** are a lesbian couple in their late twenties, friends of ours, and a great source of conversation and insight.

Annotated Bibliography

Transformations: Crossdressers and Those Who Love Them
Mariette Pathy Allen
This looks like a photography book, and it is that, but the essays—which are basically autobiographies written by the crossdressers themselves—are what really moves this book. By allowing the CDs to speak in their own words, Ms. Allen has given them not only their humanity but their own voices, their own thoughts, their dignity. In addition, there are brief pieces by the significant others of some of the CDs. This is the book—of all of them—that I found most interesting and helpful to me as a brand-new girlfriend of a CD. It gave me hope that love can conquer all, and I think gave me some realistic expectation of what my life would be like. You have to read between the lines a little bit to find that, but it's there, in lived lives, on the page. Allen has other photographs which focus on transgender people, some of which can be found at her website: www.mariettepathyallen.com

The Lazy Crossdresser
Charles Anders
I didn't understand from the title of this book what the point of it was, and I didn't really understand that much better after I finished reading it. There are some funny parts, and some enlightening funny parts, but otherwise I didn't get much out of it. A crossdresser might, the wife of one won't.

Normal
Amy Bloom
Ah, the controversial book of last year! The buzz in the TG community was pretty intense, and no one liked it. I think it was significant that a mainstream writer like Ms. Bloom wrote the book for a mainstream press—and a mainstream magazine. My problem with it was that it really was just three magazine articles, and to be honest I felt a little ripped off. I think she had

some great insights to make about TGism and gender in general, but not enough to justify the book. You'd get better insight into the Intersex from ISNA, better info on FTMs from almost any transmen site, and better info on crossdressing from someone who's not such an outsider to the community—which is so secretive to begin with. I think she found crossdressers who were willing to speak for the entire community without looking into the ones who didn't get any representation, unfortunately, and so created a very distorted picture of the crossdressing community.

Gender Outlaw
Kate Bornstein
Absolutely brilliant, a must-read. Read it slowly, think between paragraphs. There's more in here about gender and its construction than in any other book on gender I've read. And humor, to boot.

Crossdressing, Sex, and Gender
Vern L. and Bonnie Bullough
Overall, the most fact-filled, non-judgmental overview of crossdressing available. This book covers history (like The Abby de Choisy, and other "famous" crossdressers), covers social history and acceptance, the medical/psychological community's history with crossdressing, and pretty much everything else you've ever wanted to know about crossdressing in its cultural and historical context. It's not a "hands on" type of book, but one that might help CDs and their partners see where they fit in the larger scheme of things.

Gender Trouble
Judith Butler
If you don't have an advanced degree in gender theory, forget this. On the very first page she refers to Foucault, and a lot of the book is academic otherwise. Again, I would highly recommend it for anyone pretty well versed in gender theory, but otherwise it's not going to do you a whole lot of good.

Wives, Partners, and Others: Living with Cross-Dressing
Jan and Diane Dixon, Eds.
This is a publication of IFGE (International Foundation for Gender Education). There are contributions here from crossdressers, wives, partners, professionals, and even the children of crossdressers. The selection of letters and essays is comprehensive but a little repetitive. I do wish there

had been more commentary on the pieces written by a gender professional in order to put the comments of the individual in context. It's dry, humorless, but educational.

Transvestites and Transsexuals
Richard F. Docter

This is a book by a psychologist, on the subject of crossdressing as a psychological issue. It is not warm, but it is informative. The author attempts to break down what is currently a rather simplistic view of CDs by the psychological community—and does a fine job. First off, he separates the gay men who crossdress from the straight ones, and then tries to identify commonalities in the various groups. It gets a little dry, but there is an invaluable chapter toward the end that are the results of polls/conversations with the significant others of CDs. That chapter was the only reason I bought the book.

Psychopathia Sexualis
Havelock Ellis

If you can get over the fact that this book was written in 1897 and presents "transvestites" within a broad range of deviants, this is a fascinating piece of history. It should be appreciated at an almost cultish level for its stunningly honest language. It's important to note that a lot of crossdressers, in their mad search for clues, found this book in their local public library, and in it a few case histories of transvestites. I'm sure for a lot of CDs it was the first moment of realization that they were not, in fact, the only man in the universe that had ever put on women's clothes. It may not have been complimentary, but at least it was there.

Transgender Warriors
Leslie Feinberg

I can't say this book is about crossdressing per se, but more about the whole of the transgender community: identity, personal pride, history and activism all rolled into one. It's also a pretty good read, inspirational and informative at once. Leslie is hirself transgendered, and so for once it's a book straight from the horse's mouth—not by a doctor or an academic, but rather about a real person and his/her own explorations into his/her own transgendered life. Highly recommended for everyone—not just those interested in CD/TG/TS issues. Again, no practical advice per se, but a great deal of enthusiasm that's good for the soul!

Transvestites and Transsexuals
Deborah Feinbloom
I won't speak for the second half of the book about transsexuals, but the first half, on crossdressers, was very insightful and fair. Aside from her negative assumptions about wives who stay with crossdressers, Ms. Feinbloom really paints a very respectful and sympathetic portrait without glossing over the rough spots. She also does an excellent job of describing what an average Tri-Ess meeting is like (even though she didn't attend a Tri-Ess meeting per se.) Recommended for wives and CDs.

Vested Interests
Marjorie Garber
This is a well thought-out and remarkably well-documented piece of rather academic writing. If you haven't got at least a little background in contemporary theory/philosophy you might just find it abstruse and difficult. I found it to be enlightening, funny, and very very informative. Since it's broken up into chapters that are essentially essays, you can read one you're particularly interested in (say, the one on race and crossdressing, or the one on the history of sumptuary laws, or the ones on crossdressed characters in Shakespeare's plays) and leave the rest. It's an excellent guidebook: that is, it's not just a great resource for films and art and history regarding crossdressing, but it also gives you a theoretical context in which to think about it all. Brilliant, but with little practical advice whatsoever. I think wives and girlfriends generally get more out of this, especially if they've read any books about gender previously.

Transvestites
Magnus Hirschfield
Like Ellis' *Psychopathia Sexualis*, *Transvestites* is an article of history. It was published in 1910. Magnus Hirschfield was the first to study transvestites as a group unto themselves, and correctly separated them from the homosexuals (probably because he himself was a homosexual, and found he had nothing in common with most transvestites). He also coined the term transvestite for this study, founding it in Latin (*trans* = across, *vestire* = to dress) so as to give the transvestite a name that brought them some respect. (I think it's important to note that both Ellis and Hirschfield conducted their studies in order to enlighten the general public. Their goal was greater understanding, and they were not curiosity-seekers. They were trying to do what the average TG activist group does

now: getting the information out there to a wider audience, in hopes of increased tolerance.) Ironically, this is one of the most empathetic books on transvestites to this day, and explores both the sexual arousal experienced by CD/TVs, and their gender dysphoria as well.

Walk on the Wild Side
Jones, Jeannette
Nice photographs of various kinds of TG women: drag queens, crossdressers, transvestites, transgendered women, transsexuals. Not much else.

Out and About
Lacey Leigh
A great practical guide for a crossdresser who wants out of the closet. This book has an upbeat attitude, practical advice, funny anecdotes about Ms. Leigh's own experiences, and charm. The section on safety was especially valuable, both for CDs and their significant others. Mostly, I found Ms. Leigh's advice on how to defuse an uncomfortable situation with humor and directness especially worthwhile. Great for CDs.

The Transvestite and His Wife
Virginia Prince
I'll start by saying Virginia Prince is a damned remarkable person. She came out so many years ago it's hard to imagine what life was like when she did. Ms. Prince formed the first crossdresser association in America (the one which became Tri-Ess) and these early publications were her attempt to reach out to crossdressers and their partners, as she did also with *Transvestia* magazine. That said, this is pretty much propaganda, and propaganda from nearly four decades ago. The book is rife with homophobia, condescending about wives, and otherwise difficult to read. (The section on "Grades for Wives" gets an F from me.) Keeping all that in mind, however, there are some basic issues brought up that are still valid, like the fact that it's better for a wife to know than not. If you're a crossdresser looking for your history or a wife looking for perspective, this one is worth it.

Coping with Crossdressing
JoAnn Roberts
This book was probably named most frequently as having been a useful aid for a crossdresser who is telling his wife for the first time. It provides sound advice, but it's so brief on some subjects that the advice is hard to

follow. There is exactly one paragraph on sex with a crossdressing partner which is woefully inadequate for the problems so many couples face when the husband is a CD. Overall, however, there is a lot of information here that's presented in a concise, easy-to-read format: a perfect primer. Recommended for both crossdressers and their partners.

Miss Vera's Finishing School for Boys Who Want to Be Girls
Veronica Vera

One of the wives who answered my questionnaire sent this book through the shredder, but I actually enjoyed it. It's a good book for the "light side" of crossdressing, and one of the few published by a GW who is—in her own way—within the crossdressing community. Miss Vera has met crossdressers for years now, and has been making their dreams come true (in exchange for cash, of course). What I liked about it is that she has no "vested interest" in shielding anyone from the truth, and it was in this book that I found the first reference to the fact that CDs are often sexually active with men while en femme . . . which led me to wonder about it, do more research, and uncover the truth. Sometimes it's just a little too cute, a little too corny, but otherwise it presents crossdressing with a "no judgments" attitude, especially about the sexual aspects, which I think any CD would appreciate. Probably for CDs only.

Me and Bobbi and the Gyrls
George Wilkerson/Bobbi Williams

George Wilkerson and Bobbi Williams are the same person—Bobbi is the femme half of George. These fictionalized stories feel like memoirs in that they are deeply personal and focused specifically on the experiences of a crossdresser. Bobbi takes us to bars, to the mirror in his bedroom, to the Southern Comfort conference, and manages to describe some of the most important internal difficulties of being a closeted CD. There are a few inventive and surreal stories, and others that focus more on aspects of the CD community. This wasn't an easy read as an SO, but it was incredibly enlightening. Recommended for CDs and SOs who are ready to learn not just about crossdressing, but about the struggles so many go through in accepting their femme selves.

The Beauty Myth
Naomi Wolf

Recommended as a good feminist text on appearance, beauty, and the politics of beauty. I consider this a must-read for women and for any crossdresser who doesn't understand why his wife or girlfriend has an issue with his feminine presentation. Well written, well documented, and not lost in theory-lingo. Highly recommended.

Fantastic Women
Annie Woodhouse
This book should be handed to any woman who has just walked into a Tri-Ess meeting. It's honest, it's not too dated, and it makes a lot of very interesting points. This is the only (before mine) attempt to present an honest and unbiased look at the difficulties wives of crossdressers go through, without judging them and only mildly judging the CDs themselves. Feminist in perspective, it was my favorite of all the books I read.

The New Male Sexuality
Bernie Zilbergeld
I recommend this not because it has anything whatsoever to do with crossdressing, but more so because it discusses some of the realities of men in their sexual lives. I found that reading about men who avoid sex, prefer masturbation over sex with a partner, and experiences erectile dysfunction or performance anxiety put the sexual problems that crossdressers can experience into perspective. Zilbergeld makes clear that men are not, as mythology declares, ready for sex all the time with no emotional or psychological baggage of their own. Many men want to feel they are loving and loved, and some of Dr. Zilbergeld's points about men's sexual desires—and emotions—are very valid for the sexual lives of crossdressers and their partners. Recommended for everyone.

BIBLIOGRAPHY

Allen, Mariette Pathy. *Transformations: Crossdressers and Those Who Love Them*. Boston: Dutton, 1990.

Anders, Charles. *The Lazy Crossdresser*. Emeryville: Greenery Press, 2002.

Aucoin, Kevyn. *Making Faces*. New York: Little, Brown, and Co., 1997.

Bailey, Michael J. *The Man Who Would Be Queen: The Science of Gender-Bending and Transsexualism*. Washington D.C.: Joseph Henry Press, 2003.

Bloom, Amy. *Normal.* New York: Random House, 2002.

Bornstein, Kate. *Gender Outlaw.* New York: Vintage Books, 1995.

———— *My Gender Workbook.*

Boylan, Jennifer Finney. *She's Not There.* New York: Broadway Books, 2003.

Brooks, Gary R. *The Centerfold Syndrome.* San Francisco: Jossey-Bass Publishers, 1995.

Brubach, Holly. *Girlfriend: Men, Women, and Drag.* New York: Random House, 1999.

Bullough, Vern and Bonnie. *Crossdressing, Sex, and Gender.* Philadelphia: University of Pennsylvania Press, 1993.

Burke, Phyllis. *Gender Shock.* New York: Anchor, 1996.

Butler, Judith. *Gender Trouble.* New York: Routledge, 1999.

Clunis, Merilee, and G. Dorsey Green. *Lesbian Couples.* Seattle: Seal Press, 2000.

Devor, Holly. *Gender Blending.* Indianapolis: Indiana University Press, 1989.

Dixon, Jan & Diane, Eds. *Wives, Partners, and Others: Living with Crossdressing.* Waltham: Educational Resources, 1991.

Docter, Richard. *Transvestites and Transsexuals: Toward a Theory of Cross-Gender Behavior.* New York: Plenum Pub. Corp., 1988.

Ekins, Richard, and Dave King. *Blending Genders: Social Aspects of Cross-Dressing and Sex-Changing.* New York: Routledge, 1996.

Evelyn, Just. *Mom, I Need to Be a Girl.* San Diego: Just Evelyn, 1998.

Feinberg, Leslie. *Stone Butch Blues.* New York: Firebrand Books, 1993.

———— *Transgender Warriors*. New York: Beacon Press, 1997.

Feinbloom, Deborah Heller. *Transvestites & Transsexuals*. New York: Dell Publishing, 1977.

Garber, Marjorie. *Vested Interests: Crossdressing and Cultural Anxiety*. New York: Routledge, 1997.

Hirschfield, Magnus. *Transvestites*. Buffalo: Prometheus Books, 1991.

Jones, Jeanette. *Walk on the Wild Side*. New York: Barricade Books, 1995.

Kimmel, Michael S. *The Gendered Society*. New York: Oxford University Press, 2000.

Krafft-Ebing, Richard von. *Psychopathia Sexualis*. London: Velvet Publications, 1997.

Leigh, Laccy. *Out & About: The Emancipated Crossdresser*. Double Star Press, 2001.

Prince, Virginia. *The Transvestite and His Wife*. Los Angeles: Chevalier Publications, 1967.

Raynor, Darrell G. *A Year Among the Girls*. New York: Lancer Books, 1968.

Roberts, JoAnn. *Coping with Crossdressing*. CDS Publications, 1995.

Rowe, Robert J. *Bert & Lori: The Autobiography of a Crossdresser*. Amherst: Prometheus Books, 1997.

Rudd, Peggy J. *My Husband Wears My Clothes*. Katy: PM Publishers, 1999.

Vera, Veronica. *Miss Vera's Finishing School for Boys Who Want to be Girls*. New York: Bantam Doubleday Dell, 1997.

Wilkerson, George, and Bobbi Williams. *Me And Bobbi And The Gyrls*. Xlibiris, 2000.

Wolf, Naomi. *The Beauty Myth*. New York: William Morrow, 1991.

Woodhouse, Annie. *Fantastic Women*. New Brunswick: Rutgers University Press, 1989.

Zilbergeld, Bernie. *The New Male Sexuality*. New York: Bantam Books, 1992.

Resources

THIS IS A listing of resources for the crossdresser and his partner. Listings are alphabetized within categories. Contact National Organizations for help with local support. The descriptions are taken primarily from the literature or website of the organization.

NATIONAL

Gender Education and Advocacy (GEA) is a national organization focused on the needs, issues and concerns of gender variant people in human society. We seek to educate and advocate, not only for ourselves and others like us, but for all human beings who suffer from gender-based oppression in all of its many forms.
www.gender.org
   They also maintain the memorial site for transgendered people who have been murdered:
http://www.gender.org/remember/

GenderPAC, the Gender Public Advocacy Coalition, works to end discrimination and violence caused by gender stereotypes by changing public attitudes, educating elected officials and expanding legal rights. GenderPAC also promotes understanding of the connection between discrimination based on gender stereotypes and sex, sexual orientation, age, race, class.
http://www.gpac.org/

IFGE, or the **International Foundation for Gender Education** is a leading advocate and educational organization for promoting the self-definition and free expression of individual gender identity. IFGE is not a support group, it is an information provider and clearinghouse for referrals about all things

which are transgressive of established social gender norms. IFGE maintains the most complete bookstore on the subject of transgenderism available any-where. It also publishes the leading magazine providing reasoned discussion of issues of gender expression and identity, including crossdressing, trans-sexualism, FTM and MTF issues spanning health, family, medical, legal, workplace issues, and more.
www.ifge.org

NTAC (National Transgender Advocacy Coalition) works for the advancement of understanding and the attainment of civil rights for all transgendered and intersexed people in every aspect of society.
www.ntac.org

NOW (The National Organization for Women) is the largest organiza-tion of feminist activists in the United States. NOW has 500,000 contribut-ing members and 550 chapters in all fifty states and the District of Columbia. Since its founding in 1966, NOW's goal has been "to take action" to bring about equality for all women. Both the actions NOW takes and its position on the issues are often unorthodox, uncompromising and ahead of their time.
www.now.org

Renaissance Transgender Association, or Renaissance, is an organization whose mission is to provide the very best comprehensive education and car-ing support to Transgendered individuals and those close to them. This is accomplished through offering a variety of carefully selected programs and resources focused on the factors affecting their lives.
http://www.ren.org/

Tri-Ess is an international support and social organization for heterosexual crossdressers, their spouses, partners, children and friends.
www.tri-ess.org

PUBLICATIONS

The Femme Mirror is the monthly magazine of Tri-Ess, and comes with membership
http://www.tri-ess.org/

Girl Talk magazine, created by Gina Lance and Bijoux Deluxe, focuses on the upbeat side of the transgender world in all its many facets. Articles include gorgeous fashion editorial/runway report, beauty trend, celebrity interview, and personal reinforcement social commentary all geared toward the savvy TG reader. Take *People* magazine, throw in a dash of *Harper's Bazaar* and *Allure,* and you have *Girl Talk.* Available in bookstores and newsstands globally.
Girl Talk Magazine, PO Box 4915, N. Hollywood, CA 91617, 888.288.2115
www.girltalkmag.com

Transgender Community News is the monthly magazine of the Renaissance Transgender Association
http://www.ren.org/tcn.html

Transgender Tapestry is the IFGE's quarterly publication, by, for, and about all things trans, including crossdressing, transsexualism, intersexuality, FTM, MTF, butch, femme, drag kings and drag queens, androgyny, female and male impersonation, and more. It is a leading source for stimulating dialogue covering a wide range of gender topics, from medical and psychological care to family and partner issues, to film and book reviews, and much more. It is the *only* trans publication with a complete listing of trans support groups.
http://www.ifge.org/tgmag/tgmagtop.htm

VACATIONS AND CONFERENCES

Eureka En Femme Getaway is, according to the website, "is a vacation not a convention and will be quite different from the vast majority of the "T" community events that you may have attended in the past. You will enjoy an elegant and relaxing weekend: There will be no structured seminars or events to attend, no rubber chicken banquets, and none of that *big* hotel communal "closet" feeling. However, we will have a complete schedule of activities which can be done as individuals, as couples, as small groups, and as large groups, all at your choosing. Boredom is simply not possible."
http://www.femmegetaway.com/

Fantasia Fair is one of the longest-running activities in the Transgendered community. Started in 1975, "FanFair" (as many call it) has grown every year in its scope, character, and assistance to the gender explorer. Fan Fair

continues to be the leading annual program which promotes an individual's ability to function in a real-life town, and receive positive reinforcement and encouragement. This allows the cross-gender, crossdresser, MTF transsexual, and FTM transsexual to experience their preferred lifestyle in an open and caring environment—something unique in a world that typically has difficulty understanding and accepting gender options.
http://www.fantasiafair.org/fair/

Paradise in the Poconos is produced by JoAnn Roberts. From the website: "We have made every effort to create an event that will be a memorable experience for everyone involved. The weekend is designed to give you an opportunity to live out your fantasies. Dress to your heart's content. Bring your entire wardrobe! The people you'll meet at the Poconos are some of the nicest you'll ever meet anywhere. They come from different backgrounds, but they all share the same desire: to get away and let "her" roam free. We also encourage and welcome couples to attend and we usually get a large group of them at the weekend. If your partner wonders "Are there other women who deal with this?" then here's where she'll meet them. This is a great place to get to know your partner better."
http://www.cdspub.com/Poco.html

Rainbow Mountain is a gay-owned and operated resort, restaurant and nightclub that has been serving the gay, lesbian, bisexual, and transgender communities for twenty years.
http://www.rainbowmountain.com/

Southern Comfort Conference "prides itself on being an all-inclusive conference. Whatever your connection to the transgender community—whether you are transsexual, cross dresser or in between; spouse, partner or family member; straight, gay, bi or omni sexual; post-op, pre-op or non-op; young or old; married or single; FtM or MtF; or of any variance—if transgender is an issue in your life, you are welcome at Southern Comfort Conference."
http://www.sccatl.org/

S.P.I.C.E. is the yearly conference for the wives of crossdressers. It is sponsored by Tri-Ess and no crossdressing is allowed.
http://www.rainbowtrail.info/spice/

*   *   *

NEW YORK CITY AND ENVIRONS

The Center's Mission Statement reads: "The Lesbian, Gay, Bisexual & Transgender Community Center provides a home for the birth, nurture and celebration of our organizations, institutions and culture; cares for our individuals and groups in need; educates the public and our community; and empowers our individuals and groups to achieve their fullest potential." http://www.gaycenter.org/
(212) 620-7310

Chi Delta Mu is the New York tri-state area's Tri-Ess Chapter. http://www.geocities.com/WestHollywood/Heights/7396/

Chi Epsilon Sigma is the mid-Atlantic states' Tri-Ess chapter. http://members.tripod.com/~Chesapeake_Tri_Ess/

CDI (CrossDressers International) is a local group for NYC crossdressers http://www.cdinyc.org/

Femme Fever is an organization and transformation service for crossdressers, located in Long Island, NY.
http://www.femmefever.com/

Mid-Hudson Valley TransgenderAssociation (MHVTA) is a local Renaissance chapter in upstate New York.

Now Bar is a NYC bar that runs a few tranny nights. Call for details.

Silver Swan is a German restaurant by day, a crossdresser's nightclub on Saturday evenings.

Veronica Vera's Finishing School for Boys Who Want to Be Girls is exactly what it says it is.
www.missvera.com

*   *   *

RECOMMENDED WEBSITES

CDSO
http://www.tri-ess.org/spice/CDSO/CDSO.html
is an online support group for wives of crossdressers, but focuses primarily
on those who are having a hard time accepting crossdressing.

CD-WSOS
http://groups.yahoo.com/group/CDWSOS/
is an online support group for the wives and girlfriends of crossdressers.

CDS
http://www.cdspub.com/index.html
JoAnn Roberts' site, CDS, has a wealth of information, an online bookstore,
links to *LadyLike* magazine, and registration information for a yearly event,
Paradise in the Poconos.

A Crossdresser's Secret Garden
http://cdsecretgarden.femmegetaway.com/survey.html
is the homepage of the Crossdressers' Secret Garden group, run by Becca
and Dixie Nettle.

Dana's site for SOs
http://www.webdotgal.com/main/html/soforum.html
is a list of experiences by the genetic female partners of CD/TGs.

Fictionmania
www.fictionmania.com
is a collection of online, user-contributed stories

GLBTQ Encyclopedia
http://www.glbtq.com/
is an online encyclopedia of gay, lesbian, bisexual, transgendered and queer
culture.

GID Reform
http://www.transgender.org/tg/gidr/gid30285.html
is a page dedicated to reforming the definition of Gender Identity Disorder,
or GID, for the next DSM.

Girls Club Reporter
http://www.tenview.com/gcreporter
is an online magazine that brings the best of the other transgender magazines to its pages, and, of course, reports on the club scene on the local level as well.

Human Rights Campaign
http://www.hrc.org/newsreleases/2002/020930transgender.asp
is the website of Human Rights Campaign, an organization working for gay, lesbian, bi and transgender rights.

Kath & Melissa's Tea Time
http://www.geocities.com/westhollywood/heights/9072/PAGETWO.html
The last I heard, Melissa and Kath are no longer active in the CD community, but they have left their pages up which have some good articles and links.

Lynn Conway
www.lynnconway.com
features information about all aspects of transgenderism. Her pages are a regularly updated resource for the entire community.

Renee Reyes
http://www.reneereyes.com/
is one of the few "personal" websites I like, because Renee has some great information, essays, information on admirers, types of t-girls, etc.

San Francisco's Human Rights Commission
http://www.sfgov.org/site/sfhumanrights_page.asp?id=6274
Useful information on Gender Identity Discrimination, and some good definitions.

Support for Wives and Significant Others of Crossdressers
http://groups.yahoo.com/group/SFWaSOCDs/
is a support group for the genetic female partners of crossdressers, run by Cheryl and Angie.

TG Forum
www.tgforum.com
is a weekly online magazine, featuring news, entertainment and information

for the transgender community. There are both free and subscriber versions of the site.

Transgender Law and Policy Institute
http://www.transgenderlaw.org/
is the website of The Transgender Law and Policy Institute, which describes itself as a non-profit organization dedicated to engaging in effective advocacy for transgender people in our society. The TLPI brings experts and advocates together to work on law and policy initiatives designed to advance transgender equality.

Transsexual Women's Resources
http://www.annelawrence.com/
Anne Lawrence is a transitioned woman who provides resources for transsexual woman.

Yvonne's Place
http://www.yvonnesplace.net/yvonne/meet_me.htm
Yvonne maintains a good site for crossdressers, and has some useful essays on her site.

SEX RESOURCES

Good Vibrations
http://www.goodvibes.com/
Good Vibrations' online site welcomes you with this message: "At Good Vibrations, we believe that sexual pleasure is everyone's birthright, and that access to sexual materials and accurate sex information promotes health and happiness. As a worker-owned, women-owned cooperative, we believe that progressive business goes hand-in-hand with open communication about sexuality and the philosophy that sex is fun and natural. We hope you'll join us in our pursuit of pleasure!"

Savage Love
www.thestranger.com
is a great place to find archived Savage Love columns, written by sex advisor Dan Savage. Always brilliant, often hilarious.

Toys in Babeland
http://www.babeland.com/
A sex toy store run by women whose mission is to promote and celebrate sexual vitality by providing an honest, open, and fun environment, encouraging personal empowerment, educating our community, and supporting a more passionate world for all of us.

Tristan Taormino
http://www.puckerup.com/
It's all about sex, and features her columns for the *Village Voice,* information about sex toys, anal sex, and erotica.

Swan Song

My husband and I went to a trans party at a bar called Meow Mix, and a musician named Lisa Jackson got onstage. Lisa flipped her blonde hair, stroked her guitar's strings with manicured nails, and opened red lips to sing a song called "Fabulously Done." I stood toward the back, watching the FTMs, MTFs, gays, straights, and lesbians cheer her on. In that worn-out lesbian bar, Lisa Jackson was singing an anthem for t-girls everywhere; every time she sang "I'm not the only one" she drew cheers: she's *not* the only one.

Fabulously Done

Lyrics & Music by Lisa Jackson

The makeup and the clothes I wear,
The fancy do and the underwear,
It's a mystery, you see, to anyone who's not like me.

So please retract those words of hate
'Cause I'm the boy you used to date.
Yes I'm your lover and I'm your son. I'm your brother; we've just begun.

Somehow around the age of eight
I learned that I should hate
The fairies and the queers—you know they're just so fucking weird.
But little did my siblings know that I was putting on a little show
In the mirror of the bathroom as my mother ran the vacuum.

I'm not the only one. I'm not the only one
Who wants to be painted, and pretty, and shining and fabulously done.

It has taken some 20 years
For me to learn to ignore the fear
That there are people who will hate you, and people who will shame you.
But be the first to cast your stone, 'cause I would rather be all alone.
Yes if I am gonna be living, then I am gonna be giving all I can.

I'm not the only one. I'm not the only one
Who wants to be painted, and pretty, and shining and fabulously done.

I told that girl, but that girl went away.
And I told my brother, but my brother thinks I'm gay.
I told my sister, but my sister could not hear.
And I told the world, 'cause I am tired of this fear.

The makeup and the clothes I wear,
The fancy do and the underwear,
It's a mystery, you see, to anyone who's not like me.

I'm not the only one. I'm not the only one
Who wants to be painted, and pretty, and shining and fabulously done.